*ELEMENTARY*
*PRINCIPLES OF*
***LABORATORY***
***INSTRUMENTS***

# ELEMENTARY PRINCIPLES OF
# LABORATORY INSTRUMENTS

## LESLIE W. LEE, B.S., M.T.(ASCP)

Joint Commission on Accreditation of Hospitals, Chicago, Illinois;
Formerly Administrative Director of Laboratories,
Orlando Regional Medical Center, Orlando, Florida;
Clinical Assistant Professor of Allied Health Sciences,
Florida Technical University, Orlando, Florida

## L.M. SCHMIDT, D.A., M.T.(ASCP)

Product Manager, Microbiological Systems, DuPont Company,
Instrument Products, Wilmington, Delaware

**FIFTH EDITION**

*with* **476** *illustrations*

## The C. V. Mosby Company

ST. LOUIS   TORONTO   1983

**MOSBY**

A TRADITION OF PUBLISHING EXCELLENCE

Editor: Don E. Ladig
Assistant editor: Rosa L. Kasper
Manuscript editor: Rebecca A. Reece
Book design: Jeanne Bush
Cover design: Suzanne Oberholtzer
Production: Carol O'Leary, Barbara Merritt, Jeanne A. Gulledge

**FIFTH EDITION**

Previous editions copyrighted 1970, 1974, 1978

First edition published privately by Mr. Leslie W. Lee

Printed in the United States of America

The C.V. Mosby Company
11830 Westline Industrial Drive, St. Louis, Missouri 63141

**Library of Congress Cataloging in Publication Data**

Lee, Leslie W.
   Elementary principles of laboratory instruments.

   Bibliography: p. 360
   Includes index.
   1.  Medical laboratories—Equipment and supplies.
I.  Schmidt, L.M.  II.  Title.
[DNLM: 1.  Equipment and supplies.  2.  Laboratories.
3.  Technology, Medical—Instrumentation.   W 26  L478e]
RB36.2.L43  1983       616.07′5′028       82-22942
ISBN 0-8016-2918-7

GW/VH/VH  9  8  7  6  5  4  3  2  1       02/B/255

# Preface

The first edition of this book was published in 1967. In the intervening years we have seen such advances as ion-selective electrodes, transistorized circuits, computers and microprocessors, greatly improved fluidics, practical gas and liquid chromatography, widespread use of radiochemistry, automation of bacteriology, and differential cell counting by pattern recognition. The laboratory equipment industry has grown from a few small companies to a $20 billion per year colossus.

In 1967 it was practical for the laboratory worker to service and repair many instruments. Today it would be imprudent for most of us to do more than routine maintenance and the replacement of specifically designated and easily accessible elements. This trend parallels other aspects of our highly specialized society. A generation ago many people could do many of their own car repairs and adjustments. Today a trained mechanic with sophisticated testing equipment and tools is required. Even the preparation of income tax statements, once a simple chore, now often requires the services of a trained accountant.

This trend toward complexity and the resulting specialization require some change in the way we work and hence in the way we teach people to work. Considerable thought has gone into the changes made in this fifth edition of *Elementary Principles of Laboratory Instruments*.

To give the student some appreciation of the many changes that have occurred in the laboratory, a short historical chapter has been added and some comments made about possible future developments.

Since it has become impractical for the technologist to do much detailed repair and since the number of instruments nearly precludes detailed discussion, repair procedures have been minimized. At the same time, it is felt that the electrical and photometric principles involved are important to the understanding of instruments. Chapters on electronics and light measurement have been expanded somewhat.

With the advances of the past decade, accuracy, precision, and reliability have been enhanced, and with proper attention, accurate and reproducible test results can be achieved with few instrument failures. Quality control has become the major concern in instrument operation; therefore a chapter has been added to emphasize its importance and to direct the student's thinking about this important aspect of testing. Throughout the book, attention is directed to instrument maintenance and to other steps necessary to guarantee the validity of the reports generated.

In 1967 it was possible to catalog most of the instruments in general use in medical laboratories. With the tremendous increase in the variety, number, and complexity of instruments, this is no longer practical. The general principles of each type of instrument are discussed, and only a few examples of each are presented.

Perhaps one of the most important additions to this new fifth edition is my new co-author, Lois Schmidt, who brings to the book a great deal of experience in teaching and writing in the general area of electronics and instrumentation.

We hope that students of the biological and physical sciences, as well as medical technology, will find this new edition informative and enjoyable.

We are indebted to many instrument manufacturers and their representatives, as well as to numerous friends and associates, for helpful advice and encouragement.

**Leslie W. Lee**

# *Introduction*

During the performance of qualitative or quantitative automated procedures, an instrument operator can be a slave or a master. To be a slave is the easier and perhaps the more popular of the two choices. Samples are placed in the well labeled "sample well." A glowing "start" button is pushed. The "read" switch is thrown. A sounding alarm indicates malfunction, and illuminated immediately is the telephone number of the nearest service representative. Thus the flashing lights, buzzing alarms, numbered buttons, and driving gears lead, direct, and essentially command the ordered manipulations to be performed on the instrument by its assigned servant. Unhappiness does not necessarily plague this instrument operator who, in the bliss for which ignorance has been credited, believes himself or herself to be in control.

To be master over the instrument is a position not to be bought, scheduled, bestowed, or pretended but rather to be earned through study and application. Study and comprehension of operational principles of instrumentation provide the knowledge required for making judgments. Many decisions must be made in establishing a preventive maintenance schedule and a parts supply, in recognizing and repairing instrument malfunctions, and in selecting, designing, and executing an effective mode of instruction for instrument operators.

During the operation of a properly functioning instrument, there is no apparent difference between the slave and the master. However, this appearance ends the similarity. The master *is* in control. Pushing a button or throwing a switch is accompanied by the ability to intelligently interpret the effect each such manipulation has on instrument functions. As a result, less than optimal instrument performance may be accepted obliviously by the slave but will be perceived keenly by the master.

It is naive to think that knowledge of instrumental principles will transform a laboratory analyst into a troubleshooting wizard capable of pinpointing and repairing all instrumental deficiencies. This is certainly not the case. The operator of analytical instruments should be able to recognize when an instrument is not functioning properly, identify the problem, and evaluate the availability of resources required for repair. If parts are at hand for a minor repair, an individual capable of performing this repair could do so. Immediate repair could avoid expenditure of time, money, and effort needed to implement a backup method. However, if instrument malfunction diagnosis or repair is problematic, expert assistance should be requested. Of utmost importance is the ability to evaluate both the extent of an instrumental problem and the extent of one's own capabilities to rectify the problem. It is better to keep hands off than to approach a malfunctioning instrument with irresponsible overconfidence.

Confidence derived from knowledge of instrumental principles is required for the analyst to control and operate analytical instruments. These instruments are made up of functional units, the majority of which are electronic. Electronic units are composed of an assortment of electronic devices, such as resistors, capacitors, diodes, transistors, operational amplifiers, transformers, choppers, inductors, switches, and potentiometers. It is, therefore, difficult to comprehend principles of analytical instruments without first having a basic vocabulary and a fundamental understanding of electronic devices and their functional principles.

The purpose of this text is to provide a foundation of knowledge in basic electronics and instrumentation. To link the abstract to the concrete, this book applies the theoretical principles of electronics to the functional units of instruments. Six basic functional units of analytical instruments can serve as a tangible framework to which electronic principles can be related. These six functional units, as shown in Fig. 2-1, are the power source, the excitation or signal source, the sample compartment, the detector, the signal processing unit, and the readout device. Each of these units is described briefly in Section One and serves as a reference base for the description of functional principles of analytical instruments in Section Three.

# Contents

*ELEMENTARY*
*PRINCIPLES OF*
***LABORATORY***
***INSTRUMENTS***

# *INTRODUCTION*

# CHAPTER 1

# *Instruments over the years*

When we think of instruments, we generally think of black boxes with dials and knobs that perform mysterious tasks using sophisticated electronics. Actually, instruments are tools that enable us to do our work better or more easily. The cave-dweller forming a stone ax with which to kill animals may have been the first instrument maker. Today, instruments are still tools that improve our ability to perform tasks. Like a carpenter, mechanic, or surgeon, we can work better if we understand our tools and know how best to use them.

For thousands of years tools were simple. Wheels, levers, pulleys, wedges, and plows made physical work easier. Observations were made that affected navigation, metallurgy, chemistry, and medicine. These observations led to new hypotheses and new experiments, which in turn produced new observations. As people worked with new ideas, the combination of two or three of these in different perspective revealed a whole new area of investigation.

Two digits can be arranged in only two sequences. That is, the number *1* and the number *2* can be written together only as 12 and 21. Four numbers can be arranged in 16 different sequences. The popular Rubik's Cube, made of 20 small, colored cubes, can be arranged in 43 quintillion ways. This may provide some idea of how many ways the scientific knowledge now possessed can be rearranged and restructured to produce new discoveries, ideas, and devices. Largely because of the logarithmic increase in knowledge, we now have a veritable cascade of new instruments with which to work. Each new concept leads to new devices.

Communication has also improved with the introduction of the printing press, telephone, radio, television, moving pictures, and communication satellites. Old national barriers have fallen, and there is virtually one scientific community in the world. It is now practical for a manufacturer to produce highly specialized instruments used by only a few people in each country because the total market is large. Once produced, the instruments come into common use and add to the flood of instruments that we want to try to understand.

## Development of laboratory instrumentation

In the medical laboratory field, the variety of instruments is so large that merely cataloging them becomes a large task, and describing each in detail becomes nearly impossible. If we are to understand these tools or instruments, we must somehow grasp their basic concept and learn what they can do for us. A look backward at how medical laboratory instruments have developed may facilitate better understanding of the development of new instruments. Most new devices are refinements on older ideas, and the older, simpler tools were easier to understand.

*Before 1930.* Before 1930, only a few simple medical laboratory tests were performed. These were most often done by the doctor or an office helper. Such tests might include the examination of a drop of urine under the microscope, a stained smear from a wound or sore throat, a test for sugar or albumin in urine, or a rough estimate of hemoglobin in the blood. The instruments needed were simple and primitive by today's standards—a

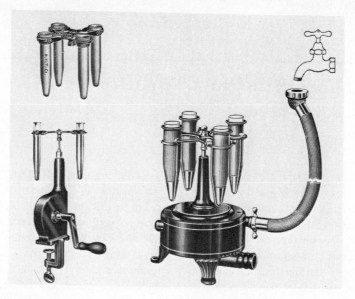

*Fig. 1-1.* Hand-cranked centrifuge and a water-powered unit. (From the 1931 Arthur H. Thomas catalog. Courtesy Arthur H. Thomas Co.)

monocular microscope, a Bunsen burner, test tubes with their wire holders, and a Tallqvist hemoglobin comparator. All these items are probably familiar, except for the hemoglobin comparator, which made use of a color chart with bands of red-brown color printed on a card. Each color represented a percentage of normal hemoglobin in blood. There was a hole in each color band. To perform the test, a drop of the patient's blood was blotted with a strip of blotter paper. The spot of blood was then placed behind the holes in the color strips until the best color match was found. It would be charitable to state that a rough estimate of the hemoglobin value was obtained.

*After 1930.* By around 1930, a number of office helpers were being trained to do laboratory work, sterilize instruments, and perform other chores around the office. Training programs soon evolved. During this period the American Society of Medical Technologists was formed to advance the knowledge and status of laboratory workers. More tests were gradually added, and the

laboratory soon became an accepted element of all respectable hospitals.

New equipment was developed. A hand-cranked centrifuge for spinning urine and blood could be clamped to the corner of a table like a kitchen meat grinder (Fig. 1-1). A set of gears allowed two tubes to be spun at a speed of several hundred revolutions per minute. Copper water baths sat on ring-stands over Bunsen burners for boiling urine albumin and blood sugar tests.

Bacteriology became more widely practiced. Media were prepared from basic ingredients. A bit of beef, for example, might be boiled to make a boullion for addition to agar to make a culture media for bacteria. The autoclave for sterilizing media and equipment was most often a vertical cylinder heated by a gas burner under its base (Fig. 1-2). A lid was bolted to the top with thumb screws and was provided with a thermometer to indicate when the desired temperature had been reached. These were awesome devices that were prone to accidents such as explosions caused by

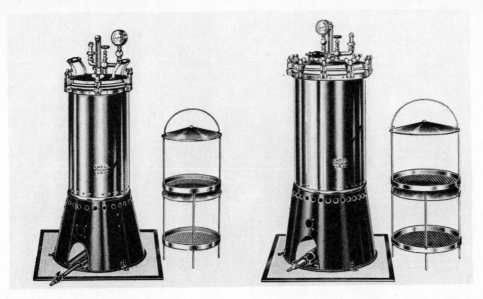

*Fig. 1-2.* Vertical gas-fired autoclave. (From the 1931 Arthus H. Thomas catalog. Courtesy Arthur H. Thomas Co.)

accumulated gas under the cylinder, scalding, and occasionally overheating, since there were no thermostatic or pressure controls. Consequently, they were generally treated with considerable respect.

Most chemistry tests were colorimetric, and colors were compared visually with standards by holding the tubes up to the light and deciding which standard most nearly matched the color of the test. Methods were not yet standardized, and it was a mark of sophistication to develop one's own tests. Reagents and standards were at times of questionable quality, and glassware and balances were often inaccurate; therefore, results were not uniformly accurate.

To alleviate some of these problems, kits were developed. One type of kit contained the ready-made reagents for the test and a wooden comparator block containing a series of colored tubes corresponding to standards of various levels. For example, the blood sugar kit might have tubes representing, 50, 100, 150, 200, and 250 mg/dl

of glucose. When the test was completed, it was matched to the closest standard and reported as that concentration. This provided a reasonable estimate and was probably somewhat more accurate than the earlier methods used in most laboratories, since the reagents, standards, and methodology were consistent.

*DuBoscq colorimeter.* Within a few years the DuBoscq visual colorimeter was introduced (Fig. 1-3). This instrument made use of Lambert's law, comparing the intensity of color at different depths of solution. It had the appearance of a monocular microscope. At the top was an eyepiece, and below this was a set of prisms. Below the prisms were two glass rods mounted on rack and pinion, which allowed each rod to be raised and lowered. A scale, graduated in millimeters on each side, indicated the displacement as the glass rod was raised and lowered into glass cups that were positioned over a mirror. When one looked into the eyepiece, a split field could be seen. The left side of the field showed the light reflected from the mir-

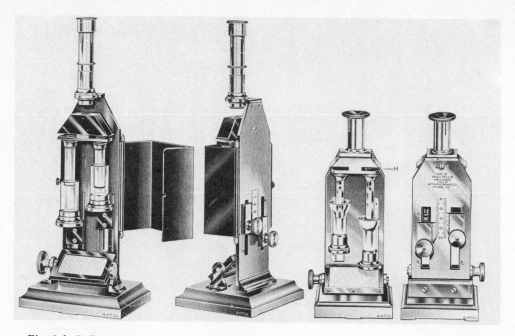

*Fig. 1-3.* DuBoscq colorimeters, original French models as constructed in the factory of the successor of Jules DuBoscq, who first announced the DuBoscq colorimeters in 1854. Scale is divided in millimeters, reading by Vernier acuity to 0.1 mm. Each instrument is furnished with a set of eight glass ray filters, which divide the visible spectrum into eight zones, permitting the examination of samples by a beam of light restricted to the wavelengths transmitted by each filter. Within the limitations of these wavelength zones, the comparison becomes spectrophotometric, with some of the advantages in accuracy offered by a more elaborate spectrophotometer illuminated by light of a chosen wavelength. (From the 1931 Arthur H. Thomas catalog. Courtesy Arthur H. Thomas Co.)

ror up through the cup, the glass rod (plunger) into the left prism, and into the eyepiece. The right side of the field was identical but passed through the right cup, plunger, and prism. According to Lambert's law, the amount of light absorbed by a colored solution is directly proportional to the distance it travels through that solution. If a standard solution is placed in 1 cup of the visual colorimeter just described and the test solution is placed in the other cup, the light intensity, or depth, of color can be compared. If both plungers are set so that the light path on either side is 20 mm and the colors exactly match, we would conclude that the patient sample and the standard had the same concentration of the analyte being tested. If, however, the standard light path were set at 20 mm and the colors matched when the test plunger was at 10 mm, the patient's level would be twice that of the standard.

The DuBoscq colorimeter was one of the first real measuring instruments in the laboratory, since it provided a reasonably precise measurement rather than simply matching the closest standard. Now the long search for ever-greater precision really began. The methods and equipment for weighing and measuring, the purity of reagents and standards, and the minute details of methodologies were increasingly scrutinized, and accuracy and precision improved accordingly.

*Photoelectric colorimeter*. A basic problem still persisted with the visual colorimeter, since color comparison depended on the subjective judgment of the analyst. Everyone was not equally able to match colors, and a few people were even color-blind. A way was needed to completely remove personal judgment from the measuring process. This was found when the photoelectric colorimeter was introduced.

The photoelectric cell produces a small electric current when exposed to light. The strength of the current is proportional to the intensity of the light. Beer's law states that light is absorbed by a solution in direct proportion to the number of molecules of a given species in the solution. The photoelectric colorimeter can compare the concentration of two colored solutions by measuring the light absorbed as indicated by the current a photocell produces. Since one specific component, which is characterized by a specific color, is being measured, other colors are eliminated by the use of light of one color (monochromatic light). In the early colorimeters, monochromatic light was produced by passing light from a tungsten light bulb through colored glass.

One of the early photoelectric colorimeters was called a *null-balance instrument*. The light from a bulb passed through two identical filters, and one light path continued through a standard solution and onto a photocell while the other light path passed through the test solution and onto an identical photocell. The current produced by the two photocells was equalized or balanced by passing the larger current through a variable resistor. The resistance required to balance the two currents was proportional to the light absorbed by the solution and hence to the concentration of the analyte.

Many of the instruments discussed in this book depend on the measurement of light by using photosensitive devices, and much of the recent history of instrument development has to do with improvements in the ability to accurately measure monochromatic light. The chapters dealing with light measurement follow these developments in considerable detail.

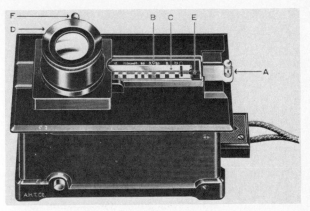

**Fig. 1-4.** Haden-Hausser hemoglobinometer used for the colorimetric determination of hemoglobin with a dilution ratio of 1:20. The direct reading gram scale is based on and coincides throughout its range with the hemoglobin content as determined by the oxygen-combining capacity method of Van Slyke, using the Hüfner conversion factor of 1.34 ml of oxygen per gram of hemoglobin. A simple, compact, sturdy, and easily cleaned instrument, the hemoglobinometer consists of a molded Bakelite case for the illuminating lamp and Daylite filter, on the lid of which is mounted a movable carrier, *A*, holding the comparator slide, *B*, with its cover glass, *C*, and a reading microscope, *D*. The diluted sample is introduced at point *E*, and the button, *F*, controls the light shutter. The comparator slide has a hemoglobin-gram scale with total range from 7.5 to 19 g in the following intervals: 7.5, 8, 8.5, 9, 9.5, 10, 11, 12, 13, 14, 15, 16, 17, 18, and 19 g. This scale was established by determining the oxygen-combining capacity of many blood samples throughout the range of the scale by the Van Slyke manometric blood gas methods and converted into hemoglobin content by the use of the Hüfner factor of 1.34 ml of oxygen per gram of hemoglobin. (From the 1931 Arthur H. Thomas catalog. Courtesy Arthur H. Thomas Co.)

*Hemoglobin measurement*. It was several years before devices for measuring hemoglobins electronically were generally used. In the meantime, some better methods were developed. The Sahli method was the favorite for many years. The Sahli comparator consisted of a plastic block with two tubes of acid hematin solution. Between these tubes was a space for the tube in which the test was performed. In this tube, 0.1 ml of blood was mixed with a few drops of hydrochloric acid to convert hemoglobin to acid hematin. Water was then added, drop by drop, until the test solution appeared to be identical to the acid hematin standard tubes. The dilution necessary to match the solutions bore a direct relationship to the concentration of hemoglobin in the blood. To make the calculation easy, a scale was printed on the test tube from which hemoglobin concentration could be read directly in grams per deciliter, or percentage of normal.

Shortly thereafter, the Haden-Hausser hemoglobinometer was introduced (Fig. 1-4). This device used Lambert's law. A fixed dilution of blood was acidified to produce acid hematin, which was introduced into a glass channel that varied in depth from very shallow on one end to deeper on the opposite end. The deeper end obviously would appear darker. The point along the channel at which the solution appeared to be identical to a standard was found, and the hemoglobin concentration was read from a scale attached to the test channel.

By the 1950s most laboratories began to read hemoglobin concentration on visual colorimeters, and within a few years photoelectric hemoglobinometers began to make their appearance.

## Development of chemistry instrumentation

A number of problems retarded the development of chemistry instrumentation. Some of these were mechanical in nature, but some were chemical. One of these had to do with protein interference. Plasma and serum contain large quantities of protein that, when heated or acidified, coagulates or becomes opalescent. Almost any chemical change makes photometric measurement impossible. The standard method of eliminating the problem for many years required production of a protein-free filtrate. Blood was acidified and coagulated and then filtered. The filtrate contained nearly all the glucose, urea, and many other analytes, but others were retained to some degree in the coagulum. The process of making the filtrate introduced some potential errors and was time consuming and awkward.

Some methods avoided the protein problem. Calcium, for example, could be precipitated as calcium oxalate and the protein washed away. Carbon dioxide could be released from plasma as a gas and measured directly. Most tests, however, depended on the protein-free filtrate preparation for many years, and automation of chemistry testing never developed until the protein problem was solved.

In the late 1950s, the Technicon Corporation came upon the idea of dialyzing most analytes through a membrane, leaving the protein behind. The idea, along with the "flowing stream" concept, opened the way for the automation of chemistry which is discussed in detail in Chapter 13.

As was noted earlier, the measurement of carbon dioxide was a special problem that was approached differently. The principle of the Van Slyke measurement of carbon dioxide is simple. Plasma is saturated with carbon dioxide by blowing bubbles of expired air through a pipette into the plasma. When lactic acid is added, the carbon dioxide is released as a gas. Subjecting the plasma to a vacuum guarantees that all of the carbon dioxide is drawn out. The released gas is then brought to room temperature and atmospheric pressure, and the volume is measured. After correction for ambient temperature and atmospheric pressure, the carbon dioxide "combining power" is calculated. The Van Slyke apparatus and procedure are fearsome to most technologists. The apparatus consists of a rather complex burette arrangement with a mercury reservoir (Fig. 1-5). When the mercury is drawn from the burette by lowering the reservoir, a vacuum is produced. If the reservoir is raised too suddenly, the mercury races into the vacuum in the burette, breaking the glass or causing stop-

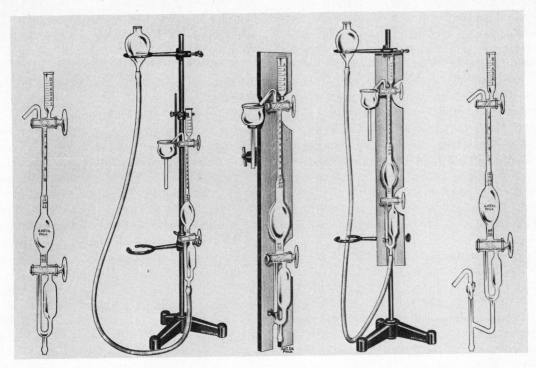

*Fig. 1-5.* Several configurations of the Van Slyke blood gas apparatus. (From the 1931 Arthur H. Thomas catalog. Courtesy Arthur H. Thomas Co.)

cocks to dislodge, showering beads of mercury over the workbench. Although the method was generally accurate when properly performed, it was difficult, expensive, and hazardous and was replaced by the Kopp-Natelson microgasometer, which worked on the same general principle but used smaller volumes of plasma and mercury and was easier to operate.

*Chemically pure reagents.* The lack of chemically pure reagent chemicals and precisely defined standards impeded the development of accurate and reproducible methods and equipment. This was a general problem, but a few typical examples are of interest.

Amylase is the enzyme that hydrolyzes starch into sugar. The type of starch used makes a great deal of difference. For many years, the source of

starch was not standardized. The process by which it is prepared alters test results almost as much as the type used. For many years, the starch solution was prepared in the laboratory. Even with a standard source and a standardized procedure for its preparation, results are often not reproducible. A commercially prepared starch is now generally used and has proved to be more reliable.

Thromboplastin for the prothrombin time test presented another problem in standardization. The brain from a freshly killed rabbit was stripped of all blood vessels and ground up with ether in a mortar. After repeated trituration with ether, a white powder was produced. When resuspended in saline, the thromboplastin solution was ready for use. Details of the procedure, temperatures, measurements, and storage had to be precisely repeated each time if the activity of the thromboplastin was to be comparable from batch to batch. Because of the inherent problems of reproducibility, commercially prepared and standardized thromboplastin is now universally used.

When photoelectric colorimeters first came into common use, it was common practice for a manufacturer to produce an instrument and all reagents for the various tests. A notebook of methods and a chart could then be provided for each that gave the concentration of the analyte for each meter reading. No standard was generally run. If one could assume that the reagents had not deteriorated, that all measurements and temperatures had been correct, and that the instrument was working correctly, the results could probably be accepted as accurate. Of course, this was often not the case. In spite of the possible sources of error, however, these instruments that provided uniform procedures and standardized reagents probably contributed to accuracy. Today many instrument manufacturers provide their own uniformly manufactured reagents for their systems to enhance accuracy and reproducibility. Even after several decades of improvement and standardization, there are still problems in the production of reagents that always give reproducible results.

*Fluid-volume accuracy.* A problem that retarded the development of automated equipment was the lack of a reliable means of dispensing accurate fluid volumes. Initially all fluid volumes were measured in pipettes, burettes, or volumetric flasks. These were generally fairly accurate if they were in good condition and properly used, but as automation developed, the means of automatically reproducing the same measurement hundreds of times became a major problem. Syringelike devices would wear, seals would leak, and deposits would build up on measuring parts, all of which produced inaccuracies. There was also a constant problem of carryover between specimens. The development of special materials and segmented stream devices and the use of continuous flow analysis have largely obviated the problem, but

continual monitoring of measurement accuracy and repeatability is still very important.

### Developments in electronics

Certainly the most important factor in the development of modern medical laboratory instrumentation and automation has been modern electronics. Fifty years ago the only practical means of measuring pH was by using indicators such as litmus to see if a solution was acid or alkaline or by titrating the solution using a chemically prepared titrant solution. This was a rather tedious procedure, which was not highly accurate compared with our modern means. It was known that an electrical potential difference existed between solutions of different pH, but there was no accurate way of measuring this difference. When the vacuum tube was introduced, a practical means was found to amplify this potential difference to a level that could be easily and accurately measured with a meter.

The development of more sophisticated electronic devices for measuring light has been important in improving medical laboratory equipment. Photoemissive and photoconductive cells have been refined to increase their sensitivity, specificity, and response time. Following the introduction of the vacuum tube, the phototube and later the photomultiplier tube were developed, which made possible the measurement of very faint light signals. This made it practical to measure very slight differences in monochromatic light, and this has revolutionized spectrophotometry.

Solid-state electronics have now virtually replaced vacuum tubes. The use of equipment such as transistor devices, photodiodes, thermistors, integrated circuits, and crystal oscillators has now made possible miniaturization of instruments, automation, and computerization beyond the wildest dreams of even a decade ago.

There have been many other notable inventions, developments, and refinements that have advanced the field. The development of specialized plastics; improvement in optics, prisms, and diffraction gratings; refinements in electrode design; and the use of radioactive materials have immeasurably increased the accuracy, reliability, sensitivity, and selectivity of the instruments with which we work.

As mentioned before, the pace of development can only increase as time goes on, and we can only wonder what direction these developments may take. Since the way we work and plan may be affected, it is appropriate to try to imagine what the future may hold.

## Costs of health care

It has been said that modern science and engineering can perform any task of which the mind can conceive. This has been demonstrated during the past decade by the achievements in space. The limiting factors, of course, are the resources that can be brought to bear on the problem. Indeed, it has become apparent that we must decide what goals we wish to set and what problems need to be solved with the money that can be spent. Medical care in the United States now uses about 10% of the gross national product, and each year the portion required is increasing. Much of this increase in cost has occurred because of the ability to diagnose better, cure faster, and save more lives. These improvements have come about because of better (and more expensive) instruments, drugs, and procedures. Not only are the results better, but we are caring more intensively for an ever-larger segment of the population.

All of this is, of course, good, but we now approach a time when decisions must be made as to whether food, clothing, housing, defense, and education must receive less funding and attention so that our resources can be applied to medicine. It is becoming apparent that the cost of medical care delivery must be reduced. The problem is how this reduction should be effected. Its solution will lend insight to the direction new instrument development will take.

*Pretesting and profiling.* Several viable approaches to reducing medical costs have been proposed or initiated. One idea is to reduce the length of each hospital stay by preadmission diagnostic testing. Some of this pretesting will be done by the hospital laboratories, but as cost competition becomes more acute, much of it may go to centralized laboratories where the maximum economy of large batch testing can be achieved. This would tend to favor the development of economical batch-testing instruments. Many laboratories are already examining their test catalogs to find which tests can reasonably be sent to outside laboratories where they can be done more economically.

*Single-test instruments.* Another approach calls for faster diagnosis and definitive treatment to shorten the hospital stay. The very fastest result reporting that can be achieved is desirable. This tends to stimulate development of single-test stat-mode instruments and computerized reporting. There is also some tendency away from profiling or testing each patient with a list of 12 or 18 of 20 tests. This trend also tends to favor the development of single-test instruments.

Another trend is toward the concentration of seriously ill patients in intensive care areas with testing facilities in the care environment. Since it is not economically feasible to keep laboratory personnel in these areas, instruments are designed to be more or less "idiot-proof," that is, to be run by personnel with little or no specific training.

*Preventive medicine.* Another approach is to improve our diagnostic capability to allow earlier diagnosis and prevention of less obvious disease states to eventually reduce the need for hospitalization. This approach requires the development of more sophisticated and sensitive instruments and more research-oriented activity.

*Batch testing.* The seemingly contradictory trends just discussed suggest several probable directions new instrument development may take. Batch testing by large centralized laboratories seems certain to increase. Highly organized, rapid collection of samples and computerized reporting to in-hospital printing terminals has proved to be practical and economical. Even the very effective systems now seen will no doubt be made more economical, rapid, and versatile. The fixed profile may give way, however, to more selectivity. The market for these large expensive supersystems would seem to be fairly limited, and it would not be surprising if only a very few companies were successful with their development.

*"Stat" systems.* The versatile "stat" systems that can perform a large variety of tests and report each in a very short time will probably get much attention. In many hospitals, the time needed to convey a report to the patient's record is greater than the analysis time; therefore, these stat systems will include the capability of producing a complete, typed report in the laboratory or in the nursing unit. Since quality control is such an important and time-consuming part of any analysis, self-calibration and statistical analysis will certainly be built into most of these systems. Naturally, economy will be of prime importance.

Because of the physical size and complexity of many hospitals, it has become very difficult for a centralized laboratory to receive an order, collect a sample, and process, analyze, and report it without an appreciable lapse of time. In response to this problem, special-purpose instruments that analyze a single analyte, such as glucose, blood urea nitrogen, calcium, or chloride, have been developed. Many of these analytes can be injected by needle with whole blood from a syringe. The instruments standardize themselves, test, and print results into a computerized patient record. The whole process

from the drawing of the blood sample may require less than a minute and be performed by the physician or nurse or phlebotomist. The inclination is to question the accuracy, precision, or reliability of such a system, but many of these instruments are proving themselves with a minimum of expert maintenance performed at long intervals. It seems to be part of the American genius to mass-produce radios, can openers, electric razors, or TV games at a low price if there is a large market. It is quite possible that the future laboratory may change drastically as common tests become available via the black box that automates the entire procedure. Less common tests would then be sent out to central laboratories.

What then might become of the laboratory and the laboratorian? Laboratories have always been places of experimentation and development and probably always will. As quickly as a test is developed, standardized, and automated, another will appear that needs to be examined, tried, and developed. The process will most likely continue as our knowledge of physiology, microbiology, chemistry, and immunology continues to grow.

As our knowledge increases, there is a growing demand for professionals who have an overview of several disciplines, and the future leader in the laboratory may need to know all the basic laboratory sciences plus radiochemistry, pulmonary physiology, physical medicine, and, above all, instrumentation.

# CHAPTER 2

# *Basic functional units of analytical instruments*

The basic functional units of analytical instruments, as shown in Fig. 2-1, are the power source, excitation or signal source, sample compartment, detector, signal processing unit, and readout device.

## Sample compartment

The sample compartment is described first because it is the functional unit with which laboratory scientists are most familiar. The sample compartment holds the sample to be analyzed. Delivery of the sample into the sample compartment occurs after the sample has been prepared according to instrument and methodology requirements. The sample form required for analysis may be gaseous, liquid, or solid. Gas chromatographs and mass spectrophotometers, for example, quantitatively analyze gaseous samples. Spectrophotometers, emission flame photometers, atomic absorption spectrophotometers, osmometers, pH meters, titrators, and automatic cell counters analyze liquid samples. Solid samples can be analyzed with electron microscopes and x-ray spectrometers.

## Power source

The power source supplies power to all electrical units of the instrument. Batteries and commercially generated power supplies are two sources of power.

Batteries generate direct current as a product of electrochemical reactions. They are not generally used as the sole source of power in analytical instruments but occasionally are used within a particular circuit of an instrument to perform a specific function. Use of batteries as a power source is limited because they are heavy, may be destructive if caustic agents leak into an instrument, and may be expensive and troublesome, since replacements are required. However, they do provide the advantage of portability. If instrumental analyses are needed in locations not accessible to

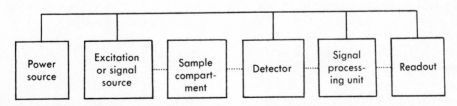

*Fig. 2-1.* Basic functional units of analytical instruments. Electrical connections from the power source are indicated by solid lines. Physical and/or electrical interconnections between units are designated by dotted lines.

electrical generators, battery-operated instruments can be used.

The diversified power requirements of instrument circuits are in most cases fulfilled by a power supply. Commercially generated alternating current is fed from a wall outlet through a power cord into an instrument's power supply. The electrical needs of each component within an instrument are not necessarily the same. One component may require alternating current (ac), whereas another may require direct current (dc). Requirements for regulation of voltage, current, and stability also may differ from one component to another. The power supply must fulfill the specific electrical requirement of each electronic unit. Therefore, the power supply must:

1. *Transform* ac voltage to higher and/or lower voltages than the 115 volts ac (Vac) input voltage
2. *Rectify* alternating current to direct current
3. *Regulate* the stability of direct current to meet the specified requirements of dc-operated components (Electronic drift within an instrument's circuit could result in erroneous readout signals and incorrect test results.)

## Excitation or signal source

Sample analyses are performed by instruments that expose the sample to some type of energy. Quantification of a constituent within a sample can be accomplished by measuring the effect the sample constituent has on a preset energy signal or the effect certain energy has on the physical and/or chemical properties of the sample constituent.

The sample may cause a measurable change in an energy signal. In spectrophotometry, a light signal is detected and measured. A sample is then placed between the light source and the detector, causing the amount of light hitting the detector to be diminished. The change in the amount of light reaching the detector before and after sample introduction is related to the concentration of a radiant energy–absorbing constituent in the sample.

An electrical potential may be used as a signal source as in the coulometric titration of chloride. A steady current is applied between two silver generator electrodes immersed in a sample containing chloride. The current causes constant generation of silver ions into the sample solution. Silver ions combine with chloride ions until all the chloride has precipitated as silver chloride and an excess of silver ion is generated. This excess of silver ions increases the conductivity of the solution. With increased conductivity, the current between the two indicator electrodes increases to a preset level that turns off a timer. The time required for excess silver ions to be detected as an increase in conductivity is related to chloride concentration.

An excitation source may change a property of the sample. This change may be physically or electronically measured and related to the concentration of a sample constituent. An example of an excitation source is the flame in an emission flame photometer. Heat from the flame excites the atoms from their unexcited ground state to a higher energy level. As the atoms return to their original ground state, light is emitted. The emitted light can be used to identify and quantitate elements in a sample. Excitation of a sample can be caused by various forms of energy, including heat and light (for example, in fluorometry).

## Detector

The function of the detector is to generate an analog signal (electrical signal) from energy derived from the signal source or from an excited, electrochemically active sample.

A transducer is a detector that changes one form of energy into another form. Generally the detectors in analytical instruments convert chemical or physical energy (for example, pressure, temperature, and light) into an electrical signal. Chemical properties of a blood sample are detected for blood gas and blood pH determinations. The pH is determined by an electrode that converts hydrogen ion activity into an electrical signal. Two examples of physical signals used in analytical instruments and their transducers are:

1. Light (spectrophotometer, emission flame photometer, atomic absorption spectrophotometer, and fluorometer): transducers used for converting light to an electrical signal include barrier-layer cells, phototubes, and photomultiplier tubes.
2. Temperature (freezing point depression osmometer): a thermistor reflects a change of temperature as a change in an electrical signal.

## Signal processing unit

The detector generates an electrical signal that must be converted into understandable data related to concentration of a sample constituent for display on the readout device. This conversion is executed by the signal processing unit. The signal processing unit may be simple or complex, depending on the sophistication of the instrument. In most cases, the signal from the detector is amplified before being fed into the readout device. Several functions performed by signal processing electronics are:

1. Signal amplification
2. Conversion of current to voltage
3. Comparison of signal to reference signal
4. Division of one signal by another
5. Addition or subtraction of two signals
6. Logarithmic conversion of signal
7. Zero adjustment
8. Calibration
9. Conversion of analog to digital signal
10. Integration and/or differentiation of signal

## Readout device

The readout device presents in visible form data obtained from sample analyses. These data should be easily read and understood. In most analytical instruments, the output data represent concentrations of specific sample constituents. The readout device in a sense translates the electrical signals from the detector and the signal processing electronics into physical or concentration values. The most frequently seen readout devices on clinical analytical instruments include:

1. Meter
2. Digital display
3. Recorder
4. Printout
5. Cathode ray tube

## From the general to the specific

The general view of instruments' functional units can be applied to specific instruments to allow for quick, logical modular disassembly into comprehensible working units. The student of instrumentation should practice identifying the six basic functional units of instruments.

This brief overview of the building blocks of instruments serves as the portal through which the material in the following chapters is viewed. Knowledge of electronic concepts, components, modules, and rules of safety strengthens theoretical and practical proficiency in instrumentation.

# BASICS OF ELECTRONICS

# CHAPTER 3

# *Fundamentals of electronics*

Fundamental to knowledge of electronics is an understanding of terms. The establishment of a basic electronics vocabulary is essential for an appreciation of electronic concepts and principles. In this chapter, electricity is defined in terms of the interrelated values of current, voltage, resistance, and power. Conductors and insulators are described in terms of the atomic structures of materials. Sources and characteristics of direct and alternating current are briefly discussed.

## *Basic concepts of electricity*

Comprehension of electrical principles begins with an understanding of the structure of the atom, which determines the availability of movable charges. Atoms of insulators restrict movement of electrical charges, whereas those of conductors allow easy passage when electromotive force is applied to a closed circuit. Current, voltage, and resistance are interdependent electrical parameters, their interrelatedness being expressed in Ohm's law. Voltage drop, voltage division, power, and electrical grounding are important fundamental electronic concepts. The definitions and principles presented in this chapter are prerequisite to developing a basic understanding of what is happening in electric circuits.

*The atom.* A discussion of electricity must begin somewhere, and the most logical starting point is the atom. The atom is the basic building block of all matter, including the matter of understanding electricity. Details of atomic structure have been studied in general chemistry and physics courses.

Therefore, atomic structure is reviewed only briefly.

Atoms are composed of an electrically positive *nucleus,* around which *electrons* move in orbits at varying distances. The simplest element is *hydrogen,* which has only one *proton* or positive charge in the nucleus and one electron or negative charge orbiting around it. Other elements have a larger number of protons in the nucleus and always an equal number of electrons in orbit around it. There may also be electrically neutral *neutrons* in the nucleus, but the net charge of the stable atom is neutral. The negative charge of an electron is exactly equal to the positive charge of a proton. An atom with an equal number of protons and electrons is electrically neutral. If an atom loses an electron, a proton excess—or more accurately, an electron deficiency—results. This atom carries a positive charge and is called a *positive ion.* If the atom gains an electron, the atom carries a negative charge and is called a *negative ion.*

Each element has a characteristic number of electrons and protons. The proton has a measurable weight, and all protons weigh the same. Almost all the weight of the atom is in its protons and neutrons. The *atomic number* is the number of protons in the atom; the *atomic weight* is roughly the number of protons and neutrons combined. See Appendix B, p. 347, for a table of the elements, giving for each element its atomic number, appropriate atomic weight, and chemical symbol. The electrons have a great deal of energy and rep-

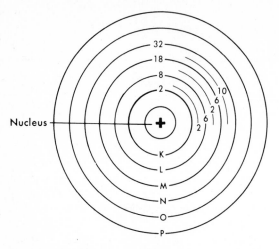

*Fig. 3-1*. Schematic representation of an atom, showing electron shells and their capacities. Note subshells of *L* and *M*.

resent practically the entire energy of the atom, but they have essentially no weight.

The electrons are characteristically arranged in *shells,* or orbits, around the nucleus. These shells are designated as *K, L, M, N,* etc., lettering from the center outward. Each shell has a maximum number of electrons that it can hold, and these shell capacities are indicated in Fig. 3-1. Each shell's capacity must be satisfied before electrons will be found in the next more distant shell. Thus sodium, with eleven electrons, will have two electrons in the *K* shell, eight in the *L* shell, and its one remaining electron in the *M* shell. There will be no electrons in the shells farther out.

As the temperature of an atom increases, the electrons move farther from the nucleus, and the distance between atoms increases. When the atoms become far apart, the substance becomes a gas. If the atoms approach each other to the point where the distance between nuclei is about the same as the diameter of the atom, the substance will become a liquid. As the atoms get still closer together, their outer electron orbits begin to overlap, and a solid is formed. These outer electrons are called *valence electrons.* If the valence electrons match each other, as do the parts of a puzzle, a

series of atoms occurs, with atoms connected in each plane in the same way, and a crystal is formed. This crystal will be *symmetrical* and, since the same configuration occurs over and over, we say it is *periodic* in nature. The outer electron orbit of most atoms has a radius in the order of 1 angstrom (Å) about one ten millionth of a millimeter). Since the outer orbits of electrons in a crystal overlap, we would expect the atoms in a crystal to be about 2 Å apart. These distances may vary somewhat, and orbits may be distorted and overlapped to the point that no single electron can be identified as belonging to a specific atom. Electrons may be shared and may adopt some new systematic pattern of motion.

In metals there are usually many electrons in the valence orbit. In the solid state, then, many of the electrons are located in the overlapping, distorted outer shells, and many electrons are shared. As many as $10^{23}$ electrons may be present in a cubic centimeter of metal. Electrons in such a situation can be considered an *electron cloud,* or sea of electrons in motion. Free charges moving about suggest electricity—that is, the capacity for electron flow. Thus, the outermost shell of the atom is recognized as the orbit most important in electronics.

As previously stated, most metals are made up of atoms with loosely bound electrons in the outer shells. These electrons may be so loosely bound that they are constantly moving randomly from one atom to another. Picture a metal wire in which many electrons are moving about aimlessly. These electrons can be made to move in one direction by placing an excess of electrons (negative charge) at one end of the wire and a deficiency of electrons (positive charge) at the other end. The loose electrons in the wire will be repelled by the extra electrons entering the wire at the negative end and attracted to the positive charge at the other end. This electron flow is diagrammed in Fig. 3-2. A stepwise description of what is happening in the wire follows:

1. An electron is introduced at the negative end of the wire.

*Fig. 3-2.* Electron flow through a metal wire.

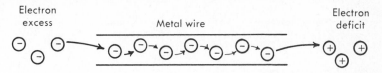

2. This electron replaces a loose electron in an atom.
3. The now free electron is repelled by the newly introduced electron and moves to another atom.
4. Here it replaces another loose electron, repels this replaced electron, and moves on.
5. This chain reaction continues until the extra electron reaches the other end of the wire, where it is accepted by a positively charged atom.

The process as described may sound slow, but it occurs at the speed of light (approximately 186,000 miles per second).

*Conductors and insulators.* Materials composed of atoms with weakly bound electrons in the outer orbits make good pathways for electron flow. Such materials are called *conductors*. The more loosely bound the outer electrons of the atoms of a material, the better the material conducts electron flow (for example, silver is the best conductor, followed by copper and gold).

Substances that give up their electrons only under great stress are nonconductors and may be called *insulators, resistors,* or *dielectrics.* As noted before, the valence electrons of atoms in a crystal are tied together in a bonding arrangement; this does not allow them to be displaced easily. Hence pure crystals are, in general, poor conductors of electricity. Examples of high-resistance or insulating materials include air, glass, plastic, and rubber.

Solids are conductors or insulators in varying degrees. What about solutions? Pure water is a relatively poor conductor but nevertheless does conduct electricity. If sodium chloride is added to pure water, the solution becomes a better conductor. When the salt is dissolved, the sodium becomes a positively charged ion ($Na^+$) and the chloride becomes a negatively charged ion ($Cl^-$). These charges will conduct electricity through the solution. The numbers and types of ions present in solution determine the conducting capacity, or conductivity, of that solution.

*Electromotive force.* For electron flow to occur, a good conducting material must serve as an unbroken pathway for electrons, and an electron excess and an electron deficit must be applied at opposite ends of the conducting pathway.

The conducting material has already been discussed. Unresolved is the source of the electron excess and the electron deficit that are applied to opposite ends of a conducting wire to initiate and maintain the flow of electrons. As shown in Fig. 3-2, it appears as though the excess electrons are pushing or forcing the free or loose electrons through the wire. In fact, this process *is* regarded as a *force.* The force exerted by the excess electrons on the loose electrons in the conductor is quite appropriately called *electromotive force* (EMF). The electromotive force is the *force* that causes *electrons* to *move* through a conductor from a negatively to a positively charged point. The unit of measure of electromotive force is the *volt.* (The definition of the volt is presented later in this chapter.)

What supplies this electromotive force? Some type of battery or generator may be the source of the required EMF. A *battery* is a dc voltage source consisting of cells that convert one form of energy (chemical, thermal, nuclear, or solar) to electrical energy. An ac *generator* is an alternating current voltage source consisting of a rotating mechanism that converts mechanical energy into electrical energy.

The batteries with which we are most familiar

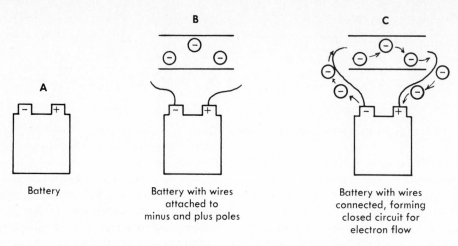

*Fig. 3-3.* Battery providing electromotive force for electron flow.

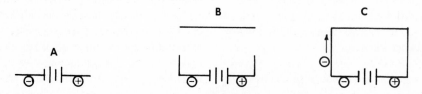

*Fig. 3-4.* Schematic representation of Fig. 3-3.

convert chemical energy to electrical energy. Different types of batteries are reviewed later in the discussion of direct current. Through a chemical reaction, an electron excess is formed at one pole (negative pole), and an electron deficit is formed at the other pole (positive pole). As shown in Fig. 3-3, if the positive and negative poles of a battery are connected with a conducting material, electrons will flow from the negative pole to the positive pole. The battery therefore provides the EMF required to move the electrons through the conductor. Fig. 3-4 is the same as Fig 3-3 but is represented with conventional schematic symbols.

*Current.* It has been established that electrons can be forced to flow through a conductor. Now relate this electron flow to electrical current. Refer to Fig. 3-5. The circuit in *A* represents electron

flow from negative to positive. Traditionally, however, current has been thought to flow from positive to negative, as represented in Fig. 3-5, *B*. This concept is considered the conventional way of perceiving current flow. In the literature both concepts of current flow may be found. Throughout this text the conventional current flow, positive to negative, is used.

*Current* (designated I) is the rate at which a *charge* moves through a conductor. What is a charge? Each electron possesses energy called a charge (designated Q). The unit for measuring this charge is the *coulomb*. Each electron carries an approximate charge of $1.6 \times 10^{-19}$ coulombs. How many electrons would it take to accumulate a charge of 1 coulomb? The charges of 6,240,000,000,000,000,000 electrons

A

B

Electron current flow                    Conventional current flow

*Fig. 3-5.* Electrical current flow.

added together would give a charge of 1 coulomb. Therefore, 1 coulomb equals $6.24 \times 10^{18}$ electrons.

The unit of measure of current is the *ampere* (A). When $6.24 \times 10^{18}$ electrons (1 coulomb) pass a point in the circuit every second, the circuit is said to be carrying a current of 1 A. For example, if the rate of flow of the electrons is $3.12 \times 10^{18}$ electrons (0.5 coulomb) per second, the current is 0.5 A. The ampere is a rather large unit. In most cases the current in circuits is in the milliampere (mA) or the microampere ($\mu$A) range. A milliampere equals one thousandth of an ampere, and a microampere equals one millionth of an ampere.

Current is the rate of electron flow in a circuit. Two factors that affect this rate of flow are: (1) the force, or *voltage* that moves the electrons through the circuit and (2) the ease with which the material in the circuit allows the electrons to pass, or in other words, the *resistance* of the circuit to current flow. Current and the two factors affecting it are interdependent phenomena. In the following discussion of the two factors, keep in mind that one cannot be defined without consideration of the other. These factors are considered separately.

*Voltage.* The force that moves electrons through a conductor is the electromotive force. The unit of measure of EMF is the volt (V). A force of one volt is required to move 1 coulomb per second (1 A) through a resistance (R) of 1 ohm ($\Omega$). Commonly used units of voltage include the kilovolt (kV), which equals 1000 V; the megavolt (MV),

1,000,000 V; the millivolt (mV), 0.001 V; and the microvolt ($\mu$V), 0.000001 V.

Electromotive force, voltage, and potential or potential difference are terms frequently used interchangeably. There are, however, subtle differences that should be noted. In the case shown in Fig. 3-3, *B*, the circuit is not closed; therefore, no electrons are moving in the conductor. No voltage is developed. However, a *potential* for current flow does exist because there are two poles of different charges, or it may be said that between the two poles there exists a *potential difference*. In Fig. 3-3, *C*, the circuit is closed, and there is a voltage or EMF forcing a current to flow.

*Resistance.* If a material is a poor conductor of electricity, it will offer resistance to current flow in a circuit. Resistance (R) to current is measured in *ohms* ($\Omega$). The kilohm (k$\Omega$) is 1000 ohms. The megohm (M$\Omega$) is 1 million ohms. One ohm is the value of resistance through which 1 V maintains a current of 1 A. The schematic symbol for resistance in a circuit is ———/\/\/\——. The types and construction of resistors are presented later during the discussion of electronic components.

What is meant by "drawing current"? If a fixed potential exists, such as in a battery, the amount of current that will flow in a closed circuit of conducting material depends on the ease with which electrons are allowed to move through the circuit. That is, if the excess electrons provided by the battery have difficulty in getting through the circuit, very few will be persistent enough to make the trip from one pole to the other. This is the case

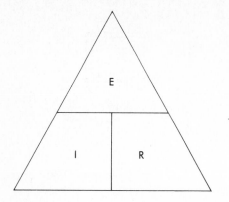

**Fig. 3-6.** Diagrammatic representation of Ohm's law.

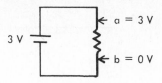

**Fig. 3-7.** Voltage drop.

when the circuit contains high resistance. Electron flow will be very small. On the other hand, when the road is easy, many electrons will take to travel. With decreased or small resistance, there is a large current.

*Ohm's law.* The relationship of voltage, current, and resistance is expressed in Ohm's law:

$$\text{Voltage} = \text{Current} \times \text{Resistance or}$$
$$\text{Volts} = \text{Amperes} \times \text{Ohms}$$

Another expression of Ohm's law can be seen in the triangular arrangement of Fig. 3-6. Any single value is equal to the other two, in the relationship that they hold in the triangle. Thus, $E = IR$, $I = E/R$, and $R = E/I$.

Voltage, current, and resistance and their interrelationships can be further explained or clarified by using an analogy to which all automobile operators will be able to relate—traffic. Think of each car as a bundle of $6.24 \times 10^{18}$ electrons or as a charge of 1 coulomb. The roads are conductors. Any degree of road blockage is a resistor. The more cars waiting to enter a roadway, the higher the potential for traffic flow (current on that roadway.

Suppose a traffic light regulates traffic so well that there are always 10 cars waiting on the entrance ramp at the beginning of a two-lane roadway. When there is no work being done on the road, traffic flows over a counting device at 10 cars

per second. Arbitrarily call the normal resistance to traffic flow 1. Now suppose that one of the two lanes is closed. Resistance to traffic flow therefore is doubled to 2.

Traffic flow before road work:

$$I = \text{Potential/resistance}$$
$$\text{Traffic flow} = 10 \text{ cars}/1 = 10 \text{ cars/second}$$

Traffic flow after road block:

$$\text{Traffic flow} = 10 \text{ cars}/2 = 5 \text{ cars/second}$$

This demonstrates that, with a constant potential for traffic flow, a change in resistance will affect that flow. The same is true of current flow in an electrical circuit.

*Voltage drop and voltage division.* Voltage has been defined as the force required to push a current through a resistance. When the current goes through this resistance, energy is given off in the form of heat. This loss of energy can be regarded as a loss of voltage or as a *voltage drop.* Frequently, voltage drop is referred to as IR drop. There is no difference in these terms, since voltage = I × R. Refer to Fig. 3-7. The voltage at point *a* is 3 V, which is supplied by a 3 V battery. The voltage at point *b* is 0 V, since 3 V were dropped or lost in going through the resistor.

The concept of voltage drop may be, and frequently is, used to obtain different voltages from one voltage source. In other words, it is possible to divide a voltage source into smaller voltage sources. This is called *voltage division.* How is this done? Refer to Fig. 3-8, *A*. The circuit shown has a 3 V battery and three 1 kΩ resistors. Three volts is dropped across three resistors of equal value. The voltage at point *a* is 3 V, and the voltage at point *d* is 0 V. Since each of the three

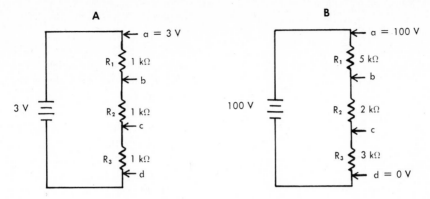

*Fig. 3-8.* Voltage division.

resistors will exert the same resistance to current flow, the voltage lost in each resistor will be the same. Thus, 1 V is lost across each resistor. With reference to the negative side of the battery, determine the voltage readings at points *b* and *c*.

Point $b = 2$ V and point $c = 1$ V

Voltage division is not always done by using resistors of equal value. A voltage may be dropped across any number of different resistances. The amount of voltage lost across a given resistor can be calculated in two ways:

1. Multiply the total voltage by the fraction that the given resistor is of the total resistance. For example, referring to Fig. 3-8, *B*, calculate the voltage lost across each resistor:

Total resistance $(R_t) = R_1 + R_2 + R_3$
$$R_t = 5\,k\Omega + 2\,k\Omega + 3\,k\Omega = 10\,k\Omega$$

Voltage drop in $R_1$: IR drop = 100 V ×
$R_1/R_t = 100$ V × 5 k$\Omega$/100 k$\Omega$ = 50 V

Voltage drop in $R_2$: IR drop = 100 V ×
$R_2/R_t = 100$ V × 2 k$\Omega$/10 k$\Omega$ = 20 V

Voltage drop in $R_3$: IR drop = 100 V ×
$R_3/R_t = 100$ V × 3 k$\Omega$/10 k$\Omega$ = 30 V

2. Multiply total current (in amperes) passing through the resistor by the value of the resistor (in ohms). For example, referring to Fig. 3-8, *B*, calculate the voltage lost across the resistor:

Total current $(I_t) = V/R_t = 100$ V/10 K $\Omega$
$$= 10\text{ mA or } 0.01\text{ A}$$

Voltage drop in $R_1$: IR drop = I × R =
(0.01 A) (5,000 $\Omega$) = 50 V

Voltage drop in $R_2$: IR drop = I × R =
(0.01 A) (2,000 $\Omega$) = 20 V

Voltage drop in $R_3$: IR drop = I × R =
(0.01 A) (3,000 $\Omega$) = 30 V

The application of voltage division is seen frequently throughout the remainder of this text. It is very important that this basic concept be understood at this time.

*Power.* Another term to be considered is *power*. When electrons are pushed through a circuit, work is done. The unit used to measure this work is the *watt* (W). One watt is the work done when 1 V moves 1 A (Joule's law):

Power = Voltage × Current or W = EI

All the normally used variations of Ohm's and Joule's laws are expressed in the circular diagram of Fig. 3-9. In each quadrant the factor in the inner circle is equal to each of the expressions in the outer circle. For example, E = I × R and I = W/E. In all these expressions:

W = Watts of power
E = Electromotive force in volts
R = Resistance in ohms
I = Current in amperes

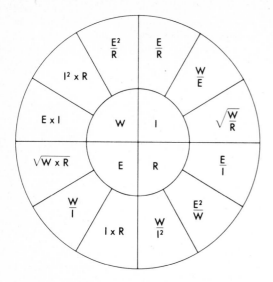

*Fig. 3-9.* Equations derived from Ohm's and Joule's laws.

Consideration of power is important in determining whether a circuit component can withstand the amount of electricity to be passed through the circuit. The energy that a battery loses is converted to heat energy in the resistance components of a circuit. If these components are not constructed to dissipate the heat generated, the component will burn or melt. Resistors have a watt rating that must be considered when a circuit is built or repaired. For example, if a 10 k$\Omega$ resistor is rated for 2 W, can it withstand a 10 mA current?

$$W = (I)(E) = (I)(IR) = (I)^2(R)$$
$$W = (0.01 \text{ A})^2 \times (10,000 \text{ }\Omega)$$
$$W = 0.0001 \times 10,000 \text{ }\Omega = 1 \text{ W}$$

Yes, 10 mA of current passing through a 10 k$\Omega$ resistance generates 1 W of energy, which can be easily dissipated by a resistor rated to dissipate twice that amount of heat.

Instruments used in the clinical laboratory are often very sophisticated and therefore expensive. In these instruments the circuits are many, complex, and intricate. With the simple insertion of a *fuse,* however, these expensive masses of electron

pathways can be protected by the principle $I^2R$ = heat.

The fuse contains a resistive element that melts at a certain temperature, causing a gap or break in the circuit. The resistive element is usually a filament of wire but can be a chemical compound, the composition of which determines its resistance and melting point. The resistance exerted by the fuse and the current through the fuse are the factors responsible for heat generation, expressed as $I^2R$. When sufficient heat is generated to melt the resistive element, the break in the element prevents further current conduction through the circuit. The voltage rating shown on fuses (for example, 32 V, 125 V, 250 V) indicates the size of the break or gap produced when the fuse's element melts. The larger the voltage rating, the wider the gap produced to ensure against arcing, that is, electrons jumping or a spark flying from one end of the break to the other.

The schematic symbol for a fuse is ⌒⌣. Refer to Fig. 3-10, which shows blown and good fuses. Fig. 3-11 is a representation of a circuit containing a fuse.

The line voltage (power from the wall outlet) entering an instrument is usually sent through a fuse. Therefore, if the instrument's circuit draws too much current, the fuse will prevent this excess from entering and damaging the instrument's circuitry. Other fuses may be located throughout the circuitry as protection for separate electronic circuits and/or components. Repeated blowing of fuses in an instrument is an indication that there is something electronically wrong, and the problem should be diagnosed and corrected.

The fuses most commonly used in laboratory instruments are called slow-blowing fuses. These fuses do not blow immediately with a surge of current; therefore, they are said to have a high time lag. However, these fuses blow quickly if the circuit is drawing abnormally high current. These slow-blowing fuses prevent unnecessary blows resulting from high starting currents when an instrument is first turned on or from the normal surges in a commercial power supply.

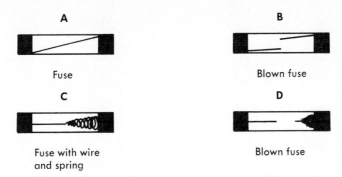

Fig. 3-10. Commonly used fuses; good fuses and blown fuses shown.

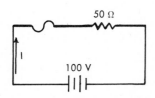

Fig. 3-11. Circuit protected with a fuse.

Standard fuses have a short time lag; that is, they blow very quickly with increased current. This type of fuse is used to protect sensitive electronic equipment and delicate meters or components within a circuit.

*Electrical ground.* A ground is a conducting material connected to the earth. Schematically a ground is represented as ⏚. The earth may be regarded as a "charge neutralizer." If a charged conductor is connected to the earth, the conductor will lose its charge to the earth. This conductor then will have a neutral or zero potential difference with reference to the earth or to ground.

The earth contains a tremendous accumulation of electrical charges. Therefore, it can gain or lose electrical charges while maintaining its electrical neutrality, that is, without itself becoming electrically charged. It is therefore reasonable that the ground is used as a reference point with which electrical measurements are made within a circuit. Voltage measurements at points in a circuit are taken in relationship to other points, called *ref-erence points.* Frequently, the reference point used is the ground or the negative side of the power source.

The chassis of an instrument may collect an electrical charge from the circuit. A connection (ground) between the metal chassis and the earth will allow the flow of the unwanted and potentially dangerous charge from the chassis to the earth. The danger in having a charge on a chassis is that an operator of that instrument may touch simultaneously the chassis and a ground (for example, a water pipe), thus becoming a conducting pathway from the chassis to earth. The resulting electrical shock is survived by the fortunate, while the less fortunate are said to have been killed by electrocution. Proper grounding is paramount in the consideration of safety.

In most modern buildings a three-pronged plug is used for electrical devices. One of the flat prongs contacts a wire in the receptacle that has zero potential. The second flat prong has a potential of about 117 V. When contact is established between the two through a lamp, a heater, or an instrument, electricity will flow. The third prong on the electric plug is used as a ground and is usually connected to any nonconducting metal surface of the appliance. When plugged into the wall, this prong makes contact with a wire that is connected to a water pipe or other conductor having immediate and good contact with the earth under the building. By this route, unwanted electrical changes are released to the earth.

## *Direct current*

Direct current is produced by batteries or by power supplies that convert alternating current to direct current. Characteristics of direct current and batteries, as a source of direct current, are described in this chapter. Instrument operators should be informed about the variety of available batteries and must be aware of the importance of required battery replacements meeting instrument specifications. Conversion of alternating current to direct current is addressed in Chapters 4 and 5 when diodes and power supplies are discussed.

*Characteristics.* *Direct current* (dc) is characterized by the fact that both the voltage level and the polarity of the electrical charges remain unchanged over time. Current as discussed earlier in this chapter was unidirectional and therefore direct current.

*Sources.* Sources of direct current include batteries and electronic power supplies. Most frequently, the direct current needed in circuits of clinical laboratory instruments is provided by the power supply circuit of that instrument. The power supply circuit converts alternating current to direct current by means of rectification. Discussion of such electronically supplied direct current is presented when power supplies are discussed in Chapter 5.

In this chapter various types of batteries are discussed. The purpose of presenting material about batteries is twofold—for theoretical understanding and for practical application.

1. Theoretical understanding: Parameters of voltage, potential, potential difference, and EMF have been defined. The various types of batteries discussed demonstrate that a potential can be generated by several different chemical reactions. The common feature shared by all batteries is that positive and negative charges are developed at two different electrodes or terminals, establishing a potential difference between these terminals.

2. Practical application: Some clinical laboratory instruments do have a battery or batteries in their circuitry. These batteries are used either as a very constant dc voltage source or as a voltage

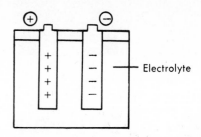

*Fig. 3-12.* Basic principle of battery. Potential difference between the two electrodes develops as a result of chemical reaction at each.

reference. A battery is a component of the circuit that a laboratory scientist may be required to replace. It is therefore very important that only the type of cell required by a particular circuit is inserted into the circuit. Many batteries are similar in size, shape, color, and general appearance and may be very easily mistaken for one another. As with fuse replacement discussed earlier, battery selection is a simple but important procedure. If a battery of incorrect specifications is installed in a circuit, the circuit may be damaged or may operate inaccurately. Batteries are common everyday items. However, they usually are not given adequate consideration by laboratory personnel who should be informed about the specifications and the advantages and disadvantages of the different types. The discussion of batteries will provide the information required for understanding specific battery selection.

Basically, a battery consists of a potential difference developed as a result of a chemical reaction, as represented in Fig. 3-12. A battery is symbolically designated: ⎯⎮ ⎮ ⎮⎯ or simply: ⎯⎮ ⎮⎯ . The longer vertical line represents the positive and the shorter vertical line the negative terminal of the voltage source. There are two general types of batteries, primary and secondary. The primary type of cell cannot be recharged; once it is dead, there is no resuscitation. The secondary type of cell, after being discharged, may be recharged by reversing the current through the cell.

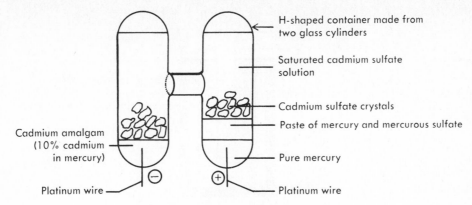

*Fig. 3-13.* Saturated standard Weston cell.

*Primary cells.* The primary cells most commonly used include the carbon-zinc, the alkaline-manganese, and the zinc–mercuric oxide dry cells. A cell used not as a source of potential to force current to flow but as a reference for voltage measurement is the cadmium sulfate cell. The discussion of primary cells includes this reference cell and the other three cells mentioned.

*Cadmium sulfate cell (standard Weston cell).* Accurate quantification requires that measurements be made with reference to a precisely known quantity or a standard. For the accurate measurement of voltage, a reference voltage or a standard voltage is used. Standard weights and measures are kept at the National Bureau of Standards, and so is a standard for voltage measurements. The Weston cell is almost universally used as a standard voltage.

The Weston reference cell can be saturated (Fig. 3-13) or unsaturated, with a potential of 1.0186 V or 1.019 V, respectively, at 20° C. The voltage decreases $4.06 \times 10^{-5}$ V for each degree the temperature rises above 20° C.

Cadmium sulfate cells produce a constant voltage for many years. To provide a stable potential difference between terminals, the chemical reaction must be constant. A constant chemical reaction can be ensured only if a cell's chemical equilibrium is maintained. The equilibrium may be altered by excessive current drain or by agitation. Severe agitation can ruin a cell by causing the contents of one tube to pass through the connecting bridge and thus contaminate the contents of the other tube. To maintain the stability of the potential, a Weston cell is usually kept at a constant temperature and in a fixed position.

*Carbon-zinc dry cell (flashlight-type battery).* An electrolyte may be absorbed by an inert material (for example, paper) or may be mixed in a paste to be used in a battery's electrochemical reaction. When such immobilized electrolyte is used in a voltage-producing cell, that cell is called a *dry cell.* A simplified representation and a cutaway view of the construction of a carbon-zinc (C-Zn) dry cell are shown in Figs. 3-14 and 3-15, respectively. At each of two electrodes, a chemical reaction occurs whereby the carbon electrode loses, and the zinc electrode gains, electrons. The end result is the development of a potential difference between the electrodes. A potential of 1.5 to 1.6 V is developed between the zinc *cathode,* or negative electrode, and the carbon *anode,* or positive electrode.

Thirty individual 1.5 V flashlight batteries could be connected in series (positive to negative) to produce a 45 V battery. This arrangement, however, would require too much space. Therefore, dry cell batteries are generally made by stacking

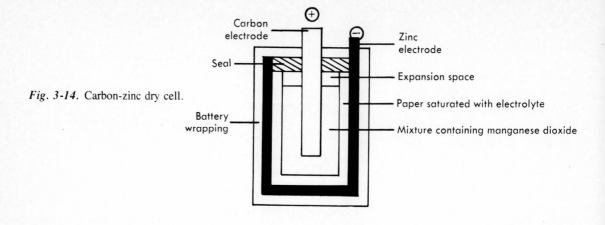

*Fig. 3-14.* Carbon-zinc dry cell.

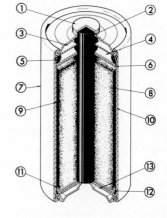

*Fig. 3-15.* Cross section of an electrochemical cell, or "dry battery." (Courtesy RCA, Electronic Components.)

1. Tin-plated steel top
2. Carbon electrode
3. Vent washer
4. Pitch seal
5. Wax-ring seal
6. Support washer
7. Plastic-coated paper jacket
8. Manganese dioxide–carbon–electrolyte cathode mix
9. Starch-flour-electrolyte gel separator
10. Zinc-anode can
11. Paper cup
12. Paperboard bottom
13. Tin-plated steel bottom

alternately a carbon plate, a layer of electrolyte paste, and a zinc plate as many times as necessary to give a desired voltage. The most common dry cell batteries have voltages of 1.5, 3.0, 7.5, 22.5, 45.0, 67.5, and 90.0 V.

Batteries discharge internally when not in use. An increase in temperature increases internal discharge, thus decreasing storage life. At room temperature, the storage life of a C-Zn dry cell ranges from 6 months to 1 year.

The length of a battery's service life depends on such factors as duration and temperature of storage before use, current drain and temperature during discharge, frequency and duration of off periods, and the quality of the battery. The service life of the C-Zn dry cell should be greater than 10 hours unless a heavy drain is placed on it. Under conditions requiring a heavy drain, frequent rest periods will extend the service life of the battery. At temperatures below freezing, this dry cell does not optimally generate a potential.

The potential of the C-Zn dry cell falls off continuously during use. The decrease in potential is caused by the change in electrolyte composition and the formation of interfering compounds during discharge. Since the potential is not constant, this battery is of little value as a reference voltage source.

The zinc casing of a C-Zn battery is the cathode (negative terminal); therefore, dissolution of zinc weakens the structure of the cell. Also, during discharge or storage, a pressure of evolved hydrogen gas builds up. This can lead to rupture of the zinc and leakage of the corrosive electrolyte into the instrument. Instruments using these dry cells should not be stored with the batteries installed.

*Alkaline-manganese dry cell (alkaline cell).* The alkaline-manganese battery is similar in mechanism to the carbon-zinc dry cell but differs in electrode materials, arrangement of electrodes, and electrolyte used. The alkaline cell consists of a zinc anode, a manganese oxide cathode, and a strong alkaline electrolyte of potassium hydroxide. The alkaline cell is four times the price of the C-Zn dry cell but provides the following advantages over the C-Zn cell: the capacity (milliampere-hours) is three to five times higher; the capacity does not decrease under heavy drain; the shelf life is about 2 years; the internal resistance is lower, yielding higher current output; and the operating temperature limit ($-40°$ C) is lower.

The battery is useful for applications requiring a relatively high current, which places a heavy drain on the battery. Considering its long shelf life and low operating temperature, it would be a good choice for an emergency power source.

*Zinc–mercuric oxide dry cell (mercury cell).* The mercury cell generates a negative charge at the zinc amalgam anode, with the oxidation of zinc to zinc oxide yielding two electrons per atom. At the mercuric oxide–carbon cathode, a positive charge results from the reduction of mercuric oxide to mercury with the acceptance of two electrons per molecule from the carbon electrode. The resulting potential is 1.35 V, which is extremely reproducible from one cell to another. Mercury cells are available in voltages ranging from 1.35 to 42 V.

Characteristics of this dry cell include a storage life of up to 2 years, a service life four to five times

that of the carbon-zinc dry cell, a very low internal resistance, a capacity that is greater than that of the alkaline cell but that is not maintained under heavy drain, a remarkably constant voltage during discharge, and a safe structure free of the effects of deterioration or evolved gas accumulation. The mercury cell costs about five times more than the alkaline cell, but the price is well worth the advantages gained. The high degree of voltage reproducibility between mercury cells and the virtually constant discharge voltage qualify this cell for such applications as providing potential for transistorized circuits and electrode biasing and serving as a secondary voltage standard.

The encasement of the mercury cell is less likely to leak corrosives. However, there is a slight amount of leakage that is not usually harmful to circuits. Therefore, mercury cells can be kept in instruments with relative safety. These batteries should be checked approximately every 6 months and any corrosive materials cleaned off.

Technologists should be aware of those instruments in which mercury cells are used (for example, the $Po_2$ measuring circuit frequently uses a 1.34 V mercury cell to impose a required potential across the $Po_2$ electrode). The voltage of this battery is constant up to the time the battery is completely discharged. This means that an instrument that is working properly may suddenly malfunction. Simple replacement of the discharged mercury cell may remedy the problem. Periodic battery replacement incorporated into a preventive maintenance schedule may prevent instrument down time resulting from battery "death." It is important not to substitute one type of battery for another. Use only the type battery specified for a particular instrument.

***Secondary cells.*** Secondary cells are also known as electrolytic cells or wet cells. Two secondary batteries discussed are the lead-acid storage battery and the nickle-cadmium battery.

*Lead-acid battery (car battery).* In their most common form lead-acid batteries contain several cells arranged in a battery to produce 6, 12, or 24 V. Each cell will produce about 2.1 V; therefore, three cells are necessary to produce 6 V. Each cell of these lead-acid batteries contains two electrodes, one lead and the other oxide. The lead is converted to lead sulfate by the electrolytic action of the liquid sulfuric acid. Two electrons are released to the lead electrode for each molecule of lead sulfate formed. The lead oxide electrode is reduced to lead sulfate, taking up two electrons. When current is applied to recharge the battery, the lead sulfate is reconverted to lead and lead oxide. This reversible process can be repeated many times during the life of the battery. The state of discharge can be measured by the specific gravity of the sulfuric acid solution containing the lead sulfate. Eventually the electrodes deteriorate so much that the battery is no longer functional, but the cycle of discharging and charging can be repeated many hundreds of times before this happens. A lead-acid battery provides a copious supply of constant direct current at an economical price. It is, of course, quite heavy and rather messy because of the sulfuric acid.

At one time these batteries were commonly used as a power source in clinical laboratories. They are no longer used to any extent. Their economy is negligible compared with the cost of today's laboratory instruments. At best, they are cumbersome and space-consuming and, at worst, dangerous around delicate electrical and optical components because of the damaging acid and acid fumes.

*Nickel-cadmium battery.* Another type of rechargeable battery that is becoming popular in the United States is the nickel-cadmium battery. This unit is completely sealed and requires no servicing other than recharging. The positive electrode is nickel hydroxide, and the negative electrode is cadmium. When the battery is discharging, the nickel hydroxide is converted to nickel, and the cadmium is oxidized. When it is recharging, the process is reversed. Each cell produces about 1.3 V and has fairly high capacity. These batteries can be stored for long periods of time either charged or discharged. They are quite expensive but are a practical source of constant current and are quite trouble free.

## Alternating current

Alternating current is generated commercially and supplied to consumers via wall outlets. Our concern with alternating current begins when it enters electrically powered instruments. The discussion of alternating current includes its description, its relationship to direct current, and its behavior in different electronic components. This presentation concentrates on the descriptive aspects of alternating current. The effects of different components on alternating current are included in the discussions of the particular components. Characteristics of alternating current include constant changing of direction of current flow, voltage variation over time, amplitude, frequency, and phase. The symbolic representation of an alternating current potential source is: —⊙— .

*Direction of alternating current flow.* Alternating current flows first in one direction and then in the opposite direction. For a more graphic description, consider the analogy of a two-lane road as a conductor and the cars as moving charges. Consider the situation in which one of the two lanes is closed. Flagmen regulate traffic flow by allowing cars (charges) to move, first in one direction and then in the other, through the constricted roadway (conductor). Thus, the direction of traffic is constantly changing. Alternating current works in the same way.

*Voltage variation over time.* There are different waveforms, of which the sinusoidal waveform (Fig. 3-16) is the most common and to which this discussion will be limited. The sine wave shown in Fig. 3-16 starts at 0 V, increases over time to 10 V, then decreases to 0 V. From 0 V the polarity is reversed, and the voltage goes to $-10$ V, then returns to 0 V again. This is considered one complete cycle of the waveform.

*Amplitude.* The amplitude of the waveform is the peak value of the voltage. Refer to Fig. 3-17. Peak-to-peak amplitude or voltage is the total voltage in both directions from 0 V. For example, in Fig. 3-17 the voltage reads 10 V in one direction and 10 V in the other direction. Therefore, the

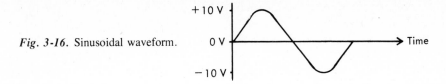

*Fig. 3-16.* Sinusoidal waveform.

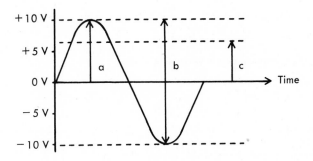

*Fig. 3-17.* Alternating current voltage: *a*, peak amplitude or peak voltage; *b*, peak-to-peak amplitude or peak-to-peak voltage; *c*, root mean square (rms) value of voltage (rms = peak voltage [×0.707]).

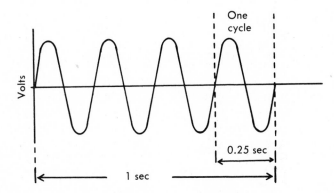

*Fig. 3-18.* Frequency and period of waveform; frequency (F) = 4 cycles per second (c/s) or hertz (Hz); period (T) = time required for 1 cycle = 0.25 second; equations: F = 1/T and T = 1/F.

total voltage, or peak-to-peak voltage, is 20 V. Peak voltage is voltage in one direction only (for example, 10 V in Fig. 3-17).

In the discussion of voltage, it would be convenient to be able to equate dc voltage with ac voltage. As a matter of fact, volt-ohm meters do read ac voltage in values equivalent to dc voltage. This equivalent dc voltage, which may be considered an average of ac voltage, is less than peak voltage by a factor of 0.707. That is:

ac peak voltage × 0.707 =
  root-mean-square (rms) voltage

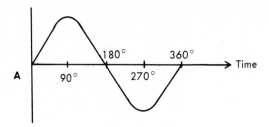

Relative degrees in ac sine wave

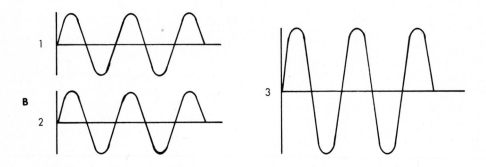

Signals 1 and 2 180° out of phase added to give signal 3

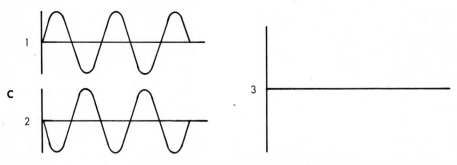

Signals 1 and 2 added to give signal 3

*Fig. 3-19.* Periodic plotting of sine wave.

The rms value of ac voltage is comparable to dc voltage in considering the amount of heat generated by ac and dc. To convert rms value to peak value:

$$rms \times 1.4 = Peak\ value$$

For example, if a voltage from a wall outlet of 110 volts ac (Vac) is the rms value, what is the peak value?

Peak value = rms value $\times$ 1.41
Peak value = 110 V $\times$ 1.41 = 155.1 Vac

*Frequency.* One complete waveform is one cycle. The number of cycles occurring each second is the frequency of the waveform. The commercially supplied ac in the United States has a frequency of 60 cycles per second (c/s), or using the preferred terminology, 60 hertz (Hz). In other countries ac current is generated at a frequency of 50 Hz.

The time required for one cycle is a period. The relationship of the period (T) and the frequency (F) of a signal is reciprocal:

Period = 1/frequency or T = 1/F
Frequency = 1/period or F = 1/T

Refer to Fig. 3-18. One cycle occurs every 0.25 second; therefore, the period is 0.25 second. The frequency is 4 Hz, since four cycles occur every second. Calculate these values:

F = 1/T = 1/0.25 sec = 4 Hz
T = 1/F = 1/4 Hz = 0.25 sec

Note: Audio frequency range = 20 Hz to 20,000 Hz
Radio frequency range = 100 kHz to 30 MHz

*Phase.* Using one signal as a reference, a time relationship (a phase difference) can be determined between that signal and another signal or signals.

Fig. 3-19, *A,* shows the periodic plotting of a waveform. Fig. 3-19, *B,* shows two waveforms, or signals, in phase. When signal 1 is at its maximum positive swing, so is signal 2, and when signal 1 is at its maximum negative swing, so is signal 2. If these two signals were added together, the resultant signal would have an amplitude equal to the sum of the amplitudes of signals 1 and 2. That is:

Amplitude of signal 1 + Amplitude of signal 2 =
Amplitude of resultant signal 3

Fig. 3-19, *C,* represents two signals that are out of phase. If two such voltages, both of equal magnitude, were introduced into a circuit, the resultant voltage felt by the circuit would be 0 V, since one signal cancels the other.

# CHAPTER 4

# *Electronic components*

Electronic circuits consist of a variety of electronic components specifically selected and purposefully arranged so as to perform particular operations. Of the commonly used components, those to be discussed in this chapter are resistors, capacitors, inductors, transformers, and diodes. Discussion of each component includes construction, function, effect on alternating and direct current, and representative electronic symbols. The collection of isolated facts and figures in this section is used in Chapter 5 to illustrate the interrelatedness of component functions in analytical instruments' functional units, for example, power supply.

## Circuit configurations

Circuit configuration is the arrangement of electronic components in a circuit. Components may be connected in series, in parallel, or in a combination of series and parallel. In this chapter different circuit configurations are illustrated by using that familiar component, the resistor.

Two commonly used methods of representing connections in an electrical circuit are shown in Fig. 4-1, *A* and *B*. Circuits may be drawn so that a node or dot at the point of intersection of lines represents an electrical connection as shown in Fig. 4-1, *A*. In this circuit representation the intersections at points *a* and *b* are not making electrical contact. In Fig. 4-1, *B*, intersecting straight lines represent electrical contact points, whereas the arched lines at points *a* and *b* indicate that these are not electrical connections. This latter type of circuit representation is used in the illustrations throughout this text.

*Series circuit.* Refer to Fig. 4-2, in which three resistors are connected in series in a circuit. A component is connected in series when it is connected to other components in such a way that current flow has only one possible pathway.

The total resistance exerted by resistors in series is calculated thus:

$$R_{total} = R_1 + R_2 + R_3 + R_4 + \ldots R_n$$

*Parallel circuits.* Fig. 4-3 shows two resistors connected in parallel. The same voltage is dropped across each resistor. However, the current flow has two alternate paths to follow. When current has a choice of pathways, the conducting pathways are connected in parallel.

The total current in a circuit is equal to the sum of the current in all parallel pathways in the circuit. The total current in the circuit shown in Fig. 4-3 is equal to the sum of the current passing through $R_1$ and $R_2$:

$$I_{total} = I_1 + I_2$$

What are the values for $I_1$ and $I_2$?

$$I_1 = V/R_1 = 25 \text{ V}/100 \ \Omega = 0.25 \text{ A}$$
$$I_2 = V/R_2 = 25 \text{ V}/50 \ \Omega = 0.50 \text{ A}$$

What is the total current in this circuit?

$$I_{total} = I_1 + I_2 = 0.25 \text{ A} + 0.50 \text{ A} = 0.75 \text{ A}$$

The resistance to current flow in this circuit is less than if these resistors were connected in series. When resistors are connected in series, the voltage from the voltage source is dropped across all of them. That is, the voltage source "sees" an "effective" resistance equal to the sum of the resistors

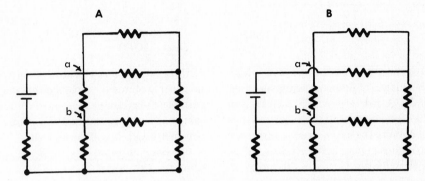

*Fig. 4-1.* Schematic representations of electrical connections.

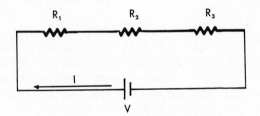

*Fig. 4-2.* Series combination of resistors.

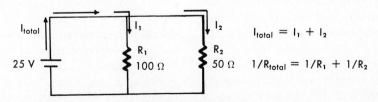

*Fig. 4-3.* Parallel circuit.

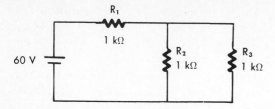

*Fig. 4-4.* Series-parallel circuit.

in series. However, when the resistors are in parallel, the full voltage is dropped across each resistor separately. A current flows in each resistor independently of the current in the other resistors in the parallel circuit. The total effective resistance in a parallel circuit is always less than the smallest resistor. The formula for calculating the total effective resistance in a parallel circuit is :

$$1/R_{total} = 1/R_1 + 1/R_2 + 1/R_3 + \ldots 1/R_n$$

Refer to the circuit in Fig. 4-3 and note the following example. What is the total "effective" resistance in this circuit?

$$1/R_{total} = 1/R_1 + 1/R_2$$
$$1/R_{total} = (R_1 + R_2)/(R_1R_2)$$
$$R_{total} + (R_1R_2)/(R_1 + R_2)$$
$$R_{total} + [(100\ \Omega)\ (50\ \Omega)]/(100\ \Omega + 50\ \Omega) =$$
$$5000\ \Omega/150\ \Omega = 33.33\ \Omega$$

If the 100 $\Omega$ and 50 $\Omega$ resistors were replaced with a 33.33 $\Omega$ resistor, what current would flow in this circuit?

$$I = E/R = 25\ V/33.33\ \Omega = 0.75\ A$$

Note that calculating total current in this circuit by adding the current flowing through each resistor results in the same value of 0.75 A.

*Series-parallel circuits.* Series circuits and parallel circuits have been discussed. A third possible variation of circuit design is a combination series-parallel circuit as shown in Fig. 4-4.

If the effective resistance of $R_2$ and $R_3$ is calculated, the two parallel limbs are essentially changed to a series with $R_1$. The effective resistance of $R_2$ and $R_3$ is:

$$1/R_{total} = 1/R_2 + 1/R_3$$
$$1/R_{total} = 1/1000\ \Omega + 1/1000\ \Omega = 2/1000\ \Omega = 1/500\ \Omega$$
$$R_{total} = 500\ \Omega$$

The total effective resistance of the entire circuit then becomes:

$$R = R_1 + (\text{effective resistance of } R_2 \text{ and } R_3)$$
$$R = 1000\ \Omega + 500\ \Omega$$
$$R = 1500\ \Omega$$

Current flow in this system is more complex than in either a series or a parallel circuit. The entire current of the circuit must flow through $R_1$. This same current then will find two paths, $R_2$ and $R_3$, between which it will be divided.

Current flow in the entire system is calculated by using the total resistance of 1500 $\Omega$.

$$I = E/R = 60\ V/1500\ \Omega = 40\ mA$$

Notice that the sum of the current in the parallel limbs is the same as that flowing through the series portion of the circuit, which must carry the total current. Using the above approach, a complex series-parallel combination of resistors can be analyzed and the effective resistance of the circuit calculated.

Voltage drop, voltage division, and current division are important electronic concepts that must be understood. Comprehension of these concepts provides a strong foundation on which other theories and concepts can be built. Therefore, it is strongly recommended that the following section, "Voltage Division and Current Division," be studied.

*Voltage division and current division.* This discussion is for those who do not yet understand the concepts of voltage division and current division. Comprehension of these two concepts in electronics is very important. The purpose of this discussion, therefore, is to present a simplified analogy to electron flow to explain and clarify these concepts.

Voltage, current, and resistance are by now familiar terms. Theoretical physicists have defined them, and students have dutifully memorized the definitions. The purpose of this section is to make these definitions more meaningful.

Three components essential for voltage division and current division are:

1. Voltage source (for example, transformer or battery)
2. Conductor
3. Resistance

Deviating from the strict definition of physicists and using simple terms, the effects resulting from the use of each of the components shown are discussed.

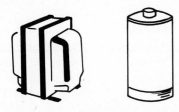

**Voltage source**

A transformer or battery can be used as a voltage source. Voltage is an electrical pressure, that is, a force that pushes electrons through wires.

The wires permit a current or passage of electrons to flow through the circuit. The wires are conductors of current.

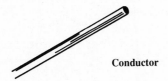

**Conductor**

Resistance is opposition to the flow of current.

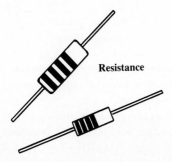

**Resistance**

Therefore, there are three components: the battery pushing the electrons, the wire allowing free passage of the electrons, and the resistor making passage of the electrons difficult.

There is one more condition that is required before any of these functions can be accomplished. These components must be connected in a closed circuit, that is, the electrons must have a continuous, unbroken pathway from one side of the battery ($-$) to the other ($+$).

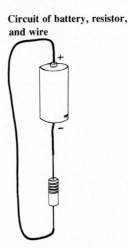

**Circuit of battery, resistor, and wire**

In this arrangement of components, the battery voltage pushes the electrons via the conducting wire through the resistor in a steady stream or a constant current.

The schematic representation of the circuit being discussed follows. The symbol for battery is: $\dashv\vdash$. The long vertical line is always the positive pole, and the short vertical line is the negative pole.

The resistor is represented as: $\longrightarrow\!\!\bigwedge\!\bigwedge\!\bigwedge\!\longrightarrow$, and the wires are designated by continuous lines.

The battery forces electrons through the circuit. Once the electrons reach the other side of the battery (+ pole), there is zero force (0 voltage) being exerted on them. This is what is meant by the expression "voltage drop." The voltage or pushing force on the electrons is used up entirely in the process of pushing the electrons through all resis-

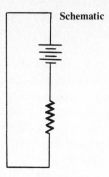

**Schematic**

tances in the circuit. This driving force is given up as heat energy as the electrons "squeeze through" the resistor.

A conceptual presentation of what occurs in this simple circuit is shown here. This is a container

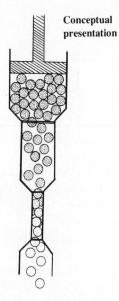

**Conceptual presentation**

filled with particles. A plunger is used to push the particles out of the container through a pathway, in which there is a constricted duct, and then on into an open area. The plunger represents the force, and the container is the reservoir of particles. Thus the container and plunger represent the battery. The passageway allowing easy flow of the particles represents the conductor or wire in

the schematic. The smaller duct represents a resistance. The open area below the duct represents the positive pole of the battery.

A constant pressure is exerted on the particles. The darkness of the stipple with which the particles are represented is directly proportional to the amount of pressure on each particle (call this "pressure energy"). Notice that as the particles pass *with difficulty* through the duct, each particle loses its "pressure energy." As the particles are pushed through the small duct, the walls of the duct become warm. The particles reaching the open area no longer have any driving force exerted on them.

With this simple circuit and the description of its operation as a basis, the circuit configurations required for current division and for voltage division are discussed.

Current division is accomplished in a parallel circuit. A parallel circuit is one in which all posi-

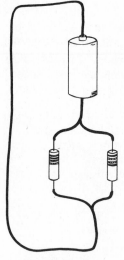

**Parallel circuit**

tive terminals are connected to a common point and all negative terminals are connected to a second common point.

Here the previous diagram is represented schematically. The only additional information added

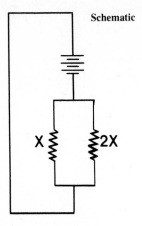

Schematic

to this schematic is that one resistor has 2× the resistance of the other resistor.

In this circuit the voltage drop over each of the resistors is the same. But the current differs. Since one resistor will resist electron flow twice as much as the other, the flow of electrons (current) through the X resistor will be greater than the current through the 2X resistor.

A conceptual view of this circuit includes the container of particles and the passageway leading from the container. The passageway is then divided into two ducts of different sizes. One duct is twice as large as the other. Note that the larger duct allows the passage of twice as many particles

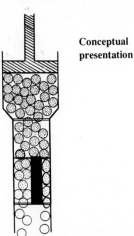

Conceptual presentation

as the smaller duct. Thus, the larger duct passes twice as much current as the smaller duct.

The particles arrive at the open area having no stipple or energy. No matter what duct they pass through, they each lose the same amount of energy, that is, there was the same voltage drop through each duct.

To achieve a division of voltage, a series configuration is used. In this series circuit, the resistances are connected end-to-end so that the same current flows throughout the circuit.

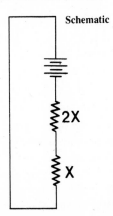

Series circuit

In this schematic, the resistances are designated X and 2X, that is, 2X has twice the resistance to current flow that X does.

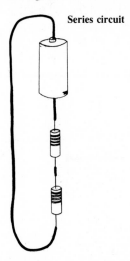

Schematic

The current is determined by the total resistance in the circuit. The current does not change in this circuit, since there is only one pathway to follow.

However, the voltage is different above the resistors and between the resistors and is zero below the resistors. The total voltage drops over the two resistors, with twice as much lost in the 2X resistor as is lost in the X resistor.

A conceptual view of voltage division is shown. The first duct through which the particles must pass is twice as narrow as the second duct. Therefore, it is twice as difficult for the particles to get by the first duct as it is for them to get by the second. Thus, twice as much voltage or force is required (lost) to get the particles through the first duct as is required to get them through the second.

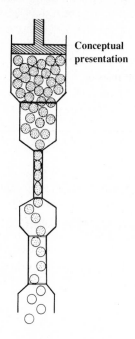

**Conceptual presentation**

Note that the current (rate of particle flow) is not greater in one duct or the other. The current is the same throughout the passageway.

The concepts of voltage division and current division are now briefly reviewed.

Voltage division occurs when resistances are in a series configuration.

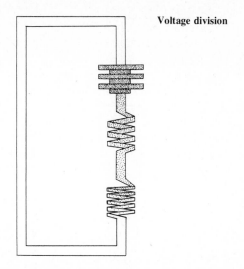

**Voltage division**

The stipple in the figure indicates voltage; more stipple means higher voltage.

The battery forces electrons through the circuit. The energy of force (voltage) is used up entirely in pushing the electrons through the resistances. The smaller the resistance to electron flow, the smaller the force required to push the electrons through the resistor. The greater the resistance, the greater the voltage required to get the electrons through the resistor. In this figure, the first resistor offers less resistance than the second resistor.

Current division occurs when resistances are in a parallel configuration.

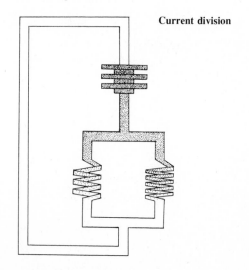

**Current division**

Note that the two resistances are not the same. The one on the left allows easier passage of current than the one on the right. Most electrons will take the route of least resistance; therefore, there will be greater current through the left resistor than through the right resistor.

Note that the force at the top of each of the resistances is the same and that the force at the bottom of each of the resistances is zero. Therefore, the same amount of force was used to push the electrons through each of the resistors.

### Resistors

As shown previously, strategically placed resistors of specifically selected values can regulate voltages and current flow in a circuit. A resistor is an electronic component that serves the useful function of providing circuits with resistance or hindrance to current flow. Thus, current limitation is achieved through the use of resistors. Resistors come in various types of construction and in many sizes and shapes. Resistors may be classified as fixed or variable. A fixed resistor has only one specified value that is unchanged during normal operation. A variable resistor allows for a selection of resistance within the specified range of the resistor. The most common types of fixed and variable resistors are discussed.

*Fixed resistors.* The symbol for a fixed value resistor is ———/\/\/\———.

*Carbon resistors.* The construction of carbon resistors is shown in Fig. 4-5. This resistor is made up of a resistive element, wire leads, an insulative casing, and an outer coating of a moisture-proof-

ing material. The resistive element is composed of a mixture of a conducting material (carbon) and a nonconducting material (resin). The resistance is determined by the proportions of carbon and resin used. With more carbon and less resin, a small amount of resistance is created. A small amount of carbon with a large amount of resin produces a large resistance. It is easy to understand why these carbon resistors are also known as composition resistors, since the resistance depends on the composition of the resistive element. The composition, not the size, of the resistor determines the value of resistance.

The carbon resistor is constructed in such a way that thickened, fan-shaped ends of the lead wires make good contact with the resistive element and secure the lead wire in place within the insulative casing of the resistor. The casing consists of resin or ceramic. A moisture-proof material (for example, wax or lacquer) is used to coat the exterior surface of the resistor.

The physical size of a composition resistor is related not to its resistance value but rather to its wattage rating. The larger the diameter of a resistor, the higher the wattage rating. Increased insulative material and surface area contribute to a resistor's ability to dissipate greater amounts of heat. The relationship between resistor diameter and wattage rating is apparent when you consider that a $1/8$ inch resistor has a rating of $1/2$ W, a $1/4$ inch resistor 1 W, and a $5/16$ inch resistor 2 W.

Fixed-value carbon resistors are generally used where power dissipation is low and where precise values of resistance are not needed. The range of

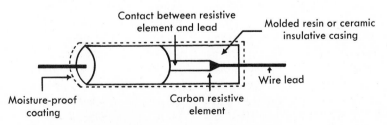

*Fig. 4-5.* Cutaway view of carbon resistor.

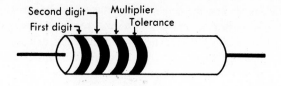

| Color | Value | | Tolerance | |
|-------|-------|--|-----------|--|
| Black | 0 | | Gold | ± 5% |
| Brown | 1 | | Silver | ±10% |
| Red | 2 | | No band | ±20% |
| Orange | 3 | | | |
| Yellow | 4 | | | |
| Green | 5 | | | |
| Blue | 6 | | Multiplier is the number of zeros | |
| Violet | 7 | | added to the first two digits | |
| Gray | 8 | | | |
| White | 9 | | | |

*Fig. 4-6.* Resistor color code.

values available is approximately 5 Ω to 22 MΩ, with tolerance values of ±5%, ±10%, or ±20%.

An internationally accepted series of colored bands is printed on most resistors to indicate the value of the resistance and the degree of tolerance (Fig. 4-6). Therefore, the value of a resistor can be interpreted from its colorful striped jacket. The tolerance of a color-coded resistor indicates the maximum percent of deviation from the given value of the resistor that can be expected. The fourth stripe of the color code gives the tolerance, as shown in Fig. 4-6.

*Wire-wound resistors.* Wire offers a certain amount of resistance to the flow of current. The resistance (ohms) can be calculated if a few dimensions and properties of the wire are known, including radius (r) or cross sectional area ($A = \pi r^2$) in centimeters, length (l) in centimeters, and resistivity ($\rho$) in ohms. The resistance of a given length of wire of a specific metal composition can be calculated with the equation: $R = \rho l / A$. Thus, if a resistor of a specified value is needed, it can be made by using a calculated length of wire. For space considerations, the length of wire can be compactly arranged by winding the wire tightly around an insulating material.

A wire-wound resistor (Fig. 4-7) consists of nickel-chromium wire tightly wrapped around a central insulating core, leads attached to each end of the nickel-chromium wire, and a casing of insulating and moisture-proofing material (for example, silicone or vitreous enamel). This type of resistor is used where precise values of resistance are needed and/or high power dissipation is required. Wire-wound resistors have excellent stability, can be made with power ratings greater than

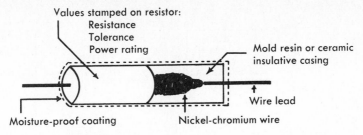

*Fig. 4-7.* Cutaway view of wire-wound resistor.

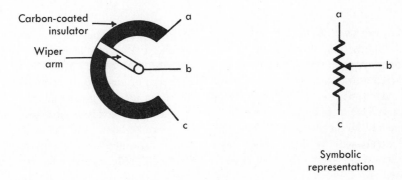

*Fig. 4-8.* Carbon potentiometer.

200 W, and are available in values up to about 100 kΩ. The values, tolerances, and power ratings are stamped on the resistor.

*Variable resistors.* Some resistors are designed so that a variable amount of the total resistance can be used. Commonly called *potentiometers,* variable resistors are also known as *rheostats.* In common electronic jargon, a potentiometer is called a "pot," and its symbol is ——/\/\/\——. There are two types of potentiometers generally available, nickel-chromium and carbon.

*Carbon potentiometer.* A carbon potentiometer is constructed by depositing a layer of carbon on a circular strip of insulation (Fig. 4-8). A metal wiper arm that slides on the carbon surface provides the point at which the desired resistance is selected. Commonly a specified voltage or a spec-

ified current is wanted. The potentiometer can be arranged in a circuit configuration for current selection, voltage selection, or both.

Shown in Fig. 4-9, *A,* is a potentiometer connected so as to absolutely change the resistance in the circuit. As the wiper arm is moved downward, the resistance increases. However, voltage at points *a* and *b* remains constant, point *a* at the voltage of the battery and point *b* at 0 V. Since the voltage drop across the resistor is constant and the resistance is increased, it follows from Ohm's law that the current is decreased. On the other hand, if the wiper arm is moved upward, the resistance will decrease, the voltage drop across the resistor will remain unchanged, and the current will increase.

Fig. 4-9, *B,* represents the more common application of a potentiometer. When the wiper arm is

**A**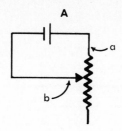

**B**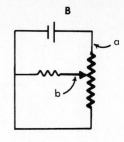

*Fig. 4-9.* Potentiometers in circuit.

"Absolute" variable
resistor

Variable resistor to obtain
wanted voltage and/or current

moved, the total resistance of the potentiometer does not change, but the total effective resistance in the circuit does change. For example, if the wiper arm is moved downward, the resistance between points *a* and *b* is increased, which will result in a decrease in voltage at point *b*. The total effective resistance will be increased; therefore, the current in the circuit will be decreased. Thus, when the wiper arm of the potentiometer is moved, changes in current and voltage result.

Carbon potentiometers are limited to applications requiring low power dissipation and to regulating large resistances. These potentiometers tend to become electrically "noisy" after considerable use. This occurs when the carbon surfaces become rough and the wiper arms become dirty because of loose carbon. In time, some areas of the carbon surface may wear away so that bald patches occur. The carbon surfaces can be cleaned of dirt and loose carbon patches, but the bald spots cannot be repaired. However, replacement carbon potentiometers are relatively inexpensive and easily installed.

Normally the contact between the carbon strip and the wiper arm is not as good as that in a wire-wound potentiometer. Poor contact can result in increased resistance. Therefore, when close regulation of resistance is essential in a circuit, a wire-wound potentiometer is used.

*Wire-wound potentiometer.* Wire-wound potentiometers are made by closely winding a coil of nickel-chromium wire around a strip of insulating material, all of which is bent into a circular form similar to that of the carbon potentiometer just described. An oxide coating on the wire insulates each turn of the wire, but bare metal is exposed to the wiper arm for good contact.

In addition to this usual shape, the resistive element can be bent into a spiral shape. If the wiper arm is mounted on a screw-threaded shaft, the shaft will gradually move the wiper arm down the spiral. By allowing the entire range of resistance to be covered in many turns (10 or more) of the shaft rather than just one, very small changes in resistance are possible.

Wire-wound potentiometers are made in a vast array of physical sizes and shapes. They are available in values ranging from a few ohms to about 100 kΩ. Power ratings usually vary up to about 3 W. Tolerances range from ±20% to ±1%. The increased stability and accuracy of wire-wound potentiometers make their use desirable.

*Resistors in dc and ac circuits.* Resistance is an opposition to current flow. The resistance exerted by a resistor is independent of the frequency of the electrical signal. Therefore, for all practical purposes, ac and dc are affected in the same way when passed through a resistor.

However, in alternating current circuits, another kind of opposition to current exists, which is called *reactance.* Reactance is caused by the presence of capacitors and inductors (both of which will be discussed later) and depends on the frequency of the electrical signal. The combined current-oppos-

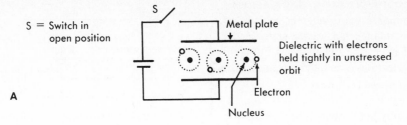

Capacitor with no charge on its plates

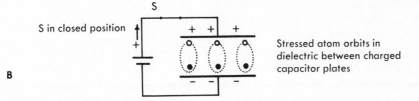

Charging of a capacitor

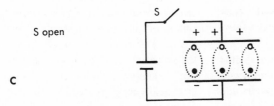

Charged capacitor in open circuit

*Fig. 4-10.* Storage of a charge on a capacitor.

ing effect of reactance and resistance in ac circuits is called *impedance*. In other words, electrical hindrance to ac is called impedance. Impedance (Z) in ac circuits is equivalent to resistance (R) in dc circuits. The ohm is the unit of measure of both impedance and resistance.

## Capacitors

A capacitor is a device used to store a quantity of electrical charge. In its simplest form, it consists of two thin sheets of conducting material separated by a layer of insulating, or dielectric, material. The simplicity of design, as with most common electronic components, is remarkable in light of the considerable importance of its function to particular circuits. Construction is only one of the many factors to be considered in the examination of capacitors. Functions and characteristics of capacitors to be presented in this section include: storage of a charge, units of and factors affecting capacitance, common types and voltage ratings of capacitors, capacitors in series and parallel, charging and discharging time constants, phase relationship, and capacitive reactance.

*How a capacitor stores a charge.* A representation of a capacitor with no potential placed across it is shown in Fig. 4-10, *A*. The switch (S) is open; therefore, current does not flow. The layer of insulation between the plates is called a *dielectric,* for which commonly used materials include air, plastic, mica, ceramic, and wax-saturated paper. As noted in Chapter 3, insulators consist of atoms in which the electrons are tightly held in their orbits.

When the switch is closed (Fig. 4-10, *B*), current flows instantly but for only a brief time. Conventional current flows from a higher positive potential to a lower positive potential. Therefore, in the wire connecting the positive terminal of the battery to the capacitor, the current flows from the battery to the capacitor plate, and in the wire connecting the capacitor to the negative terminal, the current flows from the capacitor to the negative terminal. The dielectric does not conduct a current, that is, the current does not pass through the capacitor. As a result, current flows only as long as there is a potential difference between the capacitor plates and the battery terminals to which they are connected. Once the potential on the plates equals the potential of the battery, current no longer flows and the capacitor is said to be charged.

The charge on the plates exerts a force on the atoms in the dielectric. The electrons in the dielectric atoms are attracted by the positively charged plate and repelled by the negatively charged plate, resulting in the orbital distortion shown in Fig. 4-10, *B*. The force exerted between the charged plates and the atoms in the dielectric is called an *electrostatic field* and is effective in holding the charge on the capacitor plates even after the switch is opened (Fig. 4-10, *C*). This charged capacitor is essentially a dc voltage source ready to be discharged.

The capacitor can be discharged by providing a completed pathway or shunt from the positive to the negative side of the capacitor (Fig. 4-11). The potential difference across the capacitor causes a current to flow through the wire shunt from the positive to the negative side of the capacitor. Current flows until there is no longer a potential across the capacitor. Once completely discharged, the dielectric atoms will have their original unstressed circular orbits. The charging rate of a capacitor can

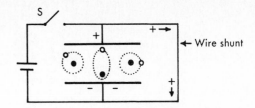

**Fig. 4-11.** Discharging capacitor.

be regulated by selecting a resistor through which to pass the charging current. Likewise, the discharging rate can be regulated by inserting a resistor in place of the wire shunt shown in Fig. 4-11. Charging and discharging rates are discussed in greater detail later in this chapter.

In summary, when a dc voltage is placed across a capacitor, current flows briefly even though there is not a completed circuit. (There is no complete circuit for dc because there is a break in the continuity of the conducting material caused by an insulator.) Current flows until the two plates attain the potential of the battery, that is, until the capacitor is charged. When the capacitor is charged, electrical energy is stored in an electrostatic field set up in the dielectric by distorting electron orbits. When the capacitor is discharging, the energy stored in the dielectric is released in the form of current flow.

**Units of capacitance.** The ability of a capacitor to store an electrical charge is called capacitance (C). The symbols used to represent capacitors in schematics are shown below. When the symbols on the right are used, the curved side represents the plate connected either to ground or to the low voltage side of the circuit.

Fixed value capacitors:  ——|⊢  or  ——|(—

Variable capacitors:  ——⫲⊢  or  ——⫲(—

The unit of capacitance is the *farad* (F). One farad is the capacitance that stores 1 coulomb of electrical energy when one volt is applied. Recall that a coulomb is a unit of measure of the quantity of an electric charge that is equal to the combined

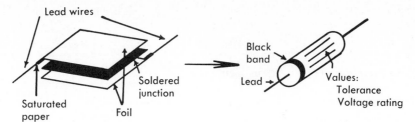

*Fig. 4-12.* Construction of a paper capacitor.

charges of $6.28 \times 10^8$ electrons. In more practical terms, a coulomb is equal to 1 A of current flowing past a point in 1 second. The equation used to calculate capacitance is:

$$C \text{ (farads)} = Q \text{ (coulombs)}/ V \text{ (volts)}$$

The farad is too large for most applications. Units commonly used are either the microfarad, designated $\mu$F (a millionth of a farad or $10^{-6}$ farad), or the picofarad, designated a pF (a millionth of a microfarad or $10^{-12}$ farad).

***Factors affecting capacitance.*** The capacitance of a capacitor is determined by the area of and the distance between the plates and by the dielectric material used. The ability of a capacitor to store electrical energy depends on the electrostatic field established between the plates and the degree of distortion of the electron orbits of the dielectric atoms. Increasing the area of the plates exposes more dielectric to the distortion effects of the electrostatic field and therefore increases the capacitance. Furthermore, if the dielectric layer is made very thin, bringing the plates closer together, the electrostatic field will be intensified, thus increasing the capacitance. Finally, the material used as a dielectric influences the amount of capacitance obtained. The degree of distortion of the electron orbits of the dielectric varies with the material used. Air is used as the reference material and is said to have a dielectric constant of 1. Other substances may have higher dielectric constants, meaning that their atoms undergo greater distortion under similar circumstances. Increased distortion yields higher capacitance for the same thick-

ness of material. For example, under similar conditions, a layer of mica will have a dielectric constant of 6 compared to the same thickness of air. Thus, a capacitor using mica as the dielectric has a capacitance six times as great as an identical capacitor using air as the dielectric. Paper has a dielectric constant of 2 or 3. Titanium oxide has a very high dielectric constant of over 150 times that of an equivalent layer of air.

***Common types of capacitors***

*Fixed capacitors.* The tubular paper capacitor is the most common type. It consists of a strip of paper saturated with any one of a variety of materials, such as petroleum jelly or paraffin wax, sandwiched between strips of metal foil. Commonly the metal foil used is aluminum.

Fig. 4-12 shows a common way of making a paper capacitor. A sheet of impregnated paper is placed between two sheets of aluminum foil. Protruding from the foil are tabs that are soldered to the lead wires for contact to the external circuit. The three sheets are rolled up to conserve space, and the entire unit is sealed to protect against moisture, to insulate, and to give mechanical stability. A black band is usually painted on the end at which the lead is connected to the outside layer of foil. Values, tolerance, and voltage rating are stamped on the surface. This type of capacitor is available in sizes from a few pF to 100 $\mu$F. Tolerances generally range from $\pm 10\%$ to $\pm 25\%$.

A mica capacitor is a fixed-value capacitor that uses mica as the dielectric between plates of metal, usually silver. These capacitors are very efficient and reliable but are expensive. Fig. 4-13 shows

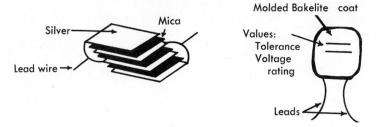

*Fig. 4-13.* Construction of a mica capacitor.

their general construction. Because mica is brittle and like a multilayered sandwich, it cannot be rolled. Alternate silver plates are connected together and attached to a lead wire. The capacitor is usually encased in molded Bakelite. Mica capacitors are usually available in values from a few pF to about 10,000 pF and can be made to a tolerance of ±2%.

The two types of capacitors described are representative of fixed-value, "dry" capacitors. When larger capacitances are needed, another type of capacitor is usually employed, the so-called "wet," or electrolytic, capacitor.

One example of the wet type of capacitor consists of a loosely rolled or folded sheet of aluminum that is immersed in a borax solution (electrolyte). The borax solution causes an extremely thin layer of aluminum oxide and oxygen gas to form on the surface of the aluminum. The aluminum sheet becomes one plate of the capacitor, and the borax solution becomes the other plate. The layer of aluminum oxide and oxygen will not conduct electricity and therefore becomes the dielectric. Because this dielectric layer is extremely thin, the capacitance is increased greatly. The aluminum plate side of the capacitor must always be connected to the positive side of the circuit. If the aluminum plate side of the capacitor is connected to the negative side of the circuit, the dielectric will be "punctured" by the current when the metal plate becomes negative, and the capacitance will be destroyed. Although "wet"-type capacitors are self-healing (in other words, if the proper connections are made, a new coating of oxide and gas will

form), once a capacitor has been misused, it should be discarded.

A variation of the above capacitor, which avoids having to handle a device containing a volume of liquid that may spill, is to replace the solution with a wet cloth. A cloth strip is saturated with borax solution, placed on the metal strip, and rolled up. Electrolytic capacitors are more expensive than the dry capacitors. Electrolytic capacitors are available in a value range of 1 to 5,000 $\mu$F and generally have tolerances of −20% to +50%.

Another type of electrolytic capacitor substitutes tantalum foil for aluminum, providing more stability, less "noise," and less "leakage current." Although made up like the aluminum type, tantalum foil capacitors rarely employ liquids, can be completely sealed, and are generally physically smaller than aluminum electrolytic capacitors of similar value.

*Variable capacitors.* Some circuit functions require capacitors with adjustable values of capacitance. There are two general types of variable capacitors. In one, the effective area of the plates can be adjusted; in the other, the distance between plates can be adjusted. Both types use metal (usually aluminum) plates and air as the dielectric.

Adjustment of plate area can be accomplished by an arrangement of stationary and movable semicircular plates positioned alternately. The movable plates are attached to a rotating shaft. As the shaft is turned, the area of the plates facing each other is changed (Fig. 4-14). Additional variable area can be obtained by increasing the number of plates used in the construction of this type of capacitor.

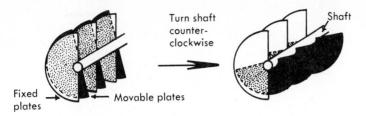

*Fig. 4-14.* Variable capacitor.

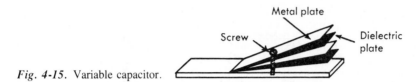

*Fig. 4-15.* Variable capacitor.

Since the area of the plates can be adjusted, the capacitance of the capacitor can be varied. (This type of capacitor is frequently used as the control to select stations on a radio.)

The other type of variable capacitor is one that changes the distance between plates. Fig. 4-15 shows the general construction. A number of metal plates are sandwiched between layers of dielectric material (air). The metal plates are constructed so they will spread apart. An insulated screw through all the plates can compress or allow the plates to flare open. Changing the distance between the plates changes the capacitance.

*Voltage rating of capacitors.* There are restrictions on the conditions under which capacitors can be used. Some of the features of the dielectric material influence the degree of capacitance. The dielectric also serves as a thin layer of insulation between the capacitor plates. All capacitors are given a voltage rating that is the maximum dc voltage that can be used safely without exceeding the insulating capability of the dielectric. When a certain level of voltage is exceeded, an arc of current will flow, causing a "breakdown" or "puncture" of the capacitor. The "working voltage" of a capacitor depends on the dielectric material used. It must be remembered that when a capacitor is used in an ac line, ac voltages are usually given

in rms values. If, for example, a capacitor is rated at 400 working V dc, 400 V ac cannot be placed across it.

*Capacitors in series and parallel.* The rules for adding capacitances in series and parallel circuits are the opposite of those for adding resistances.

Series: For any number of capacitors connected in series, the total or equivalent capacitance is:

$$1/C_{total} = 1/C_1 + 1/C_2 + 1/C_3 \ldots 1/C_n$$

Fig. 4-16 shows three capacitors connected in series across a battery. The positive charge from the positive side of the battery flows to $C_1$, placing a positive charge on the plate nearest the positive terminal of the battery. The positive charge on the left plate of $C_3$ moves to the negative side of the battery, leaving a negative charge on the left plate of $C_2$ and, therefore, a positive charge on the right plate of $C_3$ and a negative charge on the lower plate of $C_2$. The electrons move from the upper plate of $C_2$ to the right plate of $C_1$, leaving the upper plate of $C_2$ positive and the right plate of $C_1$ negative.

Parallel: For any number of capacitors connected in parallel, the total capacitance is simply the sum of all the individual capacitances:

$$C_{total} = C_1 + C_2 + C_3 \ldots C_n$$

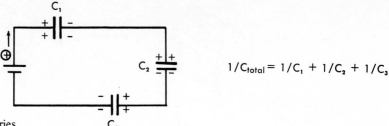

$$1/C_{total} = 1/C_1 + 1/C_2 + 1/C_3$$

*Fig. 4-16.* Three capacitors in series.

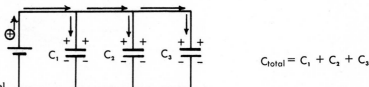

$$C_{total} = C_1 + C_2 + C_3$$

*Fig. 4-17.* Three capacitors in parallel.

Fig. 4-17 shows a parallel arrangement of capacitors.

*Resistance-capacitance time constants*

*Charging time constant.* If a capacitor is placed directly across a source of voltage with no resistance in the circuit, the capacitor is charged to its full extent in an extremely short period of time. However, a resistor placed in series with a capacitor limits the current flow and, therefore, the charging of the capacitor takes a longer period of time. (Theoretically, with resistance in the circuit, the capacitor never quite reaches full charge.)

The time constant of a capacitor is, by definition, the time in seconds required for a capacitor to reach 63% of full charge, that is, 63% of the applied voltage. The time necessary to reach this 63% level depends on the amounts of resistance and capacitance. The equation for determining the time constant is:

$$T = RC$$

where:

$T$ = Time constant in seconds
$C$ = Capacitance in farads
$R$ = Resistance in ohms

Thus, if C is expressed in farads and R in ohms, the time constant is in seconds. If C is expressed in microfarads and R in megohms, the time constant is again expressed in seconds.

Example:

$R = 4$ MΩ
$C = 0.02$ μF
$T = RC = (4$ MΩ$) (0.02$ μF$) = 0.8$ sec

Thus, in 0.08 second, a 0.02-μF capacitor will charge up to 63% of the supply voltage that is connected across it and the 4 MΩ resistor. Refer to Fig. 4-18.

*Discharging time constant.* If the charged capacitor is connected in a closed conducting circuit, the potential on the capacitor will cause a current to flow from the positive to the negative plates of the capacitor. Thus, a resistor connected in parallel with the capacitor will determine the time required for the capacitor to discharge. This RC discharge time is calculated with the same equation used to calculate the RC charging time constant (Fig. 4-19).

*Phase relationship.* With the initial application of a dc potential across an uncharged capacitor,

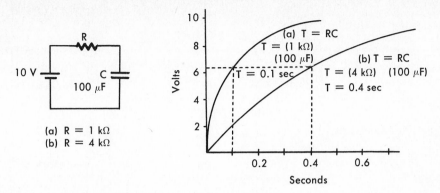

*Fig. 4-18.* RC charging time constant; affected by value of resistor in series with capacitor.

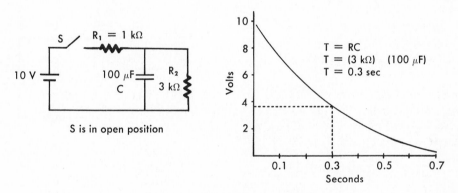

*Fig. 4-19.* Discharge of a capacitor.

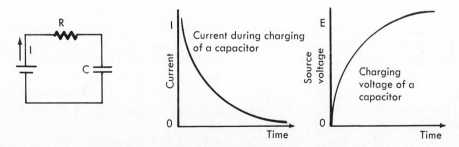

*Fig. 4-20.* Voltage and current in dc circuit during charging of a capacitor.

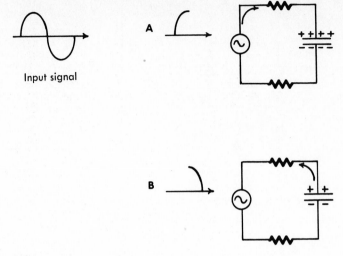

Input signal

*Fig. 4-21.* Capacitor in ac circuit; effect each quarter
sine wave has on a capacitor.

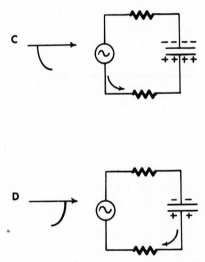

there is a maximum current flow and a minimum
potential stored on the capacitor. As a charge collects on the plates of the capacitor, the current
decreases. In other words, as voltage on the capacitor increases, it exerts a reversed force (back
EMF) that decreases current flow. When the capacitor is fully charged, the back EMF equals the
EMF of the battery, and no current flows. This
phenomenon is shown in Fig. 4-20.

When an ac voltage is applied across a capacitor, the capacitor alternately charges and discharges. The capacitor is charged by the peak voltage of the ac signal (Fig. 4-21, *A* and *D*). When
the ac signal's amplitude decreases (Fig. 4-21, *B*)
and changes polarity (Fig. 4-21, *C*), the capacitor
releases its charge in a direction opposite to the
direction of the charging current. The phase relationship of voltage and current in an ac capacitive

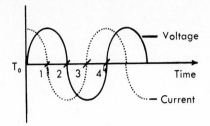

*Fig. 4-22.* Graphic presentation of voltage and current in capacitive circuit with ac voltage applied.

circuit is that current always leads voltage by 90 degrees. That is, current flows to the capacitor first, and then voltage collects on the capacitor (Fig. 4-22).

*Capacitive reactance. Capacitive reactance* ($X_c$) is the resistance to current exerted by a capacitor. As stated earlier, resistance to alternating current is called impedance (Z). Thus, capacitive reactance and impedance are interchangeable terms, and the ohm remains the unit of measurement.

A capacitor exerts infinite resistance in a dc circuit once the capacitor is charged. The charged capacitor exhibits an infinite reactance, since the back EMF of the capacitor equals the EMF of the voltage source.

In an ac circuit, just as the capacitor begins to become fully charged, the source voltage begins to drop, and the capacitor begins to discharge. If the speed at which the current changes direction is increased (increased frequency), the capacitor has less time to reach a full charge and in fact will not be able to do so. If it cannot reach full charge, it cannot establish a counter EMF equal to the source. In effect, there is less hindrance to current flow as the frequency increases. The relationship of capacitive reactance to frequency is:

$$X_c = 1/2\pi fC$$

where:

$X_c$ = Capacitive reactance in ohms
$\pi$ = A constant of 3.14
f = Frequency of current in cycles per second
C = Capacitance in farads

To fully appreciate the meaning of this equation, observe the effect on capacitive reactance when the frequency of the ac is changed.

What would the capacitive reactance of a 200 $\mu$F capacitor be if applied across it is a 120 Vac signal having a frequency of:
1. 50 Hz
2. 100 Hz
3. 200 Hz

*Solutions:*

$X_c = 1/2\pi fC$
1. $X_c = 1/(2) (3.14) (50 \text{ Hz}) (0.0002) = 15.92 \ \Omega$
2. $X_c = 1/(2) (3.14) (100 \text{ Hz}) (0.0002) = 7.96 \ \Omega$
3. $X_c = 1/(2) (3.14) (200 \text{ Hz}) (0.0002) = 3.98 \ \Omega$

In a purely capacitive circuit, capacitive reactance ($X_c$) can be substituted for the term impedance in Z = E/I, so that Ohm's law for ac circuits becomes:

$$X_c = E/I$$

In a circuit that contains both capacitors and resistors in series, the total impedance is:

$$Z = \sqrt{R^2 + X_c^2}$$

Resistance and capacitive reactance in parallel are added by using the equation:

$$Z = 1/\sqrt{(1/R)^2 + (1/X_c)^2}$$

## Inductors

A straight wire will conduct a current in a closed circuit. The current is hindered by the resistance offered by the metal wire. However, when the same straight metal wire is coiled, the resistance of the wire is not the only opposition to current flow. What mysterious change results from the new arrangement of the wire? Do charges naturally decelerate in a turn in the conducting "roadway"? Do both dc and ac meet more resistance or impedance in a coiled wire than in a straight wire? What purpose is served by coiling a wire?

*Electricity and magnetism.* Before attempting to answer any of the above questions, consider a straight conducting metal wire in which there exists an invisible force of electricity. This invisible force of electricity has an invisible partner

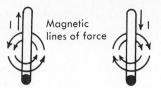

Magnetic lines of force

Right hand rule for remembering the direction of a magnetic field caused by a current passing through a wire

*Fig. 4-23.* Right hand rule.

called *magnetism*. When a current is flowing through a conductor, a *magnetic field* surrounds the conductor. The strength of this magnetic field is directly proportional to the quantity of current passing through the conductor and inversely proportional to the distance of the field from the conductor. Magnetic lines of force exist around a *conducting* wire, but when the wire stops conducting, the magnetic field collapses.

The lines of force around the current-carrying conductor travel in a clockwise or counter-clockwise direction, depending on the direction of current flow. The *right hand rule* expresses the direction of magnetic lines of force in relation to the direction of current flow (when referring to conventional current).

*Right hand rule:*  If you grasp a conductor with your right hand with the thumb pointing in the direction of current flow, your fingers will indicate the direction of the magnetic lines of force.

(*Note:* This is called the *left hand rule* if current flow is defined as electron flow. If you grasp a conductor with your left hand with the thumb pointing in the direction of electron flow, your fingers will indicate the direction of the magnetic lines of force.)

Application of the right hand rule to Fig. 4-23 illustrates that a change in the direction of current flow reverses the direction of the magnetic lines of force around the conductor.

**Induction of current.** If a current can and does cause a magnetic field, can a magnetic field cause a current? Yes. When magnetic lines of force cut across a conductor, a current is caused to flow or, in other words, a current is induced. Induction of current can be demonstrated with a magnetic field and a conductor. Fig. 4-24 shows the induction of current. The wire can be kept stationary and the magnet moved so that the magnetic lines of force cut across the conductor to induce the current. Or the magnet can be kept stationary and the conductor moved so as to cross perpendicularly the lines of magnetic force, cutting them in a downward *(A)* or an upward *(B)* motion.

Any conductor carrying a current develops magnetic lines of force around it. This magnetic field becomes stronger with increased current and weaker with decreased current and completely collapses when current ceases to flow. This "envelope of magnetic force" can be considered a package of reserved energy, which can be converted to current flow, as shown in Fig. 4-24, if the lines of force cut across a conductor. Although these magnetic lines of force exist around a current-conducting straight wire, their presence does not have any appreciable effect on current flow and therefore is ignored. However, magnetic lines of force can have desirable effects on current flow in a circuit if the current passes through a coiled conductor called an *inductor* or *coil*.

The symbol for an inductor is ⎯⎯◠◠◠⎯⎯ . This inductor does not have a central core other than air; therefore, it is called an *air-core inductor*. The symbol for an inductor with a central core of iron is ⎯⎯◠◠◠⎯⎯ . Variable inductors are shown by one of the following two symbols:

⎯⎯◠◠◠⎯⎯      or      ⎯⎯◠◠◠⎯⎯

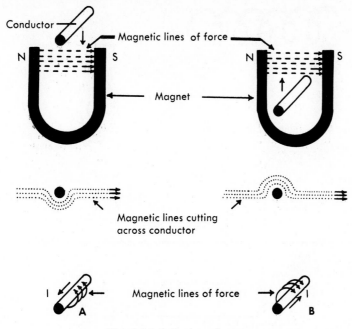

*Fig. 4-24.* Induction of current.

Capacitors and inductors are referred to as *reactors* because they do not dissipate electrical energy in the form of heat, as resistors do, but alternately store energy and then deliver it back to the circuit. Capacitors store energy in an electrostatic field. Inductors store energy in an electromagnetic field. Time is required to accumulate, store, and then release energy. This explains why reactors produce changes in phase relationships between current and voltage.

*Inductor in a dc circuit.* First consideration is given to direct current passing through an inductor. When current begins to flow through the inductor, magnetic lines of force are generated. The energy used to make this magnetic field comes from the voltage source. As magnetic lines of force are developed around each coil, they can be considered moving lines of magnetic force (just as waves radiate or move out from the disturbance caused when a pebble is dropped into a pool of water). As discussed previously, if moving magnetic lines of force cut across a conductor, a current is induced. Fig. 4-25 illustrates that current in one half of the looped wire will induce a current flow in the other half, because moving magnetic lines of force are cutting across the adjacent conducting wires. However, note that this induced current or EMF (which causes current to flow) opposes the direction of current flow from the voltage source. Or it can be said that the induced EMF is a counter EMF, that is, opposing the EMF of the source.

In a direct current circuit, the only other time the magnetic lines of force move is when the current stops and the magnetic field collapses. When the field collapses, a counter EMF is momentarily established that causes a brief counter EMF or "kickback" current in the circuit.

After the initial generation of the magnetic field around the looped conductors of an inductor in a dc circuit, there is no effect exerted on direct current flow. It is important to remember that once the lines of magnetic force are stationary, they cannot cut across a conductor. Therefore, a current

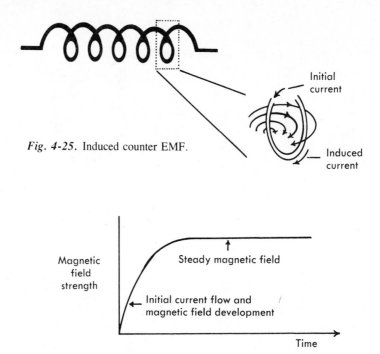

*Fig. 4-25.* Induced counter EMF.

*Fig. 4-26.* Development of magnetic field around current-carrying conductor in dc circuit.

or EMF cannot be induced. Thus, in a dc circuit, an inductor is considered to be essentially a straight wire, exerting only the effect of the resistance offered by that wire. Why not consider the effects exerted by the initial current flow and the stopping of current flow? The answer is that these effects are only momentarily exerted and do not exist during the continual operation of the circuit. Therefore, for all practical purposes, the effect of a counter EMF exerted by a coil does not exist in a dc circuit. Fig. 4-26 shows the development of a magnetic field around a conductor passing a dc current.

Direct current is essentially unaffected by an inductor. But it is given careful consideration in this chapter to express as simply as possible the development of a counter EMF in an inductor. Once this concept is understood, the effect of an inductor on alternating current can be more easily appreciated.

*Inductor in an ac circuit.* An inductor exerts an impedance to alternating current that is directly proportional to the frequency of the alternating current passing through the inductor. When an alternating current is passed through an inductor, the magnetic field produced varies at the same rate and in proportion to the magnitude of the current. The result is a constantly moving magnetic field. As the current increases, the magnetic lines of force radiate out from the conductor, and as the current decreases, the magnetic lines of force begin to collapse. This moving, or "pulsating," magnetic field cuts across the adjacent turns of the coil, thus producing a back or counter EMF. The faster the magnetic field "pulsates," the greater the counter EMF induced. Therefore, with increased frequency of an alternating current there is developed a greater counter EMF or hindrance to current flow. Impedance increases as frequency increases.

Summarized here is the development of a

counter EMF in an inductor. An important characteristic of alternating current is that voltage and current amplitude are continually changing. As the current begins to increase through the inductor, the magnetic lines of flux expand around each turn of the inductor. The expanding field cuts through the adjacent turns of the inductor, which results in a current being induced in those adjacent turns. The induced current flows in the opposite direction to the original current. This phenomenon is expressed in Lenz's law, which states: "When a current is induced in a coil as a result of any variation in the magnetic field surrounding the coil, the induced current is in such a direction as to oppose the current change that produced the magnetic variation."

*Inductance and inductive reactance.* Induction of 1 V resulting from a current variation of 1 A per second equals 1 *henry* (H). Other units of inductance are the millihenry (mH), one thousandth of a henry, and the microhenry ($\mu$H), one millionth of a henry.

The inductance of an inductor is determined by the characteristics of its construction, including number and diameter of turns, system of winding, coil length-diameter ratio, and core material. The way a coil is constructed depends on the effect it is meant to produce in the circuit. The core material contained within the center or core of the inductor may be air or a magentic material such as iron. Air-core inductors are made by winding wire on a nonmagnetic material to serve as a support or by using wire sufficiently heavy to be self-supporting. A magnetic core increases the inductance of an inductor by concentrating the magnetic field within the coil. An inductor having a movable iron core is a variable inductor, the inductance of which can be varied by adjusting the length of the iron core inside the coil.

Inductance (L) is the property that opposes change in current flow. Inductive reactance ($X_L$) is the impedance or effective resistance offered by an inductor to alternating current. Its unit of measurement is the ohm. The formula used to calculate inductive reactance is:

$$X_L = 2\pi L$$

where:

$X_L$ = Inductive reactance in ohms
$\pi$ = A constant (3.14)
f = Frequency of applied voltage in hertz
L = Inductance in henrys

Note that once a fixed inductor is constructed, the frequency of the applied voltage is the only variable capable of changing the inductive reactance.

The information derived from the above formula is better appreciated when an ac frequency change is related to the resulting change in the inductive reactance.

What would the inductive reactance be for a 200 mH inductor if applied across it is a 120 Vac signal having a frequency of:

1. 50 Hz
2. 100 Hz
3. 200 Hz

*Solutions:*

$$X_L = 2\pi f L$$

1. $X_L$ = (2) (3.14) (50 Hz) (0.2 H) = 62.8 $\Omega$
2. $X_L$ = (2) (3.14) (100 Hz) (0.2 H) = 125.6 $\Omega$
3. $X_L$ = (2) (3.14) (200 Hz) (0.2 H) = 251.2 $\Omega$

As the frequency increases, the inductive reactance increases. This is opposite to the effect frequency has on capacitive reactance, in which an increase in frequency decreases the capacitive reactance.

In a purely inductive circuit, inductive reactance ($X_L$) can be substituted for impedance (Z) so that, for ac circuits, Ohm's law is changed from Z = E/I to $X_L$ = E/I.

*Phase relationship in an inductor.* Current and voltage are in phase when an ac voltage is applied across a resistor. In other words, maximum voltage causes maximum current, and minimum voltage causes minimum current. Thus, a direct phase relationship exists between voltage and current (Fig. 4-27).

Review the phase relationship of voltage and current when an ac voltage is applied across a capacitor. Maximum current flows first; then as the voltage increases across the capacitor, the current

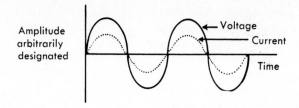

**Fig. 4-27.** Phase relationship of ac voltage and current across a resistor.

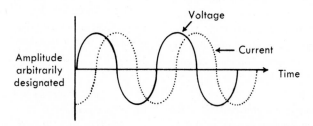

**Fig. 4-28.** Phase relationship of ac voltage and current across an inductor.

**Table 1.** A summary comparison of resistors, capacitors, and inductors in dc and ac circuits

| Circuit | Property | Resistor —/\/\/\— | Capacitor ╶┤├╴ | Inductor ╶◠◠◠╴ |
|---------|----------|----------|-----------|----------|
| dc | Resistance | Resistance (R) Unit = ohm R = E/I | Infinite resistance | Negligible resistance |
| ac | Impedance | Impedance (Z) Unit = ohm Z = E/I | Capacitive reactance $(X_c)$ Unit = ohm $X_c = 1/2\pi fC$ | Inductive reactance $(X_L)$ Unit = ohm $X_L = 2\pi fL$ |
| ac | Phase relationship between voltage and current | In phase | Current leads voltage by 90 degrees | Voltage leads current by 90 degrees |

decreases. In this case current leads voltage. The phase difference has been determined to be 90 degrees. The current leads the voltage by 90 degrees in a capacitive circuit.

In an inductive circuit, when an alternating current is applied across an inductor, the voltage leads the current by 90 degrees. As a voltage is applied to the inductor, a current starts to flow, causing the formation of a magnetic field that induces a counter EMF to oppose the increase of current flow. This hindrance to current flow delays changes in current 90 degrees behind changes in voltage (Fig. 4-28).

***Inductors in series, parallel, and series-parallel.*** Inductors in proximity in a circuit may impose the effects of their magnetic fields on each other. This is usually undesirable. Circuits may not perform effectively those functions for which they were designed if interfering, unpredictable forces are generated. Thus, the rules for determining the total effective inductive reactance of inductors connected in series, parallel, or series-parallel are applicable only if the inductors' magnetic fields cannot act on each other. The total effective inductance of inductors connected in series is calculated with this equation: $L_{total} = L_1 + L_2 + L_3 \ldots L_n$. The total effective inductance of inductors connected in parallel can be calculated with the equation: $1/L_{total} = 1/L_1 + 1/L_2 + 1/L_3 \ldots 1/L_n$.

*Resistance and impedance.* The total effective impedance exerted by an inductor and a resistor connected in series is determined by using this equation: $Z = \sqrt{R^2 + X_L^2}$. The total effective impedance exerted by an inductor and resistor connected in parallel can be determined by using the equation: $Z = (R)(X_L)/\sqrt{R^2 + X_L^2}$.

## Transformers

Transformers are extensively used in electronic instruments. They commonly function to change the level of input voltage to meet voltage level requirements of various circuits in an instrument. The input ac voltage applied across a transformer may be decreased or increased or may remain unchanged. Transformers may also serve to block unwanted direct current from passing from one circuit to another.

*Induction of current.* When an alternating current passes through a coil, the changing current causes a changing magnetic field. The expanding and collapsing of a magnetic field around a coiled, ac current-carrying wire results in the generation of a back EMF. This inductance of a back EMF in a coil is called *self-inductance*.

There is another type of current induction that plays an important role in most analytical instruments. This is the induction of a current in one coil by the current flowing in another separate coil. Two separate coils in parallel orientation and in proximity to each other are the arrangement required for this type of current induction. When ac current is passed through one of the coils (primary coil) but not through the other, a current can be measured in both coils. The coil not attached to a potential (secondary coil) has had a current induced in it by the constantly changing magnetic field generated by the alternating current in the first coil (Fig. 4-29).

Note that if a dc current were passed through the primary coil, a constant current would not be induced in the secondary coil. A current pulse in the secondary coil could be measured only during two specific times—one pulse with the initiation of dc current flow and the other with its termination. Current is induced at these two particular times because only during initiation and termination of dc current flow is there a change in the magnetic field—that is, expansion and collapse, respectively.

*Transformer construction.* The phenomenon of current induction in one coil by an ac current in another coil is employed in a transformer. The construction of a transformer allows for maximum power transfer from one coil to the other. Two factors to be considered are the proximity of the coils and the concentration of the magnetic field. The closer the coils, the greater the effectiveness of current induction. Therefore, the insulated wires can be wound over each other around a central core. A central and peripheral iron core is used to concentrate the magnetic field about the coils because current induction is directly related to the strength of the magnetic field (Fig. 4-30).

Symbolic representations of transformers are:

Air-core:          Iron-core:

*Transformer action.* Induction of current is accompanied by induction of voltage and dissipation of power. These three factors are inseparable. Voltage is the electrical factor most frequently used to describe induced energy because the input voltage on the primary coil induces a voltage in the secondary coil simultaneously with current induction.

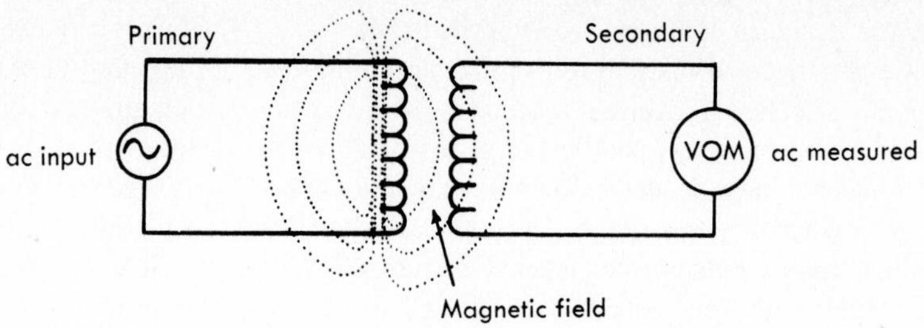

*Fig. 4-29.* Current induction.

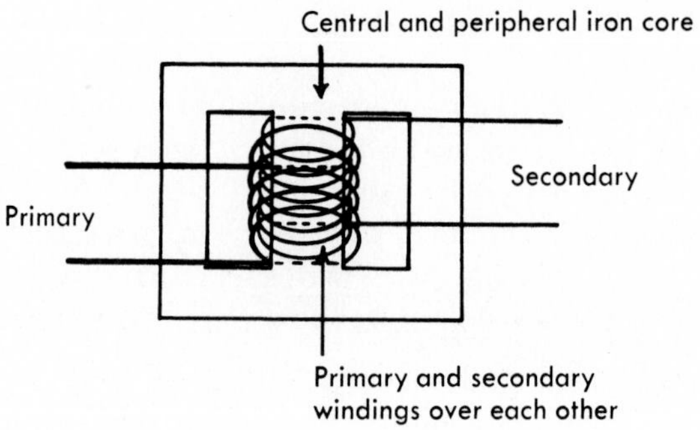

Primary                    Secondary

ac input                   VOM   ac measured

Magnetic field

*Fig. 4-30.* Iron-core transformer.

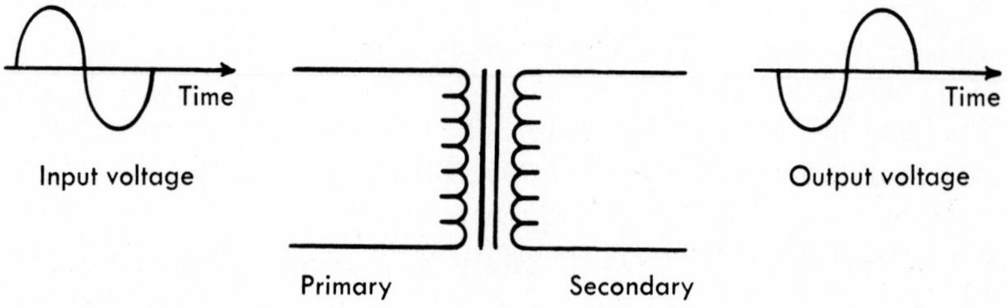

Central and peripheral iron core

Primary                    Secondary

Primary and secondary
windings over each other

*Fig. 4-31.* Transformer action.

Time

Input voltage

Primary          Secondary

Time

Output voltage

The ac voltage induced in the secondary coil is 180 degrees out of phase with the ac voltage across the primary coil. The positive half of an input sine wave generates magnetic lines of force that cut across the secondary coil in a direction opposite to the direction they are generated from the primary. Therefore, when the input voltage is positive the voltage across the secondary is negative, and when the input voltage is negative the secondary voltage is positive (Fig. 4-31).

An equation used to calculate the voltage induced in the secondary coil by the primary coil is:

$$E_s/E_p = N_s/N_p$$

where:

$E_s$ = Voltage in secondary coil
$E_p$ = Voltage in primary coil
$N_s$ = Number of turns in secondary coil
$N_p$ = Number of turns in primary coil

As seen in the equation, the voltage induced is directly related to the number of turns in the coils. If there are more turns in the secondary coil than in the primary, the magnetic field of the primary obviously will cut across more conducting wires

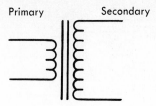

*Fig. 4-32*. Step-up transformer.

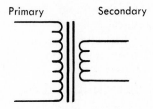

*Fig. 4-33*. Step-down transformer.

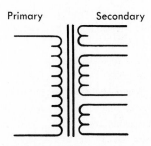

*Fig. 4-34*. Transformer with multiple secondary windings.

in the secondary, therefore inducing a larger voltage. This type of transformer is called a "step-up" transformer (Fig. 4-32). On the other hand, if there are fewer turns in the secondary coil than in the primary coil, the transformer is a "step-down" transformer (Fig. 4-33).

In another type of transformer, there are multiple secondary windings to provide several levels of induced voltages (Fig. 4-34).

The equation above is applied in the following sample problems:

1. What voltage is induced in a secondary coil of 150 turns if 120 Vac is applied across the primary of 100 turns? (Step-up transformer)

*Solution:*
$$E_s/E_p = N_s/N_p$$
$$E_s/120 \text{ Vac} = 150/100$$
$$E_s = 18000/100 = 180 \text{ Vac}$$

2. What voltage is induced in a secondary coil of 75 turns if 120 Vac is applied across the primary of 100 turns? (Step-down transformer)

*Solution:*
$$E_s/E_p = N_s/N_p$$
$$E_s/120 \text{ Vac} = 75/100$$
$$E_s = 9000/100 = 90 \text{ Vac}$$

In both step-up and step-down transformers it appears that voltage is magically magnified or diminished and that the law of conservation of energy is ignored. Not true! The energy transferred between the primary and secondary coils is power. The power in the primary coil equals the power in the secondary if the transformer is 100% efficient. Consider this ideal case:

$$P_p = P_s$$

Power is the product of current and voltage. Therefore:

$$I_p \times E_p = I_2 \times E_s$$

Thus, if voltage is stepped up, the current is proportionately stepped down, and if the voltage is stepped down, the current is stepped up. To demonstrate this concept, consider these problems:

In each of the previous problems, 1 and 2, if the power in the primary were 60 W, what would be the current in the primary and in the secondary?

$$I_s = 60 \text{ W}/180 \text{ V} = 0.333 \text{ A}$$

(Note that in the secondary coil the voltage increased and the current decreased.)

3. Current in the primary

$$I_p = P_p/E_p$$
$$I_p = 60 \text{ W}/120 \text{ V} = 0.5 \text{ A}$$

Current in the secondary

$$I_s = P_s/E_s$$
$$I_s = 60 \text{ W}/90 \text{ V} = 0.667 \text{ A}$$

(Note that in the secondary coil the current increased and the voltage decreased.)

Another useful application of transformers is the isolation of certain ac circuits and/or components from unwanted direct current. As discussed earlier, direct current is unable to induce a current. Therefore, while alternating current will be transmitted through a transformer, direct current will be blocked.

### Diodes

Diodes are electronic components with a simple design not representative of their importance. The diode (*di* meaning two and *ode* from electrode) is a two-electrode unit that plays a major role in rectification of alternating current to direct current. There are two types of diodes—vacuum tube and semiconductor. An examination of the construction and operation of each type is followed by a discussion of diode applications.

*Vacuum tube diode.* Vacuum tubes are disappearing from electronic circuits and being replaced by semiconductors. However, a consideration of vacuum tube principles of operation will contribute to the understanding of rectification and, later, amplification. The operational principles of vacuum tubes are conceptually clear and therefore easily understood. These principles can be used to aid in understanding semiconductor operational principles.

The function of vacuum tubes is based on two fundamental principles—thermionic emission and attraction and repulsion of unlike and like charges, respectively. Thermionic emission is the release of electrons caused by an increased temperature of particular metals. The rise in temperature imparts enough energy to some electrons to result in their liberation from the heated metal. The freed electrons collect at the surface of the metal, forming an electron cloud (Fig. 4-35).

A diode consists of two electrodes and a heater,

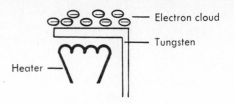

*Fig. 4-35.* Thermionic emission.

all of which are encased within an evacuated glass envelope. The electrodes are the cathode and the plate. The cathode is the electrode that is heated and from which electrons are emitted. Tungsten is commonly used for the cathode. The plate is the collector of emitted electrons.

The heater supplies heat to the cathode. The cathode can be directly or indirectly heated (Fig. 4-36). Since the heater element plays an indirect role in the function of the diode, it is frequently not shown in schematic representations of vacuum tube diodes. Regardless of whether the heater element is shown, its presence in a vacuum tube diode is understood.

Operation of a vacuum tube diode depends on the voltage at each of the two electrodes—cathode and plate. When the plate is positive in relation to the cathode, the diode is said to be "forward biased." Electrons are attracted to the plate, and a current flows. In a "reverse-biased" diode, the plate is negative with respect to the cathode. A current will not pass through this diode, since the negative charges on the plate and on the cathode will repel each other. A forward-biased diode is said to be conducting, and a reverse-biased diode is said to be nonconducting (Fig. 4-37).

Forward- and reverse-biased vacuum tube diodes in simple circuits are shown in Fig. 4-38. When the battery is connected with the negative side to the cathode and the positive side to the plate, the forward-biased diode conducts and a current flows in the circuit. The electrons emitted from the cathode and attracted to the positive side of the battery are replenished by the electrons from the negative side of the battery, and a constant current flows in the circuit (Fig. 4-38, *A*). When

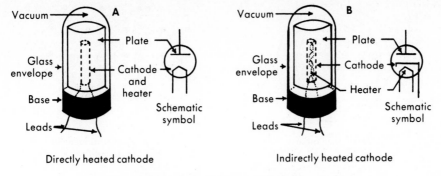

*Fig. 4-36.* Arrangement of elements in vacuum tube diode.

*Fig. 4-37.* Vacuum tube diode bias.

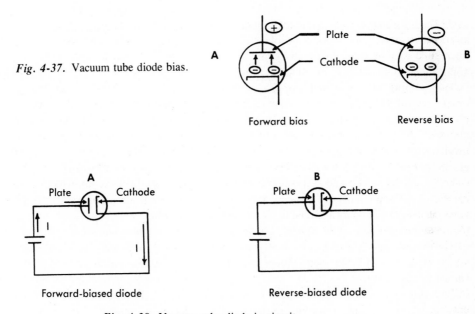

*Fig. 4-38.* Vacuum tube diode in circuit.

the battery is connected with the positive side to the cathode and the negative side to the plate, the reverse-biased diode does not conduct. The electrons emitted from the cathode are repelled by the negative charge on the plate. Since no current can pass through the diode, the circuit is not complete and current will not flow (Fig. 4-38, *B*).

Voltage and current in the anode circuit of the vacuum tube diode are designated plate voltage ($E_p$) and plate current ($I_p$), respectively. Since there is a potential difference between the cathode and the plate in a conducting diode, there is a voltage drop across the diode. According to Ohm's law, a voltage drop occurs across a resistance. The resistance of a vacuum tube diode is called *plate resistance* ($R_p$) and is calculated:

$$R_p = E_p/I_p$$

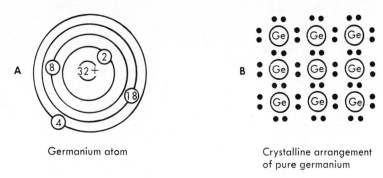

Germanium atom

Crystalline arrangement
of pure germanium

*Fig. 4-39.* Germanium atom and crystalline form.

*Semiconductor diodes.* A semiconductor electronic component is also called a *solid-state device*. Thus, the names "semiconductor diode" and "solid-state diode" are interchangeable. Semiconductor and vacuum tube diodes have similar circuit applications but different operational principles.

The operation of a semiconductor diode is based on its crystalline structure and composition. As discussed earlier, a conductor is a material whose atoms contain loosely bound electrons, and an insulator is composed of atoms that bind their electrons very tightly. Some pure crystalline substances, such as silicon and germanium, are semiconductors. The conductivity of semiconductors is between that of insulators and conductors, depending on the temperature of the crystal. Conductivity increases with increase in temperature. The crystalline structure of a pure germanium crystal is shown in Fig. 4-39.

The pure crystal can be changed to enhance conductivity by adding a specific impurity. The addition of the impurity is called "doping." The impurity must have a structure compatible with the crystalline structure of the pure crystal to allow for its incorporation into the crystal. Depending on whether the doping element is a donor or acceptor impurity, the crystal may have an excess or deficit of loosely bound electrons. A donor impurity is a pentavalent element, for example, arsenic, antimony, or phorphorus, that provides one free electron per atom incorporated. The excess electrons are not held in covalent bonds and

therefore are free to move within the crystal. An acceptor impurity is a trivalent element, such as aluminum, gallium, or boron. The acceptor impurity provides the pure crystal with an electron deficit of one electron per atom of impurity incorporated into the crystal. This electron deficit is called a "hole." Conceptually, a hole can be thought of as a positive charge.

A pure crystal doped with a pentavalent or trivalent impurity is called an extrinsic or impurity semiconductor. Impurity semiconductors are of two types, N-type and P-type. The N-type has excess electrons known as negative carriers resulting from a donor impurity (Fig. 4-40, *A*). An acceptor impurity supplies a pure crystal with excess holes known as positive carriers, thus producing a P-type semiconductor (Fig. 4-40, *B*). The addition of an impurity to a pure crystal does not give the crystal a net charge. The neutrality of the crystal is maintained, since the added atoms have an equal number of electrons and protons. The terms *electron excess* and *electron deficit* refer to the availability of or lack of mobile electrons.

When a potential is placed across an N-type or P-type semiconductor, each conducts a current. However, the method of current conduction differs in each type. A potential applied across an N-type semiconductor causes current to flow because of the negative carriers (Fig. 4-41, *A*). Current flow through a P-type semiconductor results from the apparent movement of positive carriers (holes) through the semiconductor (Fig. 4-41, *B*).

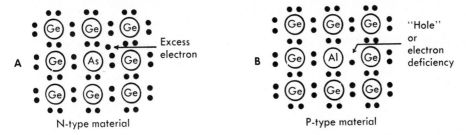

*Fig. 4-40.* Impurity semiconductor crystals.

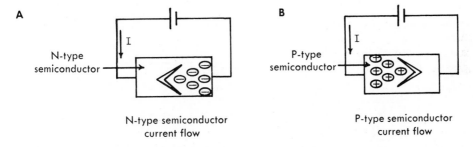

*Fig. 4-41.* Current flow through N-type and P-type semiconductors.

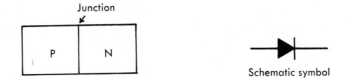

*Fig. 4-42.* P-N junction diode.

P-type and N-type semiconductor materials are used to construct a semiconductor diode, also referred to as a P-N junction diode. The P-N junction diode is made by chemically fusing a P-type crystal and an N-type crystal (Fig. 4-42). After the two materials are fused, a few majority carriers of each diffuse across the interface. The negative carriers moving into the proximal P-type crystal and the positive carriers moving into the adjacent N-type crystal result in a small potential being formed across the junction. This potential, called a *potential gradient* or *potential barrier*, impedes further charge diffusion across the junction (Fig. 4-43).

Current can be caused to flow across a P-N junction if an external potential greater than the poten-

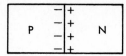

*Fig. 4-43.* Potential barrier between P-type and N-type semiconductors in semiconductor diode.

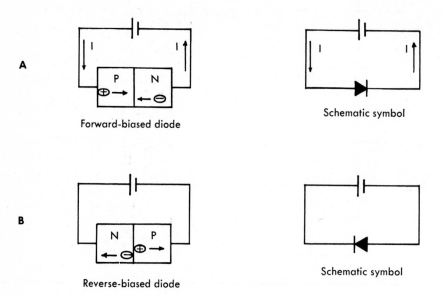

*Fig. 4-44.* P-N junction diodes in circuit.

tial barrier biases the P-N junction in a forward direction. The potential across the semiconductor diode is referred to as *bias*. The bias can be forward or reverse. Fig. 4-44, *A*, represents a circuit in which a current is conducted through a forward-biased semiconductor. The positive terminal of the battery is connected to the P-type semiconductor and the negative terminal to the N-type semiconductor. The positive and negative carriers are repelled by the battery's positive and negative charges, respectively. The holes and the electrons cross the barrier potential and recombine. Conceptually, the electrons and holes meet at the junction and neutralize each other. The net result is conventional current flow from the positive terminal to the negative terminal.

A semiconductor connected in a circuit, negative potential to P-type and positive potential to N-type semiconductor, is reverse biased (Fig. 4-44, *B*). The positive carriers in the P-type semiconductor are attracted to the negative potential, and the negative carriers are attracted to the positive potential. Since both types of carrier charges move away from the P-N junction, no current is conducted through the diode. Conceptually, the semiconductor material at the junction becomes a good insulator.

If the voltage rating of a particular semiconductor diode is exceeded, the diode can be ruined. If an excess potential is placed across a reverse-biased semiconductor diode, an avalanche current results as electrons are forced from valence bonds.

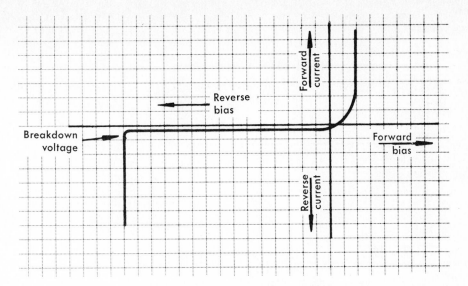

*Fig. 4-45.* Current flow through zener diode.

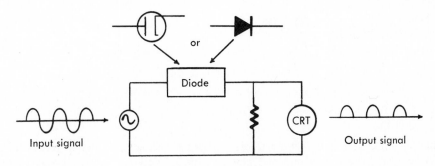

*Fig. 4-46.* Rectification.

An avalanche current destroys the integrity of the P-N junction in conventional semiconductor diodes. However, there is a class of semiconductor diodes called zener diodes (symbol: ——⊣⊢— ), which are designed to conduct only avalanche current. Zener diodes function at the reverse breakdown point and are used for regulation of voltage, although this is not their primary application. A zener diode is strategically placed in a circuit at a point where voltage level must not exceed a predetermined level. When that level is exceeded, the excess voltage is dropped through the zener diode with avalanche current flow. The zener voltage of a diode is abbreviated as $V_z$, and the amperage above which the diode will break down is indicated as $I_{MAX}$ (Fig. 4-45).

*Diode applications.* As mentioned earlier, specifically designed semiconductor diodes are used for voltage regulation. However, the primary function of diodes is to rectify alternating current to direct current. Both vacuum tube and semiconductor diodes are unidirectional current devices,

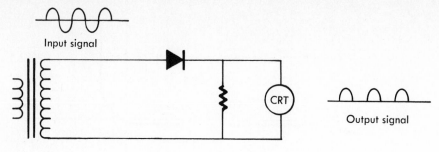

*Fig. 4-47.* Half-wave rectifier.

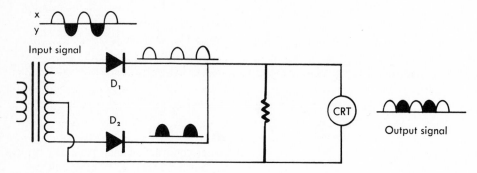

*Fig. 4-48.* Full-wave rectifier.

that is, allowing current to flow in only one direction. Each, therefore, is capable of converting ac voltage to dc voltage. Semiconductor diodes will be used in circuit diagrams for demonstrating rectification. However, in each case the semiconductor diode could be replaced with a vacuum tube diode (Fig. 4-46). Note that the output signal is monitored with an oscilloscope also called a cathode ray tube (CRT).

Rectification is shown in Fig. 4-47. During the positive half-cycle of the input ac signal at the transformer's secondary winding, the diode is forward biased. The forward-biased diode conducts, and an output voltage results. When the half-cycle of the input signal is negative, the diode is reverse biased, no current is conducted, and there is no output voltage. With each full cycle of input ac voltage, only the positive half of the cycle is conducted through the diode. This is half-wave rectification.

Fig. 4-48 shows a circuit containing two diodes functioning as a full-wave rectifier. During half-cycle X, $D_1$ is forward biased and conducts, while $D_2$ is reverse biased and does not conduct. The opposite is true during half-cycle Y. $D_2$ is forward biased and conducts, while reverse-biased $D_1$ does not. The output of a full-wave rectifier contains the voltage of both the half-cycles of the input ac voltage. Since the output voltage does not change polarity, it is dc voltage. Thus, ac voltage has been changed to dc voltage by the action of diodes.

# CHAPTER 5

# *Electronic functional units of analytical instruments*

Basic principles of electronics and descriptive detail about components are presented in earlier chapters. Isolated concepts and facts, however, carry little relevance if not put to meaningful use. Therefore, in this chapter electronic principles and component details are applied to the operation of functional electronic units. Units discussed are power supplies, detectors, amplifiers, and readout devices. These units are the basic building blocks of all analytical instruments described in later chapters.

## Power supplies

The variety of functions performed by instruments requires diverse power sources that produce an assortment of voltage levels of alternating and direct current. The power supply provides an instrument's circuit with various levels of ac voltage. This is accomplished by the transformer action previously discussed. Thus, available to the circuit are stepped-up and stepped-down voltages. The power supply also provides required direct current. Direct current is obtained through the rectification of alternating current in the power supply.

Most instruments contain within their design and construction an electronic power supply. Characteristically, electronic power supplies consist of five stages: transformer, rectifier, filter, voltage regulator, and voltage divider (Fig. 5-1).

*Transformer.* The transformer functions to step up and/or step down input ac voltage supplied from commercial power generators. This is accomplished through the induction of current in the primary winding of the transformer. Transformer construction and operational principles are detailed in Chapter 4, "Transformers."

*Rectifier.* The rectifier converts alternating current into unidirectional or direct current. Both half-wave and full-wave rectifiers produce pulsating direct current that requires additional processing to be transformed into uniformly constant direct current. Design and operation of the rectifying component, the diode, are discussed in Chapter 4, "Diodes."

*Filter.* The filter network converts pulsating direct current to smooth direct current. The variation in dc pulsating voltage is called *ripple*. When a direct current is required, ripple is undesirable and must be removed. Ripple is removed by filter-

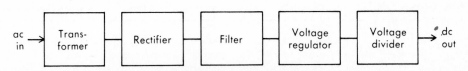

*Fig. 5-1.* Five stages of an electronic power supply.

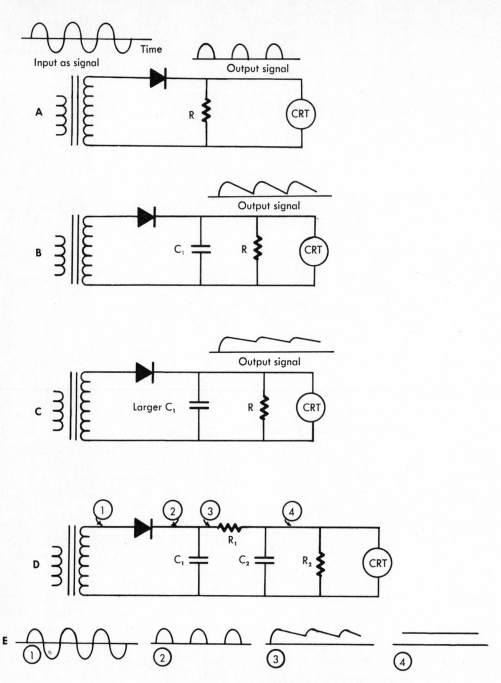

*Fig. 5-2.* Rectification and filtering.

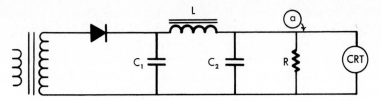

*Fig. 5-3.* Rectifier and filter.

ing. To convert pulsating direct current to smooth, constant direct current, a device is needed that will store current during the conduction part of the cycle and release it during the nonconduction part of the cycle of the diode. The capacitor is capable of storing and releasing a charge and is, therefore, an important component in the filtering process. A circuit containing a rectifier and a filtering network is shown in Fig. 5-2. Follow carefully the explanation of this circuit given below.

Refer to Fig. 5-2, *A*. Shown is a half-wave rectifier with no filtering. The output of the circuit is viewed by the cathode ray tube (CRT) connected across R. As explained in the discussion of rectification, when the diode is forward biased, it conducts and a voltage is registered on the CRT. When the diode is reverse biased, it does not conduct and in effect opens the circuit, preventing current flow. Therefore, the CRT shows no output voltage when the input ac voltage is in the negative half of the waveform.

In Fig. 5-2, *B*, to the half-wave rectifier system is added a capacitor ($C_1$) in parallel to R. When the diode is conducting, the capacitor will be charged. When the conduction of the diode begins to decline, the capacitor will discharge through R. This discharging of the capacitor will in effect "fill in the voltage gap" left when the diode is not conducting.

Now refer to Fig. 5-2, *C*. The capacitor in *B* is replaced by a larger capacitor. The larger capacitor is capable of storing a larger charge; therefore, the discharge can fill in the voltage gap better than the discharge from the first capacitor.

Refer to Fig. 5-2, *D*. Two capacitors, $C_1$ and $C_2$, are used in the filtering system. In this case, capacitance has been increased by placing two capacitors in parallel. Also, an added feature for consideration is the capability of having two different RC charging and discharging time constants. $C_1$ charges, then discharges through $R_1$. $C_2$ "sees" a pulsating current of lesser variation than was "seen" by $C_1$. It is the task of $C_2$ to further smooth out the ripple by discharging at such a rate as to fill in the "small dip" still seen in the voltage.

In Fig. 5-2, *E*, the charges occurring in the input ac voltage as it passes through the circuit in *D* are designated as numbered points in the circuit. This, in effect, represents the metamorphosis of ac voltage to dc voltage.

In Fig. 5-3, an inductor has replaced $R_1$ in Fig. 5-2, *D*. An inductor and a capacitor can be used in a power supply circuit to effect filtering. In this circuit, the current flow increasing through the inductor develops a voltage. The polarity of the voltage induced opposes the source voltage and tends to decrease the current. The magnetic field developed by the changing current flow (ripple portion of the current) in the inductor is actually stored energy that is extracted from the source. When the source voltage decreases, the magnetic field around the inductor collapses. The collapsing lines of force cut across the windings of the coil and induce current, which tends to maintain current flow in the original direction. In other words, the inductor stores energy when the diode is conducting (current increasing) and releases energy back into the circuit when the current decreases. As the magnetic field around the coils "pulsates," current is hindered or supplied to the circuit in such a way as to aid in smoothing the ripple in the dc pulsating current.

Several stages of filter networks can be used to obtain almost pure direct current, that is, direct current with extremely low values of ripple. Frequently, electrolytic capacitors are used because of their high capacitances.

For simplicity, in the foregoing examples a half-wave rectifier was used in the circuits. Capacitors and inductors must be large in these cases because of the need for stored energy over a long period of time. In other words, a large voltage gap must be filled. If a full-wave rectifier were substituted, several desirable goals would be achieved. First, both halves of the ac input sine wave would be used, thus almost doubling the efficiency of the power supply. Next, the diodes would be conducting more frequently, the total current provided by each would be less, and the diodes would last longer because of less wear. Finally, because the inductors and the capacitors would be used for filtering the power supply current for a shorter period of time, they would be smaller and less expensive.

In the above discussion about semiconductor power supplies, all points are equally applicable to vacuum tube power supplies.

*Voltage regulator.* Constant dc current output would be obtained from power supplies if the ac input were always constant. Unfortunately, line voltage fluctuations frequently occur. A fluctuation in the voltage input to the transformer results in a fluctuation in the power supply voltage output.

If instrument functional units require constant dc voltage with narrow tolerances, the voltage output from the power supply must be regulated. Voltage regulation is obtained with three types of voltage regulators: zener diode, gas-filled diode (glow tube), and electronic.

The purpose of voltage regulation is to maintain a constant voltage even during changes in current. Consider point *a* in Fig. 5-3. If voltage at this point must be maintained at a constant level, how can this be achieved if current increases in this circuit? Ohm's law provides three factors with which to work—current (I), voltage (E), and resistance (R). Therefore, if E must remain constant and I increases, then R must decrease as stipulated by the equation: $E = IR$. Thus, by replacing the resistor, R, with an electronic component with the capability of responding to current change in such a way that its effective resistance will be increased or decreased with current decrease or increase, respectively, voltage can be maintained at a constant level. This is essentially how each of the three voltage regulators operates to maintain a constant voltage at point *a*.

Fig. 5-4 shows the circuit in Fig. 5-3 with R replaced by a zener diode. The function of the zener diode was briefly discussed in Chapter 4. Current will flow through a reverse-biased zener diode when the breakdown voltage (zener voltage) is applied across the diode. Zener diodes are designed and constructed to operate at any specific breakdown voltage required. Point *a* in Fig. 5-4 is maintained at a constant voltage through the operation of the zener diode. If the voltage increases to the level of the breakdown voltage of the zener diode, current flows through the zener diode, thus dropping the excess voltage across the zener diode while maintaining a constant voltage at point *a*.

Gas-filled diodes can be used to maintain a constant voltage. The effective resistance of a gas-filled diode is determined by ionization of the gas contained within the tube. (In the symbolic representation of a gas diode shown in Fig. 5-5, the dot indicates that the tube contains a gas.) The tube exerts infinite resistance when the gas is not ionized and an extremely low resistance when the gas is ionized. Ionization of the gas occurs after a certain potential (the triggering potential level depends on the tube design) is applied across the tube. As a result of ionization, the tube conducts current, allowing a potential to be dropped across the tube. Thus, in Fig. 5-5, a constant voltage is maintained at point *a* through the responsiveness of the gas diode to an increase in voltage at point *a*.

An electronic voltage regulator will be briefly

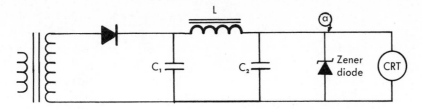

*Fig. 5-4.* Rectifier and filter with zener diode voltage regulator.

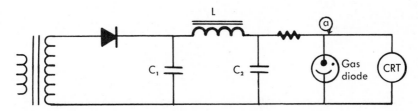

*Fig. 5-5.* Rectifier and filter with gas diode voltage regulator.

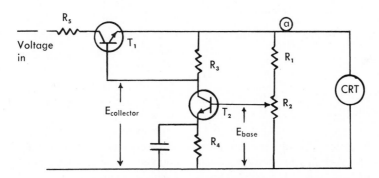

*Fig. 5-6.* Electronic voltage regulator.

described, although an understanding of its operation may not be realized fully until after the discussion of triodes and transistors in "Signal processing units." Fig. 5-6 shows an electronic voltage regulator containing two NPN transistors. An increase of voltage at point *a* results in an increased current through $R_1$ and $R_2$ and, therefore,

an increased voltage on the base of $T_2$. The more positive base causes $T_2$ to conduct more current (effective resistance decreased). As a result, the voltage on the base of $T_1$ is decreased, causing it to conduct less current (effective resistance increased). Through this type of feedback control system, a constant voltage is maintained at point *a*.

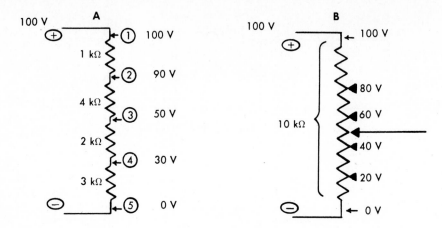

*Fig. 5-7.* Voltage divider.

*Voltage divider.* The application of voltage division enables a power supply to provide required dc voltages to different circuits within an instrument. As shown in Fig. 5-7, different voltages may be obtained by dropping voltage across a series of resistors. Voltage may also be varied by using a potentiometer. Voltage division and resistor components are discussed in detail in Chapter 3.

## Detectors

The quantification of biological fluid constituents in a sample being analyzed is based on the detection of characteristic properties of the sample. The method of detection in clinical laboratory analytical instruments is primarily photodetection, that is, detection of light or radiant energy. Other methods of detection of more limited application include temperature detection and gas composition detection. Although this list does not include all available detection methods, one of these three types of detectors is found in the majority of clinical laboratory instruments. Therefore, the discussion of detectors is limited to these three types.

Each of the three types of detectors—photosensitive, temperature, and gas composition—differs in design, construction, and operational principle. However, the three types do have one characteristic in common: they are transducers. A transducer is a device that detects one form of energy and converts it to another form of energy. The detectors in clinical laboratory instruments usually detect a physical or chemical property—for example, light, heat, and gas molecules—and convert the physical or chemical energy into electrical energy. That electrical signal is then processed by a signal handling device. For example, the signal is usually amplified before being directed to a readout display.

*Photosensitive detectors.* Photodetection is the basis of quantification in spectrophotometers, fluorometers, emission flame photometers, atomic absorption spectrophotometers, and optical cell counters. The photodetectors discussed include the barrier-layer cell, phototube, photomultiplier tube, and semiconductor photodetectors. These photodetectors use photosensitive or photoemissive materials. A photosensitive material consists of atoms that release electrons when exposed to radiant energy. When light impinges upon the surface of a photosensitive material, electrons are freed by the radiant energy. The free electrons allow for electron flow (called photocurrent) when a closed circuit is provided. This principle is applicable to each of the photosensitive detectors discussed.

The barrier-layer cell (also called a *photovoltaic*

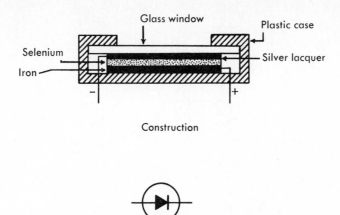

Construction

Schematic symbol

*Fig. 5-8.* Barrier-layer (photovoltaic) cell.

*cell)* generates its electrical output directly from light energy. Therefore, it needs no external power source. Construction of the barrier-layer cell is shown in Fig. 5-8. A thin layer of semiconductor, usually selenium, is deposited on a metal base, usually iron. The selenium is coated with a very thin transparent layer of silver lacquer. A glass protective window is placed over the lacquered surface, and the cell is encased in plastic. The iron acts as the positive electrode and the selenium as the negative electrode or collector. A wire lead extends through the plastic case from each of the two electrodes.

When light passes through the glass and the lacquer to impinge upon the selenium surface, enough energy is provided to the selenium to cause liberation of some electrons. The emitted electrons are collected by the silver lacquer. If the photovoltaic cell is connected in an unbroken circuit, electrons flow from the collector through the circuit to the iron electrode and finally back to the selenium. Thus, if an ammeter or a galvanometer is connected across the terminals of the photovoltaic cell, the current reading on the ammeter will be directly related to the intensity of radiant energy striking the cell's photosensitive surface.

The range of wavelengths of radiant energy to which a photodetector responds is referred to as its spectral response. The spectral response of a selenium photovoltaic cell with a protective glass window is about the same as the spectral response of the retina of the human eye. Radiant energy in the visible region (380 to 700 nm) is detected, with the greatest sensitivity being in the wavelength range of 500 to 600 nm (or the colors of green and yellow).

Radiant energy travels in a waveform and is commonly described by its wavelength, which is the distance between the peaks of adjacent waves. This distance is given in nanometers (nm) or angstroms (Å). A nanometer is $10^{-9}$ meter, and an angstrom is $10^{-10}$ meter.

The selenium barrier-layer cell is used mainly in colorimeters or spectrophotometers when relatively high levels of illumination exist. Spectrophotometers with narrow–band pass requirements cannot use a barrier-layer photodetector because of the low level of radiant energy directed to the detector. The barrier-layer cell generates an electrical signal at a level sufficient for direct readout without prior amplification.

This photodetector is rugged, inexpensive, and

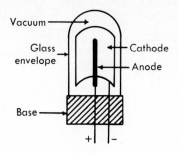

Vacuum

Glass
envelope

Cathode

Anode

Base

+  −

*Fig. 5-9*. Phototube.

Construction

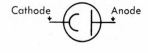

Cathode        Anode

Schematic symbol

useful for detection of relatively high levels of illumination. However, it is not suitable for use in more sophisticated instruments, because it demonstrates the undesirable characteristics of being overly subject to fatigue, a high temperature coefficient, and a poor modulation ability. With continued exposure to radiant energy, the barrier-layer cell's output gradually falls from its initial output level. High levels of illumination accentuate this fatigue effect. A fatigued cell becomes less sensitive; therefore, it may not generate a photocurrent with ordinarily detectable low levels of illumination. This disadvantage can be minimized in a spectrophotometer by using a light shutter that permits light to strike the photocell only while readings are being taken with a cuvette inserted into the cuvette well. The selenium barrier-layer cell has a high temperature coefficient. Electrons are freed from the selenium by thermal energy. In other words, with a temperature rise the photodetector's output increases. To control this effect, once the instrument is turned on, readings should be taken only after the instrument has reached a constant temperature. The modulation ability of this photodetector is poor—that is, it responds sluggishly or not at all to changes in light intensity. The barrier-layer cell cannot respond to light interruptions of only 15 to 60 cycles per second.

Another photodetector is the phototube. A phototube consists of a curved sheet of photosensitive material that serves as an emitter or cathode and a positively charged thin tube that serves as a collector or anode. Both the cathode and anode are encased in an evacuated glass envelope. A dc potential applied to each electrode is provided by the instrument's power supply. Phototubes are commonly used in many photometric instruments. The phototube construction and schematic symbol are shown in Fig. 5-9.

The cathode of the phototube is coated with a photosensitive material that emits electrons when radiant energy impinges upon it. Cesium-antimony and multialkali (Sb/K/Na/Cs) are commonly used photosensitive materials. The spectral response depends on the photosensitive material used on the cathode. Because of its positive charge, the anode attracts or collects the electrons emitted from the cathode. A proportionality exists between the intensity of the radiant energy striking the cathode and the number of electrons emitted. In other words, the greater the intensity the more electrons emitted. The amount of photocurrent generated from the phototube is very small and must undergo considerable amplification before a usable signal is obtained.

The low level of photocurrent generated by this variety of phototube is at times a disadvantage. One approach to solving this problem is to increase the gain of the amplifier, thus increasing the current to the readout device. Another approach is to modify the phototube so that it will provide considerable amplification within itself. Two types of phototube modifications have been produced.

The first type is a gas-filled phototube. The tube is filled with a gas that is ionized by the electrons emitted from the cathode. Radiant en-

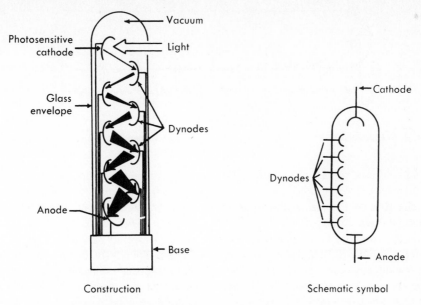

Fig. 5-10. Photomultiplier tube–linear-type design.

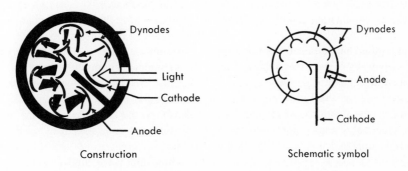

Fig. 5-11. Photomultiplier tube—circular cage–type design.

ergy striking the cathode liberates electrons that collide with, and cause ionization of, some gas atoms. The ionized gas atoms collide with and ionize other gas atoms, and the effect cascades. The overall effect of the ionization of gas atoms is to increase the total number of charged particles generated by radiant energy striking the cathode— that is, to amplify the generated signal. Gas-filled phototubes have poorer modulation ability, poorer stability, and shorter lives than vacuum photo-tubes.

The second approach to obtaining amplification within a phototube is to increase the number of electron-emitting electrodes within the tube. This modification resulted in the development of a photosensitive detector called a photomultiplier tube.

Figs. 5-10 and 5-11 show construction of, and schematic symbols for, the linear and circular design of photomultiplier tubes, respectively. The photomultiplier tube consists of a cathode, an anode, and 9 to 16 photosensitive electrodes,

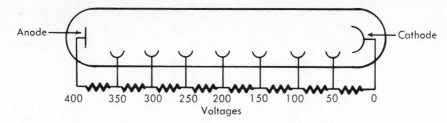

Voltages

*Fig. 5-12.* Voltage divider network supplying dynode voltages for photomultiplier tube.

called *dynodes,* encased in an evacuated glass envelope. When radiant energy strikes the cathode, emitted electrons are focused on and attracted to the first dynode. On striking the dynode, the electrons cause the emission of a greater number of electrons than the number striking it. One primary electron can yield from three to six secondary electrons. The electrons emitted from dynode 1 are then focused and attracted to dynode 2, where the process is repeated. The chain reaction continues through the entire series of dynodes until the anode is reached. Because each dynode emits more electrons than strike it, an internal amplification results.

Electrons are focused and attracted from dynode to dynode in two ways. First, the dynodes are physically placed and shaped so that electrons tend to "bounce" toward the following dynode. Second, each successive dynode is maintained at a higher positive potential than its predecessor. Successive dynodes are operated at voltages increasing in equal steps of 30 to 100 V.

The internal amplification achieved by a photomultiplier tube can be as high as $10^6$. In other words, the anode current may be as high as $10^6$ times the original current generated at the cathode. By increasing the number of dynodes, it would seem that even greater amplification could be achieved. However, each successive dynode is at a higher positive potential. Therefore, with too many dynodes, voltage levels are impractical to achieve or are so high that arcing to dynodes of lower potential will occur. Normally, the number of dynodes in a photomultiplier tube is limited to a maximum of 16.

The required dynode voltages are usually obtained from a resistor-voltage divider network across which is applied a higher positive voltage from the power supply (Fig. 5-12).

The sensitivity and the response time of the photomultiplier tube are far superior to those of the phototube. Light intensities 200 times weaker than those that can be detected by a phototube and amplifier can be measured by a photomultiplier tube. The photomultiplier tube can respond to light interruptions of $10^9$ per second.

The photoemissive surfaces in the photomultiplier tube have three general characteristics worthy of review. First, the number of emitted electrons per unit of time is directly proportional to the light intensity impinging upon the photoemissive surface. Second, the energy of the released electrons, independent of the intensity of light, depends on the frequency of the radiant energy. Therefore, a tube may respond differently at different wavelengths. A tube that responds well to visible light wavelengths may not respond satisfactorily to shorter or longer wavelengths. Photomultiplier tubes made with different photoemissive materials are selectively responsive to specific wavelengths ranges of radiant energy. Third, the delayed response in a photomultiplier tube is caused by delays encountered in the associated circuitry outside the tube. Electron emission resulting from radiant energy absorption is virtually instantaneous.

Photomultiplier tubes should not be exposed to extraneous light while voltage is being applied to them. For example, their protective covers should not be removed. If exposed to intense light, the cathode will emit more electrons than it can replace, and the tube will fatigue. The cathode may recover from the fatigue effect if stored in the dark for a period of time. However, strong intensity and prolonged exposure may destroy the integrity of the cathode.

Instruments containing phototubes or photomultiplier tubes should not be operated in an environment characterized by low temperature and high humidity. In this type of environment, condensation is likely to occur on the tube's surface. Condensation on the glass envelope will diminish the amount of light allowed to impinge upon the photoemissive cathode, resulting in erroneous output signals.

*Semiconductor detectors.* The function of semiconductors in a circuit is generally to regulate current flow. This is achieved by simply changing the resistance of the semiconductor material. A change in the potential bias across a junction between semiconductor materials effectively changes the semiconductor's resistance, or conductivity. As circuit devices, both diodes (Chapter 4, "Diodes") and transistors ("Signal processing units") are controlled through bias changes resulting from applied voltages; as photodetectors, photodiodes and phototransistors respond to bias changes resulting from absorption of radiant energy.

The simplest of semiconductor photodetectors is the photoresistor. It is an evacuated cell containing two leads attached to a thin layer of photoconductive material deposited on a transparent materials such as quartz or glass. The photoconductive material is commonly made from the sulfides or selenides of cadmium or lead. The device is connected in the circuit so that a constant potential is applied across it. When photons impinge upon the exposed photoconductive material, an increase or decrease in its resistance results. With a change in resistance there is a change in current that corresponds to the intensity of impinging light. The photoresistor's photoconductive material characteristically responds to ultraviolet, visible, and infrared radiant energy.

Junction-type semiconductors, diodes, transistors, and field effect transistors have been modified to function as photodetectors. These modifications have been successful in the development of optically controlled semiconductors. A conventional P-N junction diode is changed by adding a collimating lens positioned to focus incident light on the junction. This photodiode is reversed biased in the detection circuit. When light impinges upon the junction, the radiant energy is absorbed, electrons are freed from covalent bonds, and current flow through the circuit results. The greater the radiant energy of the incident light, the greater the resulting current.

*Transistors.* The conventional transistors and standard field effect transistors (FET) were easily converted into phototransistors and photo–field effect transistors, respectively. The collimating lens focuses incident light onto a photosensitive material at the base or gate. Transistors and FETs are appropriately biased in the circuit as described in the following section, "Signal processing units." When radiant energy strikes the photosensitive material in the base or gate, electrons are excited and move into the collector-to-emitter (in the phototransistor) or drain-to-source (in the photo–FET) conduction area. A current results that is proportional to the incident radiant energy. Since amplification is a function of transistors, it is not surprising that phototransistors characteristically exhibit a much greater gain—50 to 500 times—than do photodiodes.

***Temperature detector.*** Osmolality is a clinically useful determination of the number of particles in biological fluids. An instrument called an *osmometer* is used to determine osmolalities. Measuring the freezing point depression of specimens being analyzed is one method used in osmolality determination. A solution's freezing point decreases as the number of particles suspended in it increases. Therefore, temperature detection is used in this instrument to quantify the number of particles in a solution. The detector is called a *thermistor*.

A thermistor is a temperature measuring device consisting of a small button, constructed of a fused

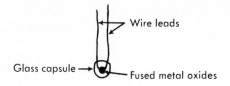

*Fig. 5-13.* Thermistor.

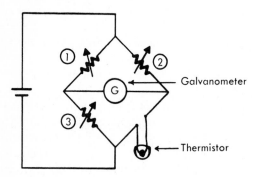

*Fig. 5-14.* Thermistor in Wheatstone bridge circuit.

mixture of metal oxides, that is attached to two leads and encapsulated in glass (Fig. 5-13). The metal oxide mixture (for example, manganese, nickel, copper, and uranium) possesses a very large negative temperature coefficient of resistance. A small decrease in temperature causes a relatively large increase in the resistance of the thermistor. For example, at 50° C a thermistor may have one fifth the resistance it had at 25° C. This large change in resistance and the thermistor's small size make this device a useful temperature detector with particular applications for small amounts of material.

A temperature change results in a proportional change in the resistance of the thermistor. Therefore, temperature can be measured by measuring the thermistor's resistance. This resistance is measured by a Wheatstone bridge circuit (Fig. 5-14). With the thermistor at a standard temperature, the three variable resistors are adjusted to balance the circuit—that is, no current is flowing through

the galvanometer. Once the circuit is balanced, the thermistor can be used to measure a temperature change. As the temperature changes, the thermistor's resistance will change and a current will flow through the galvanometer. The current then can be related to resistance change and, therefore, to temperature change.

*Gas detectors.* A gas chromatograph is an instrument used in the clinical laboratory to separate, isolate, identify, and quantify chemically related compounds in a vaporized solution. The solution to be analyzed is vaporized and carried through a column by the constant flow of an inert gas. The column is of specific design and composition and functions to delay selectively the different compounds in the sample vapor. Therefore, the compounds pass into the detector at times characteristic of their chemical and/or physical properties. Identification of the compound is based on the time required for it to reach the detector. The detector's function is only to quantify the gas molecules passing through the detector. The detectors must be very sensitive because small samples are usually used. Detection of the separated gas molecules is accomplished by using one of three general methods—thermal conductivity, flame ionization, and electron capture.

Analysis by thermal conductivity is based on the differences in thermal conductivity between a pure carrier gas and a gas containing larger and more numerous molecules. Thermal conductivity is the rate at which heat is carried through a gas. The thermal conductivity of the inert carrier gas is greater than that of the gas under analysis (effluent from the column) because the carrier gas contains faster molecules. If each of these gases were to flow at a constant rate over a heated filament, the carrier gas would cool the filament faster than the other gas would. The resistance of most metals increases with an increase in temperature. Therefore, the difference in the rates at which gases cool a metal filament can be measured as a resistance difference. This resistance difference can in turn be related to the molecular concentration of a particular vaporized sample.

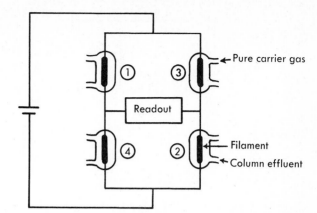

*Fig. 5-15.* Thermal conductivity detector.

Fig. 5-15 shows a thermal conductivity detector. A Wheatstone bridge circuit consists of four filaments with closely matched resistances. The pure carrier gas and the sample (effluent) from the column flow at a constant rate over filaments 3 and 4 and filaments 1 and 2, respectively. The bridge arrangement is enclosed in a temperature-regulated chamber. The filaments are heated by a constant current. When a gas containing more molecules than are found in the carrier gas passes over filaments 1 and 2, the temperature, and therefore the resistance, of these filaments increases proportionately with the number of molecules in the gas. The Wheatstone bridge will be unbalanced, and a current will be amplified and then directed to the readout device. The amount of current is directly related to the relative molecular concentration of the sample.

The flame ionization detector is represented in Fig. 5-16. The operation of this highly sensitive detector is based on the phenomenon that the combustion of organic compounds produces ionic fragmentation and free electrons. Ions and electrons between two oppositely charged electrodes will conduct a current between those electrodes.

The flame ionization detector consists of a hydrogen flame positioned between two electrodes across which is placed a high voltage. The column effluent is directed into the flame after being mixed with the hydrogen fuel. The support gas used for this flame is air. The ionic fragments and free electrons produced by the thermal energy of the flame serve as conductors of current between the two electrodes. The ions and electrons act to decrease the effective resistance between the electrodes. Therefore, with increased ions and electrons, there is decreased resistance and thus increased current through the circuit.

Current increase causes an increase in the voltage drop across R in Fig. 5-16. The output voltage is amplified before being directed to a readout device. The readout represents the amount of organic compound in the column effluent as reflected through current and voltage levels in the circuit of the flame ionization detector.

The electron-capture detector is the third type of detector used to quantify organic molecules in the column effluent. The operation of this detector is based on the ability of large organic molecules, particularly halogens, to readily capture electrons to form negatively charged ions.

The construction of the electron-capture detector is represented in Fig. 5-17. The column effluent enters the detector by passing through a screen that smooths the gas flow through the chamber. Within the chamber are a cathode, an anode, and a source of beta particles ($\beta^-$), which are high-speed electrons emitted from the nucleus of an atom. The source of beta particles is a radioactive material such as titanium tritide. As the carrier gas of nitrogen or argon flows through the detector, the beta particles cause ionization of the

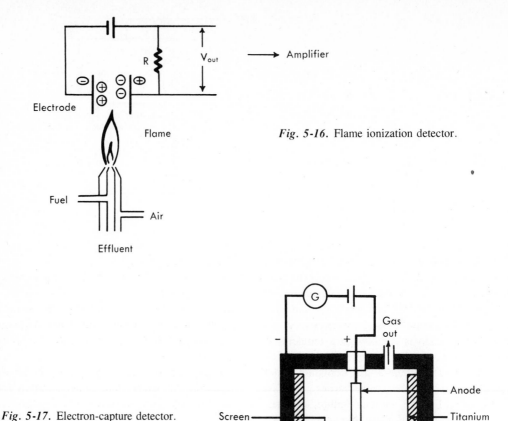

*Fig. 5-16.* Flame ionization detector.

*Fig. 5-17.* Electron-capture detector.

gas molecules, producing electrons and positive ions. The electrons are attracted to the anode, whereas the large positive ions are usually swept out of the chamber before reaching the cathode and therefore contribute minimally to the current in the circuit. Measurement of the current is represented by the galvanometer designated $G$ in Fig. 5-17. In actual practice, however, the current is amplified before being displayed on a readout device. During the flow of the carrier gas through the chamber, a constant current flows in the circuit.

When a column effluent containing organic molecules enters the chamber, the free electrons are captured by the organic molecules to form large negative ions. These large ions are slow moving and are usually swept from the chamber before reaching the anode. This results in fewer negative charges reaching the anode and, therefore, a decrease in the current in the circuit. The greater the number of organic molecules carried by the carrier gas in the effluent, the greater the number of electrons captured. With a decreased number of electrons attracted to the anode, there is a decreased current in the circuit. This method of gas molecule detection relates current indirectly to the quantity of organic molecules in the column effluent.

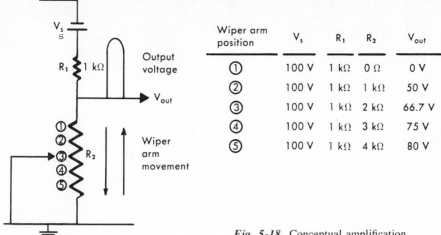

| Wiper arm position | $V_s$ | $R_1$ | $R_2$ | $V_{out}$ |
|---|---|---|---|---|
| ① | 100 V | 1 kΩ | 0 Ω | 0 V |
| ② | 100 V | 1 kΩ | 1 kΩ | 50 V |
| ③ | 100 V | 1 kΩ | 2 kΩ | 66.7 V |
| ④ | 100 V | 1 kΩ | 3 kΩ | 75 V |
| ⑤ | 100 V | 1 kΩ | 4 kΩ | 80 V |

*Fig. 5-18.* Conceptual amplification.

## Signal processing units

After conversion of physical or chemical energy to electrical energy by the detector, the electrical signal is changed to a form compatible with the appropriate readout device. The signal is changed in numerous ways by what are generally called *signal processing units*. Signal processing units specifically perform functions such as amplification and counting and mathematical manipulations include addition, subtraction, multiplication, division, integration, and differentiation. This section includes principles of amplification with vacuum tube and solid-state devices and brief descriptions of integrated circuits, printed circuit boards, operational amplifiers, and several types of signal processing circuits including amplifiers, log-to-linear converters, analog-to-digital (A-to-D) converters, integrators, discriminators, counting circuits, and feedback circuits.

*Amplification.* A frequent requirement within instruments' electronic circuitry is amplification of a signal. In this section amplification is defined, and various types of amplifiers are described and their functions discussed.

As mentioned previously, output signals from detectors may be amplified before being directed to readout devices. Amplification is simply changing a small signal into a signal of larger ampli-

tude—that is, magnifying it. A basic description of amplification is a small input signal affecting a circuit in such a way that a large output signal results.

Fig. 5-18 illustrates the concept of amplification. In the diagram, the voltage source ($V_s$) is a constant dc source, $R_1$ is a fixed resistor, and $R_2$ is a variable resistor. If the wiper arm of $R_2$ is moved upward, the $R_2$ resistance is decreased and, as a result, the output voltage ($V_{out}$) decreases. On the other hand, if the wiper arm on $R_2$ is moved downward, the resistance of $R_2$ increases and the output voltage increases. This concept of amplification is an application of voltage division discussed earlier in Chapters 3 and 4.

Consider a hypothetical situation. In Fig. 5-15 the fixed resistor value is 1 kΩ, the variable resistor can be adjusted from 0 Ω to 4 Ω in increments of 1 Ω, and the voltage source is 100 V. Calculate the output voltage for each of the five indicated positions of the wiper arm. As is clearly shown with this example, a change in the resistance of $R_2$ results in a change in voltage output.

If $R_2$ is very sensitive, a small change in the wiper arm position produces a large change in resistance. Therefore, a small movement of the $R_2$ wiper arm would result in a large voltage change at the output. This is essentially how a small input

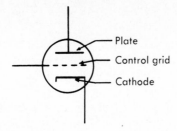

*Fig. 5-19.* Schematic symbol of triode vacuum tube.

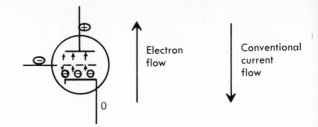

*Fig. 5-20.* Operation of tridoe vacuum tube.

voltage affects a vacuum tube or semiconductor transistor amplifier. With the change of the input voltage amplitude, there is a large change in the effective resistance of the amplifier, resulting in a large change in the output voltage. Exactly how an input voltage change is expressed as a change in effective resistance is clarified in the discussion of operational principles of amplifiers, which follows later in this chapter.

The degree of amplification of a signal by an amplifier is referred to as the *gain* of the amplifier. Gain is the ratio of output voltage to input voltage:

$$\text{Gain} = V_{out}/V_{in}$$

If an input voltage of 0.1 V results in an output voltage of 10 V, the gain of the amplifier is 100, as calculated below:

$$\text{Gain} = V_{out}/V_{in} = 10 \text{ V}/0.1 \text{ V} = 100$$

Several types of amplifiers have been developed, including vacuum tube, semiconductor, and operational amplifiers. Construction, schematic representation, and operational principles of each type are briefly discussed.

*Vacuum tubes.* Vacuum tube operational principles were included in the discussion of the acuum tube diode in Chapter 4. Since these operational principles are the basis on which vacuum tube amplifiers function, review of this previous material may be beneficial. Both rectification and amplification may be achieved through the application of these basic vacuum tube principles. Rectification results from the action of a diode. Ampli-

fication can be obtained by using vacuum tubes, including triodes, tetrodes, and pentodes.

A triode consists of the same components as a diode with the addition of one element called a *control grid*. Thus, a triode consists of a cathode, a plate, a heater, and a control grid, all of which are encased within an evacuated glass envelope. The control grid is a wire helically wound around the cathode. The grid is positioned between the cathode and plate, closer to the cathode than to the plate. Fig. 5-19 shows the schematic symbol used for a triode vacuum tube. The presence of a heater is assumed when not specifically indicated in schematic representations of vacuum tubes.

Fig. 5-20 illustrates the operation of a vacuum tube triode. As in a forward-biased vacuum tube diode, electrons are emitted from the heated cathode and are attracted to the positively charged plate. Conventional current flows through the tube from the plate to the cathode. Current through the tube is called *plate current*.

Electron flow from the cathode to the plate is controlled by the control grid. When the control grid of the triode is made increasingly more negative with respect to the cathode, repulsion of the electrons by the grid results in fewer electrons reaching the positively charged plate. Thus, with an increase of the negative grid potential, there is an increase in the effective resistance (effective resistance of a vacuum tube is called plate resistance) of the tube and a decrease in the plate current.

An operationally biased triode is one in which the plate is considerably more positive and the con-

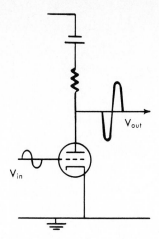

*Fig. 5-21.* Triode vacuum tube amplifier.

trol grid slightly more negative than the cathode. A small ac signal applied to the control grid continously alters the grid bias, thus changing the current through the tube and consequently the voltage on the plate. The voltage output taken at the plate will have a waveform 180 degrees out of phase with, and of greater amplitude than, the waveform of the input signal on the control grid. This production of a large output signal by a small input signal is called amplification.

Fig. 5-21 represents a triode vacuum tube amplifier that is functionally comparable to the circuit shown in Fig. 5-18. As the small input signal applied to the negatively biased control grid swings in the positive direction, the grid becomes less negative, the plate resistance decreases, the plate current increases, and the output voltage decreases. When the input signal swings in the negative direction, the grid becomes more negative, the plate resistance increases, the plate current decreases, and the output voltage increases.

In summary, the small input voltage continuously alters the control grid bias in respect to the cathode, which changes the conductivity or resistance of the tube, which affects the plate current, which determines the output voltage. The process of amplification is a dynamic expression of Ohm's law.

Two other vacuum tubes used for amplification are the tetrode and the pentode. The operational principle of each is essentially the same as that of the triode. First, the triode was modified to form a tetrode; later, a modification of the tetrode produced the pentode.

The tetrode is a four-element vacuum tube developed by adding a screen grid to the triode. The screen grid is located between the control grid and the plate (Fig. 5-22, *A*) and is maintained at a positive dc potential (Fig. 5-22, *B*). In the triode, unwanted capacitance develops between the control grid and the plate. This capacitance is called interelectrode capacitance. The screen grid has two effects: (1) it reduces the grid-to-plate interelectrode capacitance and (2) since the screen grid is at a positive potential, it attracts the electrons emitted from the cathode, serving to accelerate them toward the plate.

The impact of the highly accelerated electrons upon the plate results in the emission of electrons from the plate. The cathode emission of electrons is called *primary* emission; therefore the emission of electrons from the plate is called *secondary* emission. Electrons freed as a result of secondary emission are attracted to the electrode of highest positive potential. When the plate voltage is high, the electrons contribute to the plate current. However, when the plate voltage is at its minimum value, the electrons are attached to the screen grid, resulting in a screen grid current. This latter occurrence is undesirable, since amplification of the output signal is diminished with the decrease in possible plate current. This problem was solved by modifying the tetrode and thus developing the pentode.

The pentode vacuum tube contains a suppressor grid between the screen grid and the plate (Fig. 5-23, *A*). The suppressor grid is connected to the cathode, providing it with a potential that repels the secondary emission electrons back to the plate. Fig. 5-23, *B,* shows the bias potentials on an operational pentode. In effect, the suppressor grid eliminates excess screen grid current and enhances amplification.

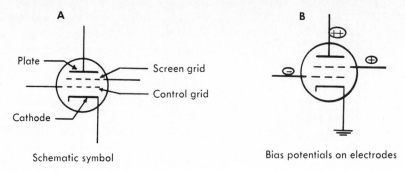

Fig. 5-22. Tetrode vacuum tube.

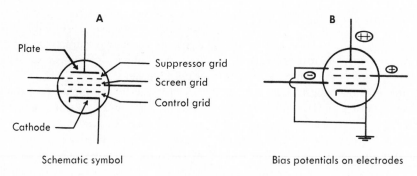

Fig. 5-23. Pentode vacuum tube.

***Semiconductor transistors.*** Vacuum tubes have been virtually eliminated with the development and use of solid-state electronic devices. Two of these, the semiconductor diode and the semiconductor transistor, have replaced the vacuum tube diode and the amplifier, respectively. This innovation brought with it a number of advantages. Transistors are much smaller than vacuum tubes and have contributed to miniaturization in electronics. Warm-up time is eliminated in solid state electronics because, unlike vacuum tubes, transistors do not require heating filaments. Lower operating voltages are needed by transistors; therefore, smaller power supplies can be used. Transistors are less susceptible to breakage than vacuum tubes. Solid-state circuits are less expensive and last longer than equivalent vacuum tube circuits.

Vacuum tubes and transistors both function in amplification; however, their principles of operation differ. The crystalline structure and conducting characteristics of semiconductor materials are discussed in Chapter 4. The P-N junction semiconductor is the simplest of semiconductor functional electronic devices. Construction, operation, and application of the semiconductor diode are described in Chapter 4 and should be reviewed prior to the presentation of semiconductor transistors.

The origin of the name "transistor" represents the operation and the functional application of the device. When this semiconductor device was

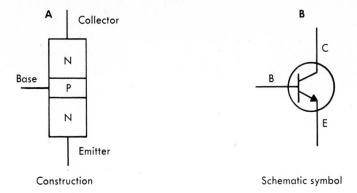

*Fig. 5-24.* NPN transistor.

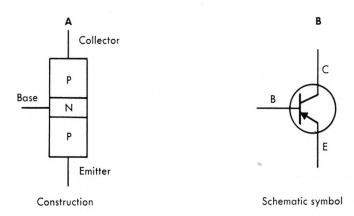

*Fig. 5-25.* PNP transistor.

first developed in 1948, it was recognized that its resistance could be changed to regulate current flow in a circuit. The device was initially called a "transfer resistor," a functional description that soon became "transistor."

The first semiconductor transistors to be developed were junction transistors of two types, NPN and PNP. These transistors are called "junction transistors" because charge movement through them is regulated at the junction between fused negative or positive semiconductor materials. An NPN transistor consists of two N-type semiconductor wafers between which is fused a P-type semiconductor (Fig. 5-24, *A*). N-type semi-

conductor material sandwiched between two P-type semiconductor wafers makes a PNP transistor (Fig. 5-25, *A*). The middle semiconductor material layer is very thin (approximately 0.001 inch thick) in each type of transistor and is called the *base* (B). The other two semiconductor elements in the transistor are called the *collector* (C) and the *emitter* (E). Schematic symbols for NPN and PNP transistors are shown in Figs. 5-24 *B*, and 5-25, *B*, respectively.

The base of the transistor is functionally equivalent to the cathode, and the collector is equivalent to the plate. The base potential regulates the current flow through the transistor as the control

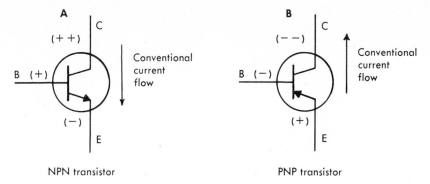

*Fig. 5-26.* Biasing of PNP and NPN transistors.

grid potential regulates the current through the vacuum tube triode, tetrode, or pentode.

The direction of conventional current flow through a transistor is indicated by the emitter arrows in the schematic symbol. Current flow through the transistor is regulated by the base-to-emitter bias potential. The base exerts its control on electron flow in the NPN transistor and on "hole" or positive charge flow in the PNP transistor. The emitter is the source of free electrons and "holes" in NPN and PNP transistors, respectively. The collector is the electrode that attracts electrons and holes in NPN and PNP transistors, respectively.

To avoid confusion, it must be emphasized that charge flow through a transistor is from emitter to collector. In the NPN transistor, electrons flow from the emitter into the base region and then to the collector. In the PNP transistor, holes, or conceptually positive charges, flow from the emitter into the base material and then to the cathode. Movement of charges in the direction indicated above is achieved by biasing the electrodes of the transistors—that is, applying fixed dc potentials of different levels on each of the three electrodes. Transistors must be correctly biased to allow current flow. If a positive potential is applied to the P-type semiconductor and a negative potential is applied to the N-type semiconductor, the P-N junction will be forward biased. The P-N junction will be reverse biased if a positive potential is

applied to the N-type semiconductor and a negative potential is applied to the P-type semiconductor. The standard operational fixed bias applied to junction semiconductor transistor amplifiers will cause the emitter-base junction to be forward biased and the base-collector junction to be reverse biased, as shown in Fig. 5-26.

Refer to Fig. 5-26, *A,* and follow the explanation of current flow through a properly biased NPN transistor. The negative potential at the emitter repels electrons toward the positively charged base. The majority of the electrons pass through the very thin base region to the collector, which is at a high positive potential. Current flow through a PNP transistor differs only slightly from that through an NPN transistor (Fig. 5-26, *B*). In the PNP transistor, the charges moved through the transistor are holes (positive charges) instead of electrons, as is the case in NPN transistors. The positive potential on the emitter of the PNP transistor repels the holes into the base region. The majority of these holes are attracted by the high negative potential on the collector and pass through the thin base region to the collector. Regulation of current flow is accomplished by regulating the emitter-base bias in both NPN and PNP transistors. Therefore, if the emitter potential remains unchanged, the potential on the base will regulate current flow through the transistor. This characteristic allows for the application of transistors to amplification.

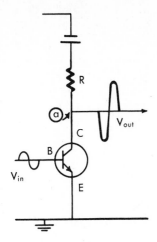

*Fig. 5-27.* NPN transistor amplifier.

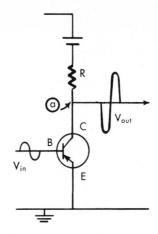

*Fig. 5-28.* PNP transistor amplifier.

The principle of amplification was considered in the presentation of vacuum tubes. Since the principle of amplification by transistors is similar to the principle of amplification by vacuum tubes, it is mentioned only briefly here. In an NPN transistor, with a change in the emitter-base bias, current flow through the transistor is changed, and with a change in current flow through the transistor, the voltage at point *a* in Fig. 5-27 (that is, output voltage) is changed. An input signal is introduced at the base. As the base becomes more positive with respect to the emitter, more electrons are attracted by the base and more current flows in the circuit. With increased current, there is a greater voltage drop over R, and the voltage at point *a* decreases. When the input signal swings negative, the emitter-base bias is decreased, decreasing current flow, and therefore less voltage is dropped across R. In this case, the voltage at point *a* increases.

Refer to Fig. 5-28, and follow the explanation of amplification using a PNP transistor. An input signal is applied to the base. As the base becomes more positive with respect to the emitter, fewer holes are attracted to the base (essentially, the transistor's effective resistance is increased) and the voltage drop across the transistor is increased, resulting in a decreased voltage at point *a*. As the input signal swings negative, holes are strongly

attracted to the base region and then to the collector. This results in decreased effective resistance of the transistor, increased current flow through the transistor, decreased voltage drop across the transistor, and increased voltage at point *a*. Note that, as is the case with the vacuum tube amplifiers, a small input signal produces an output signal of greater amplitude that is 180 degrees out of phase with the input signal.

The junction transistors discussed above are of limited usefulness when a signal must be amplified with minute current drain from the signal source. For example, a barrier-layer cell produces a photocurrent as a result of radiant energy striking a photosensitive material. To amplify the output signal from the barrier-layer cell, the amplifier must be able to produce a greater output signal without drawing much current from the barrier-layer cell. If substantial current were drawn from the barrier-layer cell, the cell would become fatigued, since the electrons would not be returned to the photosensitive material at a sufficient rate. Therefore, for limited current drain from voltage sources, an amplifier with a high input impedance must be used.

A semiconductor amplifier developed to provide a high input impedance is the field effect transistor (FET). Frequently, an FET is used as the first

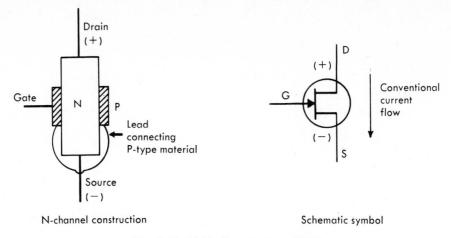

*Fig. 5-29.* Field effect transistor (FET).

stage (that is, at the input) of a multistage ampli-fier. (A multistage amplifier consists of many in-dividual amplifying transistors connected collec-tor-to-base in series, with each transistor ampli-fying the output signal of the previous one.)

Field effect transistors are of two types, N-channel and P-channel. The construction and the schematic symbol of an N-channel semiconductor FET are shown in Fig. 5-29. The FET consists of a bar of semiconductor material called the channel, which is N-type or P-type depending upon whether the FET is N-channel or P-channel. An electrode is connected to each end of the channel. These electrodes are called the source (S) and the drain (D). The N-channel is fused between two layers of P-type semiconductor that are electrically con-nected. To the P-type semiconductor is attached an electrode called the *gate* (G). Some FETs are designed with a gate consisting of a sleeve of P-type material around the N-channel.

FET operation closely parallels the operation of a vacuum tube diode. The effective resistance of the FET is controlled by the potential applied to the gate. In the N-channel, the electrons flow from the negatively charged source to the positively charged drain. When a negative voltage is applied to the gate, electron flow through the N-channel is hindered. The greater the negative potential on the gate, the greater the impedance to electron flow. Thus, current flow decreases.

The advantage of very high input impedance has been enhanced with the development of the insulated-gate FET, or the metal oxide semicon-ductor field effect transistor (MOSFET). This modified FET consists of a gate insulated from the channel by a film of insulating metal oxide. As in the FET, the gate's electrostatic field con-trols charge flow through the channel. The MOSFET exerts the highest input impedance (as high as $10^{10}$ $\Omega$) of any transistor.

*Integrated circuits.* The evolution of electronic devices, which has led to the development of the vacuum tube and the specifically designed semi-conductor, continues. Discrete transistors and as-sociated circuitry are being replaced by integrated circuits. An integrated circuit (IC) is a functional electronic circuit incorporated into a tiny piece of silicon, referred to as a "chip." Diodes, transis-tors, FETs, resistors, capacitors, and associated connections can be built into very small silicon chips. With the development of integrated circuits, miniaturization in electronics is frequently limited only by the requirement that connecting leads ex-tend to the exterior of the protective cover of the IC.

The availability of ICs for a wide variety of

applications has rapidly increased while the cost has decreased. Repair of ICs is difficult if not impossible; therefore, they are usually replaced rather than repaired. Such disposable electronic circuits are feasible because they are relatively inexpensive. Integrated circuits are being used increasingly in clinical laboratory instruments. A recent development in integrated circuits is the large-scale integrated circuit (LSI), which is an IC chip containing an entire instrument circuit or a large portion of it. LSI circuitry permits micro-miniaturization of instruments. Digital computers and small calculators are the first instruments to contain the LSI circuit.

*Printed circuit boards.* By combining these miniaturized, simplified devices on *printed circuit boards,* instruments are designed so that field repairs can be made very simply by replacing an entire board, bypassing the time-consuming and tedious task of analyzing the instrument's performance to diagnose the failure. Although many advances have been made during the past few years, there is much more to be done in designing laboratory equipment, and the next decade will probably see many more small, sophisticated instruments introduced that will make present instruments seem crude and awkward by comparison.

*Operational amplifiers.* The operational amplifier (OA or op amp) is a multistage amplifier system contained within one small unit or package. Like the solid-state devices discussed earlier, the op amp is replaced rather than repaired. The name "operational amplifier" was derived from its intended function of performing mathematical "operations" on a signal or signals. The flexibility and versatility of the op amp provide for a multitude of applications, some of which are utilized in the signal processing units of clinical laboratory instruments. A few of the many mathematical operations performed by the op amp include addition, subtraction, integration, differentiation, logarithm derivation, antilogarithm derivation, multiplication, and division.

The op amp unit is available in different shapes and sizes, each having several (8 to 16) terminals.

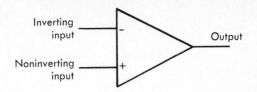

**Fig. 5-30.** Operational amplifier schematic symbol.

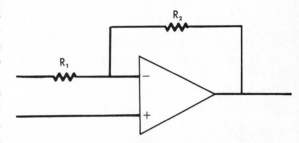

**Fig. 5-31.** Common operational amplifier circuit.

These terminals are connected to biasing voltages and associated circuitry. The terminals to be referred to in this brief discussion are the two input terminals and the one output terminal. As shown in Fig. 5-30, the output terminals are conventionally marked − and + for inverting input and noninverting input, respectively. A signal applied to the inverting input produces a signal of the opposite sign at the output—that is, the input signal is inverted. If a signal is applied to the noninverting input, the output signals have the same sign.

The function performed by an op amp is determined by the external associated circuitry. Fig. 5-31 shows a commonly used amplifier circuit that amplifies the input signal. The op amp has a large input impedance of at least $10^5$ Ω and a high gain of at least $10^4$. The gain of an operational amplifier circuit is calculated as follows:

$$\text{Gain}_{\text{op amp}} = R_2/R_1$$

where:

$R_1$ = Resistance of input resistor
$R_2$ = Feedback resistance

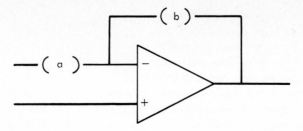

*Fig. 5-32.* Operational amplifier; optional associated circuitry for mathematical operations.

Examples of mathematical operations performed by op amp circuits are presented with reference to Fig. 5-32. A detailed understanding of the operation of each sample op amp circuit is not expected. The examples are provided only to demonstrate the versatility of the op amp in performing different functions by changing and/or rearranging associated circuit components.

Addition of signals is achieved by establishing a circuit with a resistor in the feedback loop at *b* and parallel resistors at *a,* with each resistor conducting one of the input signals to be added. The output of the op amp will be the negative sum of the input signals.

Two signals can be subtracted in an op amp circuit by placing a resistor at *b* and two parallel resistors at *a,* with one input signal having a positive sign and the other a negative sign.

Integration is achieved in an op amp circuit that has a resistor at *a* and a capacitor at *b.* Measurement of area is obtained through the operation of integration.

Differentiation is obtained by exchanging the components in the integration circuit. Thus, a differentiator op amp circuit has a capacitor at *a* and a resistor at *b.* Measurement of slope or rate change is achieved through the operation of differentiation.

A logarithmic function is obtained from a log op amp circuit, which has a resistor at *a* and a P-N junction diode in a forward-biased orientation at *b.* This operation makes possible the direct conversion of transmittance to absorbance in spectrophotometry.

Antilogarithms can be obtained from an op amp circuit with a forward-biased P-N junction diode at *a* and a resistor at *b.*

Multiplication and division are more complex operations and require the application of three op amp circuits. To multiply or divide, first the logarithms of the variables are obtained. Then these logs are added for multiplication or subtracted for division, and finally, the antilogarithms are extracted.

The modular design of modern instrumentation has developed through the use of operational amplifiers and integrated circuitry. Since operational amplifiers have a multiplicity of applications, they are found in most instruments in which signal handling, simple or complex, is required. In clinical laboratory instruments, the signal generated or affected by the sample being analyzed is processed through any number of signal manipulations before being presented to the readout device.

*Types of circuits.* In the preceeding pages many of the components that are used in electrical circuits are discussed. These are the tools with which the instrument designer works to make electricity do what is wished. Circuit design is technical, and it is not the purpose of this text to give any particular detail of this science. It is necessary, however, that the student understand what is involved in certain types of circuits and what functions they perform. The following terms are of importance in understanding instrumentation.

*Amplifiers.* It has been noted that vacuum tubes and transistors can amplify a signal. When amplifiers are referred to in a broader sense, however, all the components necessary in a rather complex circuit to amplify and condition the signal are considered. Thus, the voltage or the amperage may be amplified, or both may be amplified. The amplifier circuit may have more than one amplifying tube or transistor; if so, it is said to have more than one *stage* of amplification. Direct current amplifiers are made but are not used widely in laboratory instruments.

*Log-to-linear converters.* Discussion in Chapter 7 points out that the light absorbed by a solution depends on the concentration of the solute, if Beer's law applies. The relationship between absorbed light and concentration is not linear; if a graph is made by plotting one against the other, the curve will be logarithmic. It is possible to pass the photosignal from a light detector through a log-to-linear converter and produce an electric signal that is linear with concentration, thus allowing one to read the concentration of a solution directly on a digital meter. These converters are further discussed in the appropriate chapters.

*Analog-to-digital converters.* Whenever the current from a photocell, a pH electrode, or other type of transducer is measured, a signal that is analogous to the parameter being measured is received. It is unknown what that electric signal means except in comparison to a similar one from a standard situation. The electric signal that is comparable, or analogous, to the parameter measured is called an *analog signal.* If it is necessary to tell a computer, for example, what this signal means, the signal must be converted into numbers or digits. An *analog-to-digital* (A-to-D) converter is a circuit that performs this task.

*Integrators.* To understand what function an integrator performs, a comparison to a totally unrelated subject can be made. A restaurant serves no coffee at 10:30 AM, but by 10:45 it is serving at the rate of two cups a minute. By 11:00 it is serving five cups a minute, and at 11:30, 8 cups a minute. This rate is continued until 12:45, when it drops off to 4 a minute, and by 1:30 the restaurant is no longer serving. With only these facts how could it be determined how much coffee was served? The

serving rates could be plotted and the points connected and (if one wanted to work for many hours) the quantity could be estimated, minute by minute, and added all up. Since the change in rate of serving was a variable, one could never arrive at a definite figure, however. If somehow the area under the curve of the graph drawn could be figured, the resultant total would be fairly valid. If those minute-by-minute figures were accurate, one could have a very accurate answer. An integrator performs this type of function—one that can be defined as continuously summing the product of time versus rate to give a cumulative total. Since many of the phenomena to be measured are variables, this is an important device. Integration is accomplished electronically by a battery of capacitors that digitize a variable electric signal into units that can be counted.

*Discriminators.* Whenever a cell counter senses a blood cell or a gamma detector senses an emission, the detection may be thought of as an electrical event that produces a signal or pulse of some sort. To determine the size of the cell or the energy of the pulse, the amplitude of the pulsation must be measured, and, if one is looking for a specific size of cell or one isotope, all impulses that do not meet the criteria set must be screened out. For example, the pulse from a white blood cell will be considerably larger than that of a red blood cell. One discriminates between them by measuring their electrical pulses, using a discriminator circuit. A capacitor may be set up in the circuit in such a way that only impulses exceeding a predetermined level will pass. All smaller pulses are shorted out to ground. This arrangement would be called a *lower,* or *threshold, discriminator.*

Another capacitor arrangement may be set up to short to ground all signals that exceed a given level. This would be called an *upper discriminator.* Both of these may be used in a circuit, leaving only signals that exceed a given level but are less than a predetermined maximum. This would leave a *window* through which passes only pulses from a red blood cell, for example.

If a large number of signals are being processed

in a brief time period, there will be times when two signals occur at exactly the same instant and will appear to be one signal that is twice as large. This coincidence can be anticipated if the duration of the impulse and the approximate number occurring each second are known. Obviously the larger the number per second, the larger the number of coincidences will be. It is possible, mathematically, to calculate coincidence probability and, electronically, to make a correction for the error involved. Hence an *anticoincidence circuit* may be added to a discriminator.

*Counting circuits.* After having discriminated between pulses in the manner just described, it may be necessary to count the blood cells or gamma emissions that the pulses represent. For this a counting circuit of some sort is used. The pulses selected may be occurring so rapidly that it is difficult to count them accurately. For this reason a *scaler,* which selects only a representative number of pulses for counting may be added. Two types are common. The *binary scaler* may be set to select first every second pulse, then every second one of these, and every second again, so that we may count one out of two, four, eight, sixteen, thirty-two, etc. The *decade scaler* will count every tenth impulse, then every tenth of these, etc.; the progression is 1, 10, 100, 1000, 10,000, etc.

The sampling ratio of pulses to be counted having been selected, the pulse may be sent to a relay that mechanically causes a counter, such as a Veeder-Root tally, to turn and advance numbers on a dial. These devices are used less commonly now, however. A profusion of devices such as *glow tubes, NIXIE tubes, bar tubes,* and *light-emitting diodes* are available, which indicate the number of pulses coming to them. Readout instruments using such devices are generally referred to as *electronic displays*. This explanation is obviously an oversimplification of a fairly technical subject but should give some idea of the rationale behind these devices.

*Current-summing devices.* These circuits generally make use of capacitors to store all of the current involved in an operation, such as the count-

ing of impulses of a given size, during a selected interval. This electrical total can then be used for further operations such as averaging or integration.

*Feedback circuits.* When a part of the output of an amplifier is returned to the input side, to achieve some desirable effect, it is termed a *feedback circuit. Negative feedback* is often used in amplifiers, to stabilize the gain of the amplifier. Feedback information can also be used to inform the instrument of changes in conditions and hence cause it to modify its performance. At times amplifiers may inadvertently develop resonance from unwanted *positive feedback* causing oscillation and distortion.

## Readout devices

Readout devices used in clinical laboratory instruments have become increasingly sophisticated with the increased complexity of instruments. However, all readout systems serve the same ultimate function—to supply the operator with required data in correct, clear, and understandable form.

Signal detection and processing are discussed in earlier sections. A physical or chemical property of a sample under analysis is detected by a transducer that converts the physical property into an electrical signal. This signal is processed, which usually includes amplification, and is then presented to the readout device. It is important to note that there is a proportionality between the concentration of the detected sample component and the generated electrical signal. Thus, the electrical signal can be related to the concentration of a component. This relationship is established when an instrument is calibrated in units of concentration, transmittance, or absorbance or in arbitrarily selected units. A readout device measures the amount of current or voltage generated by a detection system, which in turn presents wanted information about the sample being analyzed.

Commonly used instrument readout (or display) devices discussed include meters, recorders, digital displays, and oscilloscopes.

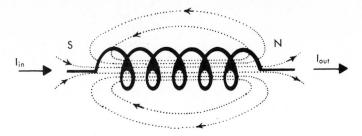

*Fig. 5-33.* Magnetic field around conducting coil.

*Meters.* Housed within a case are the meter face and the meter movement. The meter face displays a scale of units appropriate for the use of that particular meter. The meter movement is a mechanism that deflects from a preset position when current is applied. The degree of deflection is related to the amount of current flowing through the meter movement. The operation of most meter movements used in clinical laboratory instruments is based on the electromagnetic theory.

The electromagnetic theory as it applies to meter movements can be understood easily with the application of the three basic concepts listed below.

1. When a current flows through a coiled wire, the magnetic lines of force around each loop are concentrated in the center of the coil. These magnetic lines of force form closed loops traveling south to north inside the coil and north to south outside the coil (Fig. 5-33).

2. With increased current flow through the coil, the strength of the magnetic field is increased.

3. Like magnetic poles repel, and unlike magnetic poles attract.

The interaction of the poles of a permanent magnetic field with those of an electromagnetic field is the basis for current measuring devices. A current measuring device, called an *ammeter,* consists of a coiled wire positioned between the poles of a permanent magnet. The orientation of the coiled wire is such that the electromagnetic poles generated by a current are close to their corresponding poles on permanent magnet. Thus, when a current flows through the coiled wire, the like poles will repel and the coil will deflect, or

rotate. A coiled spring is attached to the coiled wire assembly to control its degree of deflection and to return it to its original position once current no longer flows through the coiled wire. This permanent magnet–moving coil assembly operates on the principle of d'Arsonval, or moving coil movement, which is the most commonly used movement in clinical laboratory instruments with meter readouts. The original d'Arsonval moving coil movement is used in the galvanometer. The d'Arsonval meter movement is a modification of the d'Arsonval moving coil movement. Both types are described, since both are still in clinical laboratory instruments.

A galvanometer is a device capable of detecting very small amounts of current. The assembly consists of a permanent magnet and a delicately suspended moving element, of which the degree of rotation is controlled by a very flexible current-carrying spiral spring. The moving element consists of a fine wire wound around a lightweight nonconducting material upon which is mounted a small mirror.

Illustrated in Figs. 5-34 and 5-35, respectively, are the galvanometer moving element assembly and the galvanometer optical arrangement for readout display. Refer to these two figures, and follow the description of how the galvanometer operates. A current generated by a detector is presented to the galvanometer. As the current flows through the suspension wire, the coil, and the spring, a magnetic field is generated around the coil. The polarity of the generated magnetic field is such that its north pole is near the permanent magnet's north

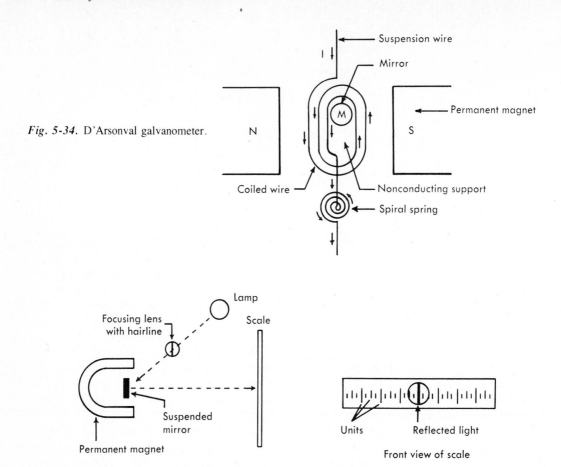

*Fig. 5-34.* D'Arsonval galvanometer.

*Fig. 5-35.* Galvanometer optical arrangement.

pole and its south pole is near the permanent magnet's south pole. The like poles repel each other, and the moving element assembly rotates. A light beam is focused onto the mirror attached to the moving assembly. The light reflected from the mirror is directed to a translucent readout scale. A hairline on the focusing lens is used to indicate the readout point on the scale. As the moving assembly rotates, the reflected light from the mirror moves across the readout scale. When the current through the coil stops, the electromagnetic field around the coil collapses and the moving assembly is returned to its initial or zero position by the spiral spring.

The "zero adjust" on the galvanometer is a delicate adjustment of the spiral spring tension to be made only when no current is flowing through the coil. The zero adjustment can be used to position the reflected image in the center of the readout scale. Using a galvanometer adjusted in this way, current flow through the coil in either direction can be detected and measured. The readout light image will deflect in one direction when current flows in one direction and in the opposite direction when current flows in the other direction. When no current is flowing and the light image is at the preset mid-scale, the image is said to be in the null position.

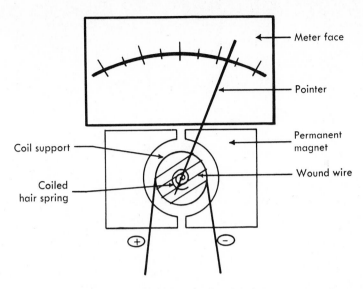

*Fig. 5-36.* D'Arsonval meter movement.

The high degree of sensitivity of the galvanometer is contributed to by the very lightweight moving coil assembly suspended by the fine phosphor bronze wire and the highly flexible spiral spring. This delicate suspension requires only a very small magnetic force to produce a deflection. The delicacy of construction contributes to the galvanometer's sensitivity; however, it also contributes to its susceptibility to damage from small mechanical shocks. Therefore, a galvanometer should be handled carefully to avoid any physical trauma. Some galvanometers found in spectrophotometers and osmometers consist of moving element assemblies with sturdier suspension to diminish the danger of mechanical damage. Although diminished, the chance of mechanical damage still exists and should be considered when relocating or moving instruments with galvanometer readouts.

The d'Arsonval meter movement is a modified galvanometer. It is not as sensitive as the galvanometer, since the movement assembly is heavier and is mounted on bearings that contribute to the friction to be overcome. Therefore, the meter movement requires more current to generate an electromagnetic field of sufficient strength to rotate

the element. The d'Arsonval meter movement is used in instruments in which the amount of current to be measured does not require the high degree of sensitivity provided by the delicate suspension of the d'Arsonval galvanometer. The operation of the meter movement is based on the same principle as the moving coil movement. The degree of deflection of the movement element assembly depends upon the amount of current flowing through the wire coiled on the element.

As shown in Fig. 5-36, the meter movement assembly is positioned between the curved magnetic poles of a permanent magnet. Linearity of the meter movement rotation is achieved using this arrangement. Magnetic force of repulsion between like magnetic poles is exerted consistently upon the moving element. Thus, the degree of element deflection is directly proportional to the amount of current flowing through the movement assembly.

The meter movement assembly consists of a coil of fine wire wound onto a support fitted with hardened-steel pivots and mounted on jeweled bearings. The jeweled bearing mounting allows the moving element to rotate with a minimum of fric-

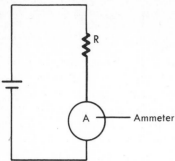
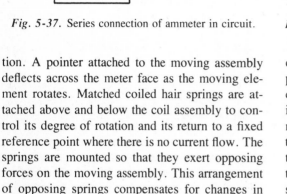

*Fig. 5-37.* Series connection of ammeter in circuit.

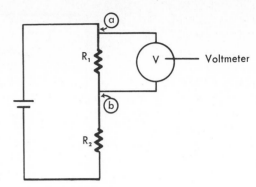

*Fig. 5-38.* Parallel connection of voltmeter in circuit.

tion. A pointer attached to the moving assembly deflects across the meter face as the moving element rotates. Matched coiled hair springs are attached above and below the coil assembly to control its degree of rotation and its return to a fixed reference point where there is no current flow. The springs are mounted so that they exert opposing forces on the moving assembly. This arrangement of opposing springs compensates for changes in the spring tension caused by thermal effects. The expansion or the contraction of one spring because of a temperature change is corrected by the identical change occurring in the opposing spring.

Meter movement damage can result from mechanical shock and/or excess current. Mechanical shock may disrupt the jeweled bearing mounting, thus hindering the smooth rotation of the movement element. Excess current applied to the meter movement assembly will drive the moving assembly beyond the limit of the control springs. This would stretch and, therefore, ruin the control function of these coiled springs.

D'Arsonval meter movements are used to measure current, voltage, and resistance, which may be displayed on the readout in units of current, voltage, and resistance or in units of other measurements, such as absorbance, transmittance, and concentration. Regardless of the units displayed on the readout scale, the meter is responding to current. It is important to note that the d'Arsonval meter movement is a current-measuring device that

can be used to relate current to a variety of other parameters. When this meter is used to measure current in a circuit, the meter must be connected in series, as shown in Fig. 5-37. A series arrangement is required in order that the total current in the circuit will flow through the meter and be registered on the meter's readout. An essential characteristic of a current meter is that it have a very small input resistance so that the meter itself does not add an additional resistance to the circuit and therefore change the current. It is important that the measuring device does not alter the value it is measuring.

If the meter is used to measure a potential difference or voltage in a circuit, a meter with a very high input resistance must be connected in parallel across the two points between which the potential difference is to be measured. This arrangement is shown in Fig. 5-38. As illustrated in this figure, if the potential difference between points *a* and *b* is to be determined, a voltmeter must be connected in parallel to $R_1$. This parallel arrangement allows for voltage measurement with minimal effect on the current flow in the circuit. The required high input resistance will prevent an appreciable current drain from the circuit. A current drain would result in the undesirable situation of the measuring device altering the value to be measured.

All meter movements have an internal resistance resulting from the resistance of the current-carrying elements. The factors of length, cross sectional diameter, and resistivity of the wire used in the construction of the coil are used to calculate the internal resistance, which is indicated on the meter face or in the specifications of the meter. Since each meter has a fixed internal resistance, Ohm's law ($E = IR$) can be applied to measure the voltage across the meter through its direct relationship to current. In this way, a current meter can be used for voltage measurement.

The amount of current required to deflect a meter movement full-scale is referred to as the sensitivity of the meter. The smaller the current required for full-scale deflection, the greater the meter's sensitivity. Sensitivity depends on two construction characteristics of the meter. First, the greater the number of turns in the coil, the smaller the amount of current required to generate an electromagnetic field strong enough to deflect the coil assembly. Second, the weight of the assembly, the friction of the bearings, and the tension of the controlling hair springs influence the amount of energy required for coil rotation. Meter sensitivity using current is expressed in amps, milliamps, or microamps. The lower the current, the higher the meter sensitivity.

Although sensitivity, in its strictest definition, is the amount of current required to produce full-scale deflection, this term is also related to meter voltage drop and meter internal resistance. Meter voltage drop, usually given in millivolts, is the amount of voltage dropped across the internal resistance when full-scale deflection current is flowing. Ohms-per-volt is another expression of meter sensitivity. This value is calculated by dividing the meter internal resistance by the full-scale voltage. The higher the ohms-per-volt ratio, the less current required for full-scale deflection, and thus the more sensitive the meter. The ohms-per-volt value is frequently indicated on the meter face.

Design and construction of a meter determine sensitivity and, therefore, the range in which a particular meter can be used. Meters with only one range are of limited use. For example, a meter with an internal resistance ($R_m$) of 100 $\Omega$ and a sensitivity of 5 mA can be used to measure currents of no more than 5 mA and voltages of no more than:

$$E = IR = (5 \text{ mA})(100 \ \Omega) = 500 \text{ mV}$$

Fortunately, the limitation of the fixed range of a meter movement can be eliminated by connecting resistors in series or parallel to the meter. The circuit configuration used depends on the use of the meter. If the meter is used as an ammeter, the resistors are connected in parallel to the meter movement. A voltmeter's range is extended by connecting the resistors in series with the meter movement.

The methods of extending the ranges of an ammeter and a voltmeter are demonstrated in the following example.

An available meter has an internal resistance of 100 $\Omega$, a sensitivity of 5 mA, and a full-scale voltage of 500 mV. This meter must be used to measure currents up to 50 mA and voltages up to 50 V.

Figs. 5-39 and 5-40 illustrate the addition of a resistor to extend the range of the meter when it is to be used as an ammeter. The resistor is connected in parallel to divert or shunt from the meter the current in excess of 5 mA. Since the range is to be extended to 50 mA, 45 mA must be shunted around the meter. From the concept of current division, it is evident that the shunt resistor ($R_s$) can be selected with a value appropriate for diverting 45 mA through the shunt. The voltage drop across the meter is the same as that across the parallel shunt—500 mV. The shunt resistor value is calculated as shown below.

$$R_s = E_{fs}/I_s$$

where:

$R_s$ = Value of shunt resistor
$E_{fs}$ = Full-scale deflection voltage
$I_s$ = Current through the shunt
$R_s$ = 500 mV/45 mA = 11.11 $\Omega$

Illustrated in Fig. 5-41 is the range extension of the meter when used as a voltmeter. In accordance with the principle of voltage division, the resistor $R_x$ (known as the "multiplier") is con-

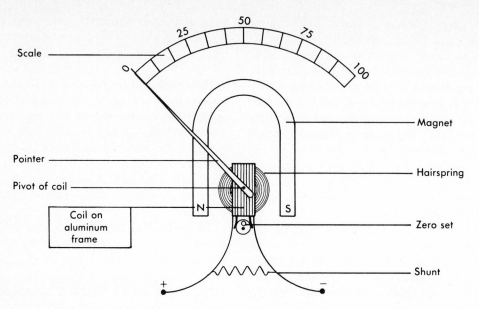

*Fig. 5-39.* Basic d'Arsonval movement. Range extension using resistor shunt.

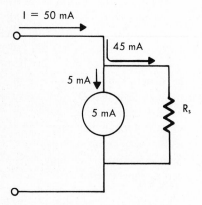

*Fig. 5-40.* Range extension of ammeter.

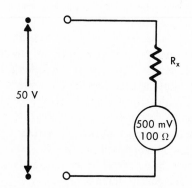

*Fig. 5-41.* Range extension of voltmeter.

nected in series with the meter so as to drop voltage in excess of 500 mV (the full-scale voltage). Since 50 V is to be measured with this meter, 49.5 V must be dropped across $R_x$. To determine the value of $R_x$, first calculate the total resistance required for a circuit with a voltage of 50 V and a current of 5 mA, and then subtract the meter resistance as shown below.

$$R_T = E/I = 50 \text{ V}/5 \text{ mA} = 10,000 \ \Omega$$
$$R_x = R_T - R_m$$
$$R_x = 10,000 \ \Omega - 100 \ \Omega = 9,900 \ \Omega$$

***Recorders.*** Recorders are readout devices used almost as much as meters in clinical laboratory instruments. Functionally, meters and recorders are the same—that is, a signal produced by the detector and processed by the signal processing unit is displayed in a form of understandable data. The advantage recorders have over meters is that the display data are presented as a permanent record.

Two major classifications of recorders are the moving coil or galvanometer recorders and the potentiometric recorders. The potentiometric recorders are most commonly used in the clinical laboratory. However, both types are discussed, the moving coil recorded briefly and the potentiometric recorder in more detail.

The electromagnetic principle on which the operation of moving coil meters is based is also applicable to moving coil or galvanometer recorders. An electromagnetic field is generated by a current passing through a conducting coiled wire on a moving coil assembly. The assembly mounted between the poles of a permanent magnet is rotated as the electromagnetic and permanent magnetic fields interact. The degree of rotation is proportional to the strength of the electromagnetic field, which is in turn related to the amount of current flowing through the coiled wire. Rotation of the assembly is recorded by some type of transcribing device. These devices are of two types, indirect writing and direct writing. The type of indicator attached to the moving coil assembly determines whether a moving coil or galvanometer recorder is indirect or direct writing.

In both types of recorders, chart paper is the permanent record. A chart drive moves at a constant rate the chart paper upon which the indicator element traces the output data. Thus, the final recorded data are presented on a time axis.

The indicator element on an indirect writing recorder can be a reflected light beam or an ink jet. Recorders using the reflected light beam are called oscillographic recorders. The moving coil assembly is similar to that of the d'Arsonval galvanometer, with a mirror attached to the moving coil. The reflected light beam is focused onto photosensitive chart paper, producing a chart tracing. This type of optical recorder has a very high frequency response of above 150 Hz and as high as 4.8 kHz. That is, this type of recorder is capable of recording signals presented to it at a rate above 150 signals per second. This frequency response is possible because the moving coil assembly, like that in the galvanometer, with its extremely low inertia, responds to very small amounts of current.

A disadvantage of the oscillographic recorder is that the chart tracing must be developed in a darkroom. To eliminate the need for photographic development, oscillographic recorders have been introduced in which ultraviolet light replaces the visible light source. The ultraviolet light beam is focused onto a self-developing chart paper that produces the permanent tracing.

The other type of indirect writing recorder uses an ink jet expelled from a capillary onto the moving chart paper. The inertia of this moving coil assembly is slightly greater than that of the optical recorders. However, the frequency response of the ink jet recorder is as high as 1 kHz.

The direct writing moving coil recorders are classified as medium frequency recorders. They respond to frequencies up to a maximum of 105 Hz. Direct writing recorders are available with an ink pen or a heated stylus attached to the moving coil assembly. The ink pen type uses untreated chart paper upon which the ink flows by capillary action to produce a permanent chart tracing. Heat-sensitive paper is used in the heated stylus type. The heated stylus produces a tracing on the heat-sensitive chart paper.

The most commonly used recorder in the clinical laboratory is the potentiometric recorder. This type of recorder is classified as a low-frequency recorder, responding to signals from 0 to approximately 5 Hz. The potentiometric recorder utilizes a null-balancing measuring system, illustrated in a simplified block diagram in Fig. 5-42. The input voltage is from an analytical instrument, for example, a spectrophotometer. The reference voltage is a constant voltage source supplied by a mercury cell or generated by the power supply within

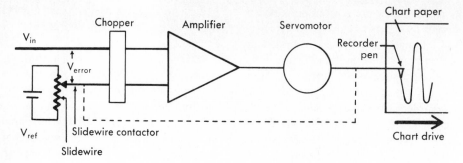

*Fig. 5-42.* Simplified block diagram of null-balancing potentiometric recorder.

the circuit. The difference between the input voltage ($V_{in}$) and the reference voltage ($V_{ref}$) is called the *error voltage* ($V_{error}$):

$$V_{in} - V_{ref} = V_{error}$$

The input voltage and reference voltage are compared, and the error voltage is converted by a chopper (a device that permits intermittent passage of two signals that are to be compared with each other) to a pulsating dc signal, which is then amplified, usually by an operational amplifier. The amplified error voltage drives a servomotor (*servo* is Latin for slave; the servomotor is a slave to the error voltage). The greater the error voltage, the faster the servomotor rotates. A smaller error voltage drives the servomotor more slowly, and an error voltage of zero provides no force to the servomotor, and the servomotor stops. The servomotor is mechanically connected to both the slidewire contactor and the recorder pen, as in indicated by the dashed line in Fig. 5-42. The servomotor drives the pen and the slidewire contactor simultaneously. The slidewire offers a resistance over which the reference voltage provided to the circuit is altered. As the servomotor drives the slidewire contactor, the reference voltage is continuously changed and compared to the input voltage. Once the slidewire contactor reaches the null position (where the reference voltage equals the input voltage), the error voltage is zero and the servomotor stops, as do the recorder pen and the slidewire contactor on the reference potentiometer. The ser-

vomotor does not operate again until a different input voltage is applied. This rebalancing is continuous and begins immediately with any change in input voltage.

Three adjustments on potentiometric recorders to be considered are the range, the zero, and the gain adjustments. These three adjustments are indicated in Fig. 5-43. The potentiometric reference circuit is more detailed than the one shown in Fig. 5-42. Since the complexity of actual recorder circuits can be confusing, overly simplified diagrams are used to present potentiometric recorder operational principles.

The range of a recorder may be indicated, for example, as 1 mV. This means that full deflection of the pen across the graph paper is equal to an input voltage of 1 mV. Thus, 10 mV and 100 mV ranges mean that full deflection of the pen is caused by the input voltages of 10 mV and 100 mV, respectively. As is indicated in Fig. 5-43, the range is determined by introducing resistances over which the input voltage will be dropped to a maximum value of 1 mV at point *a*. For example, in the 10 mV range, if 10 mV is the input voltage, the value of $R_1$ is such that there is a 9 mV voltage drop across this resistor. Therefore, point *a* is at 1 mV, and the circuit functions as if the 1 mV range were being used. The same is true for the 100 mV range. When 100 mV is the input voltage, the voltage drop over $R_2$ is 99 mV; therefore, point *a* is at 1 mV.

The range of a recorder may be specifically in-

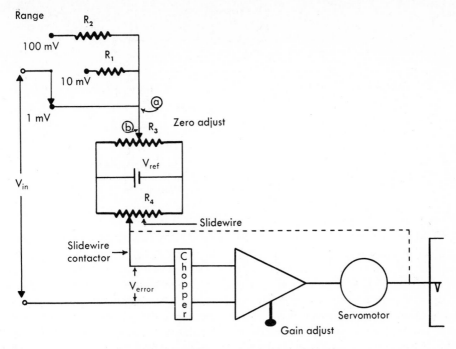

**Fig. 5-43.** Null-balancing potentiometric recorder.

dicated, as described previously, or selected from a continuous scale from 1 to 100 mV. In the latter case, the range selected could be a variable resistor as shown in Fig. 5-44 instead of a set of fixed resistors as indicated in Fig. 5-43. The variable resistor type of range selector is needed when full deflection of the pen must be set on the chart paper. For example, when using a recording spectrophotometer, the operator sets the pen at full deflection (100% transmittance) when the blank is read for a procedure using a direct color reaction, such as the procedure for determining the concentration of blood urea nitrogen (BUN). The recorder is being "told" (calibrated) that this is the maximum voltage to be recorded throughout the procedure.

The "zero adjust" is used to set the recorder pen at a baseline. In essence, the recorder is being "told" the value of the minimum voltage to be applied during a procedure. In a BUN colorimetric procedure using a recording spectrophotometer, all

the light is blocked from the photodetector. Even though no light is hitting the photodetector, a small amount of current will flow in the circuit because of free electrons thermally liberated from the photodetector. This current is called *dark current*. The dark current voltage is eliminated from the circuit by dropping it across a variable resistor, $R_3$ (Fig. 5-43). The contactor B on $R_3$ is adjusted until the pen reads zero on the chart paper.

The "gain adjust" controls signal amplification. The higher the gain of the amplifier, the greater the resulting signal amplification. Thus, the amplifier increases the error signal to a level that will drive the servomotor. If the gain, or amplification, is reduced, the amount of error signal needed to move the pen will be larger. If the gain is increased, the amount of error signal needed to move the pen will be smaller.

The gain adjust is conceptually shown in Fig. 5-43. This control is used to increase or decrease the response of the servomotor to the error volt-

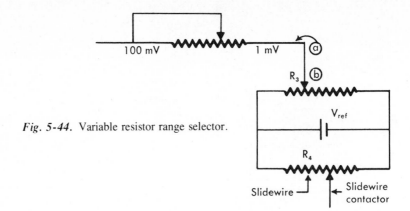

*Fig. 5-44.* Variable resistor range selector.

age. If the gain is too high, the pen will respond to such a small signal change that it will chatter, or oscillate back and forth, even though no apparent input signal is received. This is called "noise." The gain must be reduced until the noise stops. On the other hand, if the gain is too low, the pen will respond sluggishly or not at all to input signals.

In most potentiometric recorders, the chart is driven at a constant rate by a motor drive. This produces a linear time axis. Time (T) is one axis, and a variable (Y) is the other. These recorders are called *TY recorders* or, more commonly, "stripchart" recorders.

The stripchart potentiometric recorder has been modified to produce two other types of potentiometric recorders, the X-Y recorder and the linear-logarithmic recorder. The modification was the addition of another set of slidewires and servomotor. Since these potentiometric recorders are not commonly used in the clinical laboratory, they are described only briefly.

The X-Y recorder has two sets of slide wire and servomotor systems. One of these systems moves the pen along the X-axis (abcissa), while the other system moves it along the Y-axis (ordinate). Plotted on a chart are two variables, neither of which is time. In some X-Y recorders the chart moves (usually on the X-axis), and one of the variables can be recorded in relation to time—that is, the variable has a time base. A stripchart re-

corder may be used to plot enzyme activity against time, but an X-Y recorder can provide more information by plotting, for example, enzyme activity against temperature change. In this example, one of the X-Y recorder systems would be detecting enzymatic change while the other system would be monitoring temperature change over time.

The linear-logarithmic recorder contains two separate sets of slidewires and amplifiers. One set is a linear amplifier and slidewire used for plotting data in linear form. Data can be plotted in logarithmic form by using the logarithmic amplifier and slidewire.

Three important recorder characteristics in addition to frequency response, described earlier in this chapter, are chart speed, pen response, and sensitivity. Chart speed is the rate at which the chart paper moves, usually expressed in inches or centimeters per minute. Pen response is the time (in seconds or milliseconds) required for the pen to move from one edge of the chart paper to the other when full-scale voltage is applied. Recorder sensitivity is a measurement of the degree of deflection caused by a unit of current and is expressed in centimeters per microampere or milliampere.

The graphic presentation of recorders is a series of peaks on a chart. The concentration of a constituent of an analyzed sample can be determined by relating concentration to either the height of a peak or the area under a peak. Relating peak height to concentration presents no particular problems

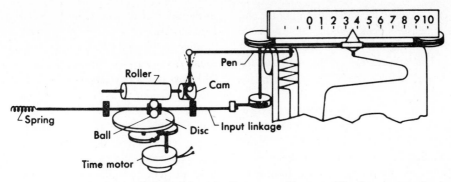

**Fig. 5-45.** Mechanical principle of the Disc Integrator. (Courtesy Disc Instruments, Inc.)

and can be done very easily. However, relating the area under the peak to concentration presents the problem of determining the area under the peak, the process called integration. If the graph paper used is divided into very small squares, the squares under each peak could be counted to determine the area. This method is not ideal. It is tedious, time consuming, and subject to inaccuracy resulting from human error. Integration of peaks has been automated by incorporating an integrator into recorders used for applications requiring peak integrations—for example, in densitometers used to quantify protein fractions separated by protein electrophoresis.

*Integrators.* Integrators are of two types, mechanical and electronic. The mechanical integrator consists of a disc rotated at a constant rate (Fig. 5-45). Upon the disc is a freely rotating ball. The rate at which the ball rotates is determined by its position on the rotating disc. If it is at the center of the disc, it does not rotate. Near the center it rotates slowly, and at the edge of the disc it rotates very rapidly. The ball is contained within a small assembly that supports two separate mechanical linkages to two separate pens, the recorder pen and an integrator pen that is positioned at the edge of the graph paper. The movement of the recorder pen determines the position of the ball on the rotating disc. When the recorder pen is at zero, the ball is in the center of the disc, and when the recorder pen is at maximum deflection, the ball is

on the edge of the rotating disc. The integrator pen responds to the rate at which the ball rotates. With each rotation or with a specified number of rotations (depending on the design of the integrator), the pen makes a stroke along the edge of the graph paper. Therefore, the greater the area under the peak, the more integration strokes will be made. Since the number of integration strokes is directly related to the area under the peak, the number of strokes can be related to sample constituent concentration.

Modern recorders use electronic integrators rather than the mechanical type. Various types of electronic integrators are available. One type consists of very accurate capacitors that store a representative portion of the output signal and then discharge into circuits, which record this current fraction as an event, such as a pen stroke. This capacitor discharge may be recorded as blips on the edge of a recorder paper, as digits on a dial, or as some other form of record. Electronic integrators possess the advantages of having very few moving parts and being trouble free.

Integrated circuits can be used to process electronic signals and integrate the area under curves. Microprocessors are then used to manipulate the collected information as the situation demands. If the actual graphic display is not needed, the recorder may be eliminated entirely and the data processed, integrated, and reported as a digital display. It is possible, using electronic devices now available, to sense the valley denoting the end of a peak, measure peak height, and measure slope sense irregularities with a high degree of accuracy and reliability. Hence the need for the rectilinear recorder with its mechanical problems is fast declining.

*Digital displays.* In clinical laboratory instruments, digital readouts are in the process of replacing conventional meters containing meter movements. This new generation of readouts is capable of displaying information in alphabetic or numeric form. Analog-to-digital conversion occurs within the digital circuitry, which changes electrical signals to digital binary form that is then converted to decimal arithmetic numbers. Digital displays require associated electronic circuitry to accept input information and apply required voltages to the appropriate readout elements. This associated circuitry is called the *drive circuitry* of the readout display device.

Digital readouts have several advantages over conventional meters. They are not susceptible to mechanical shock as the meter movement assemblies are. Digital display systems are more accurate than meters. Data presented in digital form eliminates possible reading error caused by parallax. (Parallax is an optical illusion that makes an object appear displaced when viewed from an angle. Thus, a meter pointer's position on a readout scale depends on the angle from which it is read. To eliminate such errors, the eye should be aligned directly above the meter pointer.)

Brief descriptions of common types of digital displays will be presented. Two broad classifications of digital readout systems are electromechanical and electronic. Electromechanical readouts used in clinical laboratory instruments are the coupled-wheel or drum type. This mechanical register consists of a number of wheels coupled in such a way that each can be rotated independently. Rotation of the wheels is caused by the driving force from the servomotor or electronic source. Upon each wheel are printed the digits 0 through 9. Thus, rotation of the coupled wheels can display numeric data containing a number of digits equal to the number of wheels in the electromechanical readout device.

Electromechanical readout devices have a maximum frequency of approximately 15 to 20 Hz. This low frequency response limits the use of this type of readout to those analytical instruments for which high frequency response is not required. For example, these readouts could not be used in particle counters, since rapid response to particle-produced signals and immediate digital display are required. An application for which mechanical registers commonly have been used is readouts in emission flame photometers. The continuous signals generated in this instrument are compatible with the response of the mechanical readout. This type of readout is not susceptible to damage by mechanical jarring or vibration. It is also inexpensive and operated by simple electronic circuitry. Therefore, replacement of mechanical with electronic displays in clinical laboratory instruments (for example, flame photometers) was not initiated by the limitations of mechanical registers but rather by the popularity of electronic displays.

Electronic readouts are the most popular of digital readout displays. The first to be developed was the NIXIE tube, followed by the filament segment tube. With the surge of advances in solid-state electronics, two types of solid-state displays have evolved, the light-emitting diode (LED) and the planar glow panel.

The NIXIE tube consists of a glass tube containing neon gas and a maximum of 12 stacked filaments in the form of numbers or letters. A specific number or letter is illuminated when a potential of 100 to 180 V is applied to that alphabetic or numeric filament. Although the operating voltage is high, the driving circuitry is relatively simple when compared to that of other electronic readout displays.

In the filament segment tube, the operating voltage is decreased to 15 to 25 V, while the complexity of the driving circuitry is increased. The segmented type of display, shown in Fig. 5-46, consists of seven filaments that can be selectively

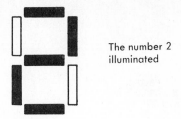

**Fig. 5-46.** Seven-segment display.

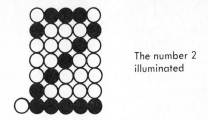

**Fig. 5-47.** X-Y array of light-emitting diodes.

illuminated for an alphabetic or numeric display.

The solid-state light emitting diode (LED) type of digital display is available as a seven-segmented display or as a 36-diode X-Y array readout. The diodes used in these readout devices are the gallium arsenide type. The advantages of this display over the earlier ones is its very low power consumption. It requires an operating voltage of 1.75 V with a current of 50 mA. The seven-segmented display consists of seven rod-shaped diodes in the configuration shown in Fig. 5-46.

The other type of LED display consists of small dot-shaped diodes arranged as illustrated in Fig. 5-47. Alphanumeric characters are displayed with the selective illumination of the diodes in the array. Only 5 to 10 mA current is required to illuminate one character in this display.

Planar glow panel or planar panel solid-state displays consist of double-anode, single-cathode gas discharge diodes arranged in an 111-dot X-Y array. The diode anodes are oriented with one of the anodes toward the front of the panel and the other toward the back. When a dot in the array is to be visible on the panel, its front anode is illuminated. Those dots not visible on the panel are diodes with their back anodes illuminated. Thus, alphanumeric characters are displayed with the illumination of the anode positioned in the front panel of the array.

*Oscilloscopes or cathode ray tubes.* The oscilloscope is a readout device used for viewing electrical waveforms; measuring voltage, current, and frequency; and determining phase relationships between signals. Another name for the oscillo-

scope is cathode ray tube (CRT). CRTs are included in clinical laboratory instruments when the visualization of electrical signals is required in monitoring sample analyses. For example, most electronic particle counters have a CRT upon which are displayed the electrical impulses produced by individual particles. The final particle counts are presented on digital readout displays.

Oscilloscopes are used to measure electrical signal parameters. To measure voltage, an operator first calibrates the oscilloscope by observing on the screen the amplitude of a known voltage. The unknown voltage is then determined by comparing its amplitude to that of the known voltage, since the ratio of amplitudes is equal to the ratio of the voltages. Current in a circuit is calculated by measuring the voltage drop across a known resistance in the circuit. To determine the frequency of a signal, the operator first calibrates the CRT screen with a signal of known frequency. The unknown frequency of the signal can then be measured on the calibrated screen of the CRT.

The cathode ray tube consists of three major parts enclosed in an evacuated tube: an electron gun, two sets of deflection plates, and a screen (Fig. 5-48). The electron gun generates a well-focused electron beam. The gun consists of a heated cathode, a control grid, a focusing anode, and an accelerating anode. Free electrons are emitted from the hot cathode. An aperture in the control grid allows a small stream of electrons to pass. The potential of the control grid is negative with respect to the cathode and therefore functions as the control grid in the vacuum tube triode func-

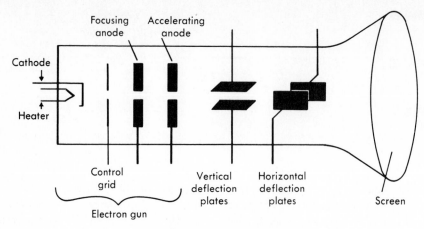

*Fig. 5-48.* Cathode ray tube.

tions—that is, to control the number of electrons passing through. The electron beam intensity is controlled by adjusting the potential on the control grid. The focusing anode is the first anode beyond the control grid. The potential of the focusing anode is very positive with respect to the cathode. Thus, the electrons are accelerated and the beam is concentrated as it passes through the anode's aperture. Adjustment of the potential on this anode controls the sharpness of the electron beam. A more positive potential on the next anode, the accelerating anode, increasingly accelerates electron flow. The electron beam produced by the electron gun is directed to the center of the screen.

Before reaching the screen, the electron beam passes through two pairs of parallel plates, the horizontal and vertical deflection plates, oriented at right angles to each other. One of each of the two sets of plates is maintained at a fixed potential, usually equal to the potential on the accelerating anode. When the other plate of a set is made positive, the electron beam is attracted toward that plate. Therefore, a positive potential applied to the variable plate of the horizontal or vertical deflection plates causes the electron beam

to be deflected horizontally or vertically. Deflection in the opposite direction is obtained with the application of a negative potential to the variable plate with respect to the fixed plate. The negative potential repels the electron beam. With application of voltages to both the vertical and horizontal deflection plates simultaneously, the electron beam can be deflected in any direction. The direction and extent of deflection depends on the relative magnitudes of the two voltages.

The interior surface of the screen is coated with a fluorescent or phosphorescent material that emits visible light when its molecules are bombarded by electrons. Thus, the deflections of the electron beam produce a highly visible trace on the CRT.

One of the associated circuits of the oscilloscope is a time base generator that applies a sawtooth voltage signal to the horizontal deflection plate. This causes the electron beam to move at a constant rate across the screen and then return rapidly to the starting position to begin another sweep across the screen. In this way, the signal displayed on a CRT is the voltage change with respect to time.

# CHAPTER 6

# *Electrical safety*

Of primary importance in working with electrical equipment is an appreciation of the possible hazards involved. Safety precautions should be taken at all times in operating or working on electrical devices. Precautions discussed in this chapter include: recognition of training limitations, adequate grounding, insulation of conductors, self-protection, circuit modifications, and extinguishing electrical fires.

The proliferation of electronic instruments in the clinical laboratory has increased recognition of the hazards associated with their operation. Laboratory personnel should be keenly aware of the danger of electric shock and informed of the precautions to be taken when working with electronic instruments.

## Electric shock

Fortunately, electric shock is not always fatal; however, it is responsible for hundreds of deaths each year. Conduction of an electrical current through human tissue results in the unpleasant sensation called electric shock. Since body fluids contain electrolytes, they are good electrical conductors. Therefore, when the body makes contact between two points of differing potential, it serves as a conducting pathway for current flow.

The severity of a shock is determined by the amount of current and its route of flow through the body. Although body fluids are conductors, the body is provided with a very effective insulation against shock. Dry, unbroken skin is a good insulating material. When the skin is wet, the resistance of the body's insulating covering decreases drastically, altering the body's resistance from the megohm range with dry skin to as low as 300 $\Omega$. Such a change in body resistance affects the magnitude of current produced by the potential applied across the body. For example, if a 60 Hz ac potential of 115 V were applied across the body when the skin is wet, the resulting current could be greater than 300 mA.

The magnitude and the pathway of current passing through the body are influential factors in determining the type and severity of damage inflicted. Current flow is accompanied by heat dissipation, which is responsible for varying degrees of burns. Electrochemical action potentials are the communicating links between the nervous and the muscular systems. Externally introduced electric current may interrupt the electrical impulses of the neuromuscular communicating network or may exert direct effects on muscles to cause contraction. Stimulation of the neuromuscular system with a 1 mA current is felt as a tingling sensation. Currents above 10 mA cause muscle contractions sufficiently severe to result in temporary paralysis. This electrically induced paralysis prevents the release of the grip on the conductor (source of electric shock). Currents passing through vital organs may interfere with their normal functions and result in death. For example, if the muscle-contracting electrical impulses propagated across the heart are altered, ventricular fibrillation and death may result. Thus, if a 60 Hz ac current of 100 mA passes through the body arm-to-arm or arm-to-opposite leg, death is a likely outcome.

The phrase "current, not voltage, kills," is significant. When working with electrical devices, operators should take every precaution to prevent current flow through the body. Therefore, the body should never be put into a position to function as a circuit-completing conductor.

## Electrical safety precautions

Safety precautions to be taken in working with electrical instruments are itemized and briefly discussed below. Simply being aware of such precautions is inadequate for effective avoidance of potential electrical hazards: these safety practices must be an integral part of daily routine.

*Recognition of training limitations.* The most important precaution that can be taken during the operation of electrical instruments is that the operator perform only those functions within his or her capabilities. Understanding Ohms' law and knowing how to use a VOM certainly do not constitute a license to probe irresponsibly into instrument circuits. The repair of electronic malfunctions should be performed only by those who are adequately trained to do so. For example, in a spectrophotometer, changing a blown fuse, a burned out light bulb, or a damaged photovoltaic cell is within the capabilities of all technical laboratory personnel, while replacing a power supply would probably require a qualified electronics technician.

*Adequate grounding.* Protection against electric shock is the primary function of grounding instruments. Usually the instrument chassis is connected to ground to drain to earth unwanted, dangerous voltage that may collect on the chassis from current leakage or from a short in the circuit. By touching two points, an ungrounded instrument upon which a potential has collected and a conductor to ground (for example, a water pipe), an individual serves as a conductor through which current will flow from the higher potential (the instrument chassis) to ground. The metal chassis of two different instruments may carry different potentials because of their differing degrees of effectiveness of grounding. Therefore, if both instruments were touched at the same time, current

would flow hand-to-hand from the higher to the lower potential. For this reason, an instrument and a ground or another instrument should never be touched simultaneously.

Protection by grounding is effective only when a good, continuous ground connection exists. Power cords on most instruments have three-prong plugs. The third (round) prong serves as the connector between the ground lead attachment to the instrument chassis and the ground conductor into the earth.

First, the adequacy of the grounding outlet should be determined by a competent electrician.

Second, a continuous ground conducting pathway from the instrument to the grounded outlet should be ensured. Removal of the ground pin on the three-prong plug breaks the grounding circuit, rendering the grounding protection ineffective. Use of ''cheater'' plugs (two-to three-prong adapters) is essentially the same as removing the grounding pin. The grounding lead on the cheater plug should be connected to a ground, but such ground attachments are not usually reliable. For example, this ground lead is frequently attached to a screw on the outlet receptable plate, but if the screw is coated with paint (an insulating material) or is not connected directly to ground, such an attachment is of no value, providing only false security. Removing a plug from outlet receptables by pulling on the cord may break or loosen the ground wire, thus diminishing the effectiveness of the grounding protection. Use of extension cords may also jeopardize grounding protection, in addition to presenting a tripping hazard. If absolutely required, extension cords should be the heavy-duty type with three-prong plugs.

Third, the ground lead should be securely attached to the instrument chassis. This connection must be metal-to-metal to provide a conducting connection. If this lead becomes loose or disconnected, grounding protection is diminished or eliminated. If an instrument is not effectively grounded and the chassis collects a charge, that charge can be transferred to a conductor that comes into contact with it. Therefore, operating instruments should not be placed on metal surfaces such as metal carts or tables.

*Insulation of conductors.* Conducting leads in an instrument should be insulated. An exposed conducting wire may result in electric shock and/or circuit damage. It should be evident from the earlier discussion of electric shock that if an exposed conducting wire were touched by a person in contact with a ground connection, electric shock would be experienced. A short in a circuit (for example, if an exposed conducting wire makes contact with the instrument chassis) will draw a large amount of current. This current will flow from the power outlet, through the circuit to the shorted connection, and then to ground. If the instrument chassis is not grounded, a large potential will be stored on the chassis. The large current passing through the circuit generates excess heat, which may damage or ruin electronic components.

To avoid electric shock and/or circuit damage caused by exposed conductors, periodically visually inspect the accessible circuit wiring for frayed wires and cracked or melted insulation coatings on electrical leads. Wires with damaged insulation should be replaced immediately. Also, a conscious effort should be made to keep electrical cables and circuit wiring in good condition. Electrical cables should not be stepped on or run over with carts. Cleaning solvents containing alcohol should not be used to clean electrical equipment, since alcohol damages most types of insulation varnishes.

*Self-protection.* Protective measures taken by an instrument operator may be lifesaving and therefore should be consistently practiced. The following self-protective practices are essential for electrical safety. Read a new instrument's instruction manual before operating the instrument. Note and observe special operating and maintenance instructions. Report immediately the slightest shock obtained from an instrument. Turn off and unplug instruments before performing repairs.

Do not assume that the circuit of an unplugged

and/or turned-off instrument is safe to probe into indiscriminately. The capacitors in the circuit may hold their charge even when the circuit is no longer energized. These capacitors are discharged in circuits designed to include "bleeder" resistors. Bleeder resistors are resistors connected in parallel to capacitors so as to discharge the capacitors to ground when the circuit is turned off. However, if the circuit design is not well understood, it is best to assume that potentials may be stored within the circuit and to approach the circuit as if it were energized.

When working on circuits, follow some key rules. Keep one hand away from conducting surfaces to avoid hand-to-hand electric shock (a lab coat pocket is a safe place for that second hand). Use only insulated tools. Keep work area, hands, and clothes dry. If you are standing on a damp surface (for example, a concrete basement floor), wear rubber-soled shoes. Do not wear metal jewelry such as rings, wristwatches, or loose necklaces and bracelets, since a short circuit may result from contact with these conducting ornaments.

Those whose capabilities and training permit them to work on high voltage circuits should not work alone, and assistance should be immediately available if required.

Those whose confidence outweighs their respect for electricity and their common sense should either reevaluate and change their attitudes or seek another pastime.

*Circuit modifications.* Circuit modifications should be left to the electrical engineer. Components replaced in an instrument should be in compliance with the instrument's specifications. Fuses should be replaced with fuses of specified ratings. Jumpers or other conducting substitutes should not be used to bypass a fuse. The fuse serves to protect the circuit from damage caused by excess current. Therefore, the fuse is an important circuit component that should be used properly.

The blowing of a fuse is a warning of an electronic problem that should be identified and corrected immediately.

*Extinguishing electrical fires.* The generation of excess heat by high current may cause an electrical fire. If smoke and/or odor indicate burning within a circuit, the instrument should be turned off and unplugged immediately. Carbon dioxide–type fire extinguishers are used on electrical fires. Water and foams are electrical conductors and therefore should not be used on electrical fires.

Poisonous selenium dioxide fumes, with a characteristic pungent odor, are liberated from a selenium rectifier when it burns out. The fumes should not be inhaled; therefore, ventilation of the instrument is of immediate importance. Replacement of the burned out rectifier should not be attempted until after it has cooled.

# *INSTRUMENTATION*

# CHAPTER 7

# Light and its measurement

A great many of the instruments discussed in this book are devices that measure light in some way. Before the actual instrumentation is approached, think about light as a form of energy. An understanding of its nature, origin, and behavior is helpful later as its emission, absorption, and quantitation in laboratory instruments are considered.

The electrons of an atom possess most of the energy of the atom. When these electrons move from one orbital position to another, there is always some energy absorbed or given up. If an element is heated in a flame, certain valence electrons will move from their normal position, which is usually referred to as *ground state,* to a new characteristic orbital position. This means that the atom has absorbed a certain, definable amount of heat energy. When the atom cools, this energy is released as light. This very specific amount of energy corresponds to an exact color or wavelength of light.

Each electron of each element has a characteristic amount of energy that is required to perform this transition. The electrons of some molecules may have more than one discrete and definable new orbital position they can occupy. The transition from each of these orbital positions to ground state is characterized by emission of a very specific amount of light energy that corresponds to a characteristic color. It is therefore common to find more than one color of light emitted when an element is burned. (Fig. 7-1).

The human eye is not able to differentiate several colors at the same time; therefore, when presented with several wavelengths, the eye will see a composite, with the most intense color predominating. This helps explain the variety of hues and colors that can be seen in a paint store. When all wavelengths of light are present at the same time, the combination is sensed as white light. When there are none present, the eye does not respond, and it is said to be "black."

The light from the sun is normally considered to be pure white light because sunlight contains all wavelengths. The large number of elements in the sun and the very intense heat energy to which they are subjected make it a near certainty that all wavelengths are produced. When white light, such as that from the sun, hits a prism, a rainbow, or *spectrum,* of colors is produced. As shall be seen, this is because the different wavelengths are diffracted (or bent) to different extents, and each color comes out separately.

The colors of the rainbow, or spectrum, go from violet, at one end, through blue, green, yellow, and orange to red, at the other end. If these colors are observed closely, it can be noted that each color is not discrete but gradually blends into the next; thus, it is impossible to say at what point one becomes another. Every shading of color represents a wavelength, and the spectrum actually represents a span of constantly decreasing wavelengths, which may be called a *continuum of energy.* On each end of this span are more wavelengths that are invisible to the human eye. These "colors" that cannot be seen can be characterized as infrared (IR) (beyond the red end of the visible span) or ultraviolet (UV) (past the violet color).

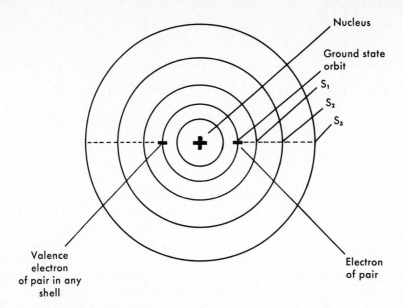

*Fig. 7-1.* Hypothetical atom to show transition of electron. Heat or light energy is generally required to move an electron from ground state to a new orbital position—$S_1$, $S_2$, or higher. As the electron returns to ground state, light is emitted; its wavelength will be determined by the energy given up. Remember, violet is of higher energy than red.

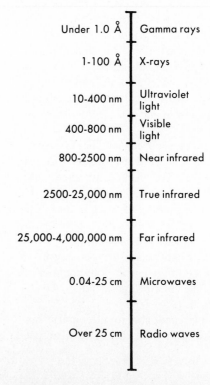

*Fig. 7-2.* Continuum of electromagnetic energy, showing the wavelength span of each segment.

| | |
|---|---|
| Under 1.0 Å | Gamma rays |
| 1-100 Å | X-rays |
| 10-400 nm | Ultraviolet light |
| 400-800 nm | Visible light |
| 800-2500 nm | Near infrared |
| 2500-25,000 nm | True infrared |
| 25,000-4,000,000 nm | Far infrared |
| 0.04-25 cm | Microwaves |
| Over 25 cm | Radio waves |

Fig. 7-2 shows the entire span of wavelengths and the name given to each particular grouping. Note that visible light is a small segment of this entire *electromagnetic spectrum*. Let us look at some characteristics of this form of energy (Table 2), which is usually thought of as "light."

*Table 2.* Electromagnetic energy

| Types of radiation | Wavelengths |
|---|---|
| Gamma rays (isotopes) | Less than 0.1 nanometer (nm) |
| X-rays and "soft" x-rays | 0.1 to 10 nm |
| Ultraviolet light | 10 to 400 nm |
| Visible light | 400 to 800 nm |
| Near infrared | 800 to 2500 nm |
| True infrared | 2500 to 25,000 nm |
| Far infrared | 25,000 to 4,000,000 nm |
| Microwaves | 0.04 to 25 cm |
| Radio waves | Over 25 cm |

Light, or radiant energy, is generally considered to travel in transverse waves. It has energy that is measurable in *photons*. Light waves have two characteristics that define them (Fig. 7-3). First, they have *wavelength,* which is the distance from crest to crest of a wave. Wavelength is the factor that determines *color*. Second, they have *amplitude,* or wave height, which determines the *intensity* of the light.

In a vacuum all light travels at a constant speed, which is about $3 \times 10^{10}$ cm, or 186,000 miles, per second. If the distance light travels in 1 second is divided by the length of 1 wave, the number of waves per second is determined. This is light's *frequency* per second. The energy of light depends on its frequency, or wavelength. The higher the frequency (the shorter the wavelength), the higher its energy (Fig. 7-4). Note that light can be defined in terms of its wavelength, its frequency, or

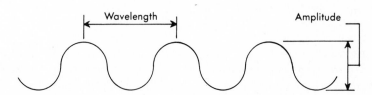

*Fig. 7-3.* Characteristics of light waves.

Violet light

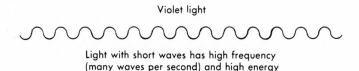

Light with short waves has high frequency
(many waves per second) and high energy

Red light

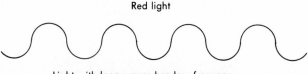

Light with long waves has low frequency
(fewer waves per second) and low energy

*Fig. 7-4.* Short and long waves.

**Table 3.** Sources of electromagnetic energy

| Wave-length | Common name | Source of energy | Fre-quency |
|---|---|---|---|
| Several meters to 25 cm | Radio waves | Electron-spin orientation | |
| | Microwaves (radar) | Molecular rotation | $10^{11}$ c/s |
| 5,000,000 nm | Infrared | Molecular vibration | $10^{12}$ c/s |
| 700 nm | Visible light | Valence electron transition | $10^{15}$ c/s |
| 375 nm | Ultraviolet (soft x-rays) | | |
| 5 nm | X-rays | Inner-shell electron transition | |
| 0.01 nm and lower | Gamma rays | Nuclear transition | $10^{17}$ c/s |

**Table 4.** Units of length in measuring electromagnetic energy

$$1 \text{ meter} = 100 \text{ cm}$$
$$1 \text{ cm} = 10 \text{ mm}$$
$$= 10,000 \ \mu\text{m}$$
$$= 10,000,000 \text{ nm}$$
$$= 100,000,000 \text{ Å}$$
$$1 \text{mm} = 1000 \ \mu\text{m}$$
$$= 1,000,000 \text{ nm}$$
$$= 10,000,000 \text{ Å}$$
$$1 \ \mu\text{m} = 1000 \text{ nm}$$
$$= 10,000 \text{ Å}$$
$$1 \text{ nm} = 10 \text{ Å}$$

its energy. Physicists and engineers often express electromagnetic energy in terms of its frequency or *cycle per second* (c/s). In discussing very short wavelengths such as gamma energy and x-rays, it is more convenient to refer to the energy. Their energy is measured in thousands of electron volts (keV) or millions of electron volts (meV). When light is transmitted through matter, whether a liquid, a gas, or a solid, its *speed is somewhat slower* than in a vacuum, but its *frequency is always constant*. The ratio of the speed of light in a vacuum to its speed in a substance is referred to as the *refractive index* of the substance. This varies slightly with the wavelength under consideration, as well as with the composition of the substance.

The energy of light may be calculated by the formula

$$E = h \ v$$

in which $E$ is the energy in photons, $h$ is Planck's constant, or $6.6 \times 10^{-27}$ erg-second, and $v$ is the frequency. This is another way of saying that the energy increases as the frequency increases. The very high-frequency gamma rays of radioactivity are quite dangerous, and considerable caution

should be exercised in exposure to x-ray. Even the lower frequencies of ultraviolet light can cause severe damage to the eye if one looks directly into the source for more than a few seconds. The low-frequency rays of the infrared and the even longer radio waves may warm or pass through a person with no damage at all unless they are very intense.

It has been noted that visible light is produced when a valence electron is involved in a transition. Other energy levels in the electromagnetic spectrum derive from other molecular energies, shown in Table 3. Gamma radiation, which is the most potent form of electromagnetic energy, derives from the transition of a proton from the nucleus of the atom—a very fundamental change indeed.

The frequency of light remains constant regardless of the medium through which it travels. The speed, however, may vary slightly and, as a consequence, the wavelength will also change. Also, the frequency may be expressed as cycles per second (c/s), but wavelength is expressed in a confusing number of units—meters, centimeters, microns, millimicrons, angstrom units, etc. It is for these reasons that physicists like to refer to the *frequency* of electromagnetic energy. In biology and medicine the *wavelength* is commonly used as the term of reference. In practice, the change in wavelength in different media mentioned before is not significant for most purposes. Furthermore, the visible and near-visible light, with which one usually works, can be described in all cases in terms of millimicrons (or nanons). Hence the wavelength designation is adequate and is easier to visualize. The Greek letter *lambda* ($\lambda$) is used as a symbol for wavelength.

Table 4 may help you remember the various units of length commonly employed in describing energy waves. Micrometer (micron) is abbreviated as $\mu$. One one thousandth of a micrometer is called a *nanometer* (nm) or a *nanon*. The symbol Å is used for angstrom unit. (Some texts may simply use the capital letter *A;* this can be confusing, since A is also used as the abbreviation for absorbance and for ampere.)

Early students of light used the intensity of a candle made in a specific way as a term of reference. The term *standard candle* is still used, although it has since been more scientifically defined. *Illumination* is measured in *footcandles*. A footcandle is the illumination provided by 1 standard candle at a distance of 1 foot. Illumination varies *inversely* with the square of the distance from the source.

The total amount of light hitting a surface at a given distance is called the *luminous flux*. A *lumen* is the luminous flux on 1 square foot of surface, all points of which are 1 foot from a light source of 1 candle.

$$\text{Total luminous flux} = \text{Candles} \times \frac{4\,R^2}{R^2}$$

$$= \text{Candles} \times 4$$

The surface of a sphere is equal to $4\,R^2$, and the flux decreases as the square of the distance (R = radius) increases.

As the number of candles (or candlepower) of a light is increased, the intensity of the light obviously increases. If a photocell is placed 1 foot from a light source and the light intensity is steadily increased, the output of electricity from the cell increases; this increase in electricity is directly proportional to the light intensity. Note that this output depends on the *intensity* of the light source, not on the wavelength or the energy level.

If the light intensity is kept constant and the cell

is located 1 inch from the light, then 2 inches, and later 3 inches, it can be seen that the output of the photocell varies *inversely with the square of the distance* from the light. This becomes a critical factor in the design of photometric instruments.

When light hits a surface that causes it to diffract, there is a tendency for the different wavelengths to bend at slightly different angles and form a spectrum. This happens because of the difference in refractive index of a substance for various wavelengths of light, mentioned previously. The colors in the spectrum normally listed are violet-blue-green-yellow-orange-red. The blue, green, and red are, of course, the primary colors that stand out. The human eye can see green, at a wavelength of around 555 nm, better than any other color. The sensitivity of the eye falls off rather symmetrically in both directions, and one cannot see much below 400 or above 700 nm.

Photosensitive devices are subject to the same sort of limitations as the eye, and most have an optimum range at which they are most sensitive. In a colorimeter, the 100% T (transmittance) reading must be reset each time the wavelength is changed. This is because of the difference in sensitivity of the photocell at different wavelengths. To compensate for this difference in sensitivity, scanning spectrophotometers may have a cam-driven slit or other device to regulate total light falling on the phototube.

Several devices are capable of breaking up white light to form a spectrum. Two that are commonly used in spectrophotometers are the *prism* and the *diffraction grating*. The prism is a piece of glass or quartz cut in such a way as to have interfaces at very precise angles. These can produce the fine quality of spectrum seen in some of the better instruments.

The diffraction grating is a highly polished surface into which a large number of parallel grooves have been cut. Such a surface is able to scatter light and produce a spectrum. The grating may either reflect light or transmit it. More detail is given later on this subject.

Since many of the instruments used in the clinical laboratory sense or measure light, a surprising number of photometric devices are in use. In addition to colorimeters and spectrophotometers, there are flame photometers, fluorometers, atomic absorption photometers, isotope-counting equipment, some cell counters, some coagulation-measuring devices, and many other instruments that are either light sensing or light measuring. Some of these are important enough to merit individual chapters. They share many features with colorimetric absorption devices, which are usually referred to as *photometers.*

Before instruments are discussed, let us clarify our thinking about terms, many of which are often misused. *Photometry* is simply the measurement of light intensity, and the simplest photometer would be a light meter such as is used in photography. This is usually a photoemissive cell and a small meter to measure its electrical output. A *colorimeter* for people in the paint industry is a meter that tells the color of paint by analyzing the light reflecting from its surface. (Of course, in the medical laboratory something different is meant.) A *spectrometer* is a device designed to break down emitted, transmitted, or reflected light into its component colors. This information tells something about the material that is emitting, transmitting, or reflecting the light. Material about measuring light of fluorescence, flame emission, flame absorption, scintillation, and so forth is found in other chapters. Devices for these functions can better be defined in the context of the chapter devoted to them.

The subject discussed in the next section is what is usually referred to as photometry or colorimetry. In reality it might better be called *absorptiometry.* After we have considered why, we can return to calling the instruments *colorimeters* and *photometers,* but first let us be definitive about the matter.

Molecules in a solution absorb light energy. The same kind of molecule will absorb the same amount of light. Thus, if one knows how much light a 1% solution absorbs, one can predict that a 2% solution will absorb twice as much. Beer's law, which is defined later, is a statement of this

fact. In order for this law to apply, light of a specific wavelength must be used because every substance absorbs more light at some wavelengths than at others. Some means of producing *monochromatic light* is necessary to measure absorption.

Next it is necessary to identify an intensity of light as a norm (100% T) and then measure how much of the light is absorbed. This is, of course, a bit more complicated. The identification of terms, establishment of standard conditions, and refinement of mechanics pertinent to this subject are considered later.

Any device for measuring the absorption of light by a solution will have certain basic components, diagrammatically shown in Fig. 7-5. A source of power of some sort is required for the exciter lamp. An exciter lamp *(A)* provides light containing many colors or wavelengths (represented by many arrows at *B*). This light passes through a filter or other device *(C)* that allows one color of light (represented by the single arrow at *D*) to impinge on the sample *(E)*. This light is called the *incidence* light. Some of the incident light is transmitted through the sample and is called *transmitted* light. The remainder of the light energy (remember that light is a form of energy) is absorbed by the molecules in the sample. This energy absorption represents energy used up in the displacement of valence electrons in the sample molecules. It is obvious that more energy would be used up if more molecules were in the path of the light. It would make little difference whether this increase in molecules were due to a longer light path through the solution or to the higher concentration of molecules in the solution.

The transmitted light, represented by the intermittent line *(F)*, impinges upon the photosensitive surface of the photocell *(G)*, where it produces an electric current that is proportional to the amount of light. This current, called the *photocurrent (H)*, flows through the meter circuit and causes the needle to move up scale on the meter *(I)*.

When a colorimeter is referred to in the clinical laboratory, it is generally meant to be an instru-

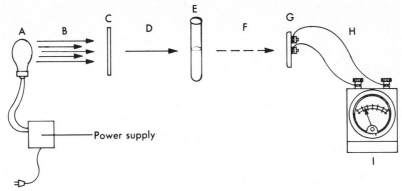

*Fig. 7-5.* Process of absorption measurement.

ment for measuring light absorption in a liquid, using a light of a particular color. Furthermore, it is implied that colored glass filters are used to produce the incident light of the color desired. The term *colorimeter* may, however, be used in a generic sense to include instruments of all types that measure light in this way.

Colorimeters (Fig. 7-5) all have essentially six parts. There are (1) power supply, (2) exciter lamp, (3) monochromator, (4) sample holder, (5) photodetector, and (6) readout. These parts may be very elementary or quite sophisticated.

Since absorptiometry is so important in the clinical laboratory, it is necessary to thoroughly understand each step and each component. Let us go through this system again, considering possible additions and refinements.

### Basic elements of colorimeters

*Power supply and exciter lamp.* Some supply of electricity to operate the exciter lamp is necessary. Details of power supplies are discussed in Chapter 5. The exciter lamp must furnish an intense, reasonably cool, constant beam of light that can be easily collimated. The filament must be small and must provide an intense light; it must be of such a design that it can be exactly aligned when replaced; and it must be highly reproducible in all respects.

As any object changes temperature, it emits a somewhat different spectrum. This is apparent if one notices what happens when house lights dim during a power failure. Lamps take on a yellow color, and if the power surges back past its normal value, the light becomes whiter. If the spectra produced by the lamp in such cases could be compared, it would be immediately obvious that the same area of the spectrum does not give the same distribution of wavelengths. Hence the temperature of the lamp is important. The quality and uniformity of construction of the exciter lamp are significant factors in the uniform performance of the spectrophotometric instrument.

For work in the visual and low infrared ranges, a tungsten lamp is a good source of radiant energy. Some light in the high UV region is emitted, but below about 360 nm this lamp is inadequate. If everything else about the system is optimal, a tungsten lamp may be used down to about 360 nm, but it is not recommended for routine use. Several other sources are available for UV work. The hydrogen lamp is probably one of the best choices. The mercury lamp has a much more uneven emission spectrum and is less desirable. A xenon lamp gives a brilliant light that is ideal for very narrow slit work but is almost too brilliant for routine application, since there is a large stray light problem with such an intense beam. The xenon lamp requires a high voltage to ignite or fire. Ozone is produced by ionization of oxygen around the lamp, in dangerous quantities, and must be dissipated in some way. Hydrogen, mercury, and xenon lamps are all vapor lamps. In lamps of this sort a high voltage is applied through the envelope that contains the "vapor" of the element named. The molecules of gas are ionized and emit a characteristic light, which will contain the same wavelengths that would be seen if the element were burned in a hot flame. There is no filament in a vapor lamp. The high firing or ionization voltage is required only initially, after which a rather low voltage is adequate to maintain ionization and cause the lamp to glow.

For IR spectrophotometers a silicone carbide rod heated to about $1200°$ C works satisfactorily.

When the exciter lamp is changed in a photometer, the calibration of the instrument should be rechecked. Calibration is included in the discussion of spectrophotometers.

Most colorimetric instruments now use a *prefocused lamp*. This is a lamp having the characteristics just discussed and a flange around the base for alignment. There are three tear-shaped holes in the flange to accept and lock in three pins on the lamp socket. Since the lamp may be locked in only one position, any lamp of the same design will be positioned and centered in the identical way. The filament in each lamp is positioned in the same place in relation to the base. Even with the prefocused lamp there may be some slight, but important, error of alignment. As shall be seen presently, the angle at which light strikes a diffraction grating determines the position of the spectrum and hence the color of light striking the sample. Recalibration is therefore necessary each time a lamp is changed.

A few newer instruments make use of light emitted by lasers. Others may use light-emitting diodes as a source of light. The use of these unusual energy sources is discussed as it applies to specific instruments.

Between the exciter lamp and the monochromator, collimating lenses are often inserted. These lenses collect the light rays and focus them in such a way that the light passing into the monochromator will be an organized beam of parallel light. A heat filter may also be placed in the light beam close to the exciter lamp to protect the monochromator from radiant heat. A heat filter is clear glass designed to absorb or reject heat-producing infrared rays while allowing visible light to pass.

*Monochromator.* A monochromator is a device for producing light of a single color from an impure source. The word *monochromatic* means "of one color." As has been noted earlier, it is difficult to identify the point at which one color begins and another ends. Monochromatic light is identified specifically when its wavelength is specified. It is unlikely, however, that a light of one uniform wavelength will be isolated. It must be explained, what range of wavelengths is being discussed. This range is the *band pass*. A monochromatic light that appears to be grass green in color would have a wavelength of about 550 nm, but wavelengths of 525 to 575 nm in length might also be present. The band pass would be from 525 to 575, or 50 nm wide.

The term *band pass* needs to be defined still more specifically. Consider the green light passing through a glass filter. All the light of 550 nm wavelength passes, but somewhat less blue-green light also passes. Blue light may pass in small amounts, and a trace of violet (400 nm) may pass. In the same way yellow-green, yellow, and orange (600 nm) may be present in decreasing amounts. If transmitted light were plotted against wavelength, there would be a curve similar to that in Fig. 7-6. Since the outer edges of the curve extend more or less to infinity, the previous explanation of band pass is quite vague. By definition, the band pass is the range of wavelengths *between the points at which transmittance is one half the peak transmittance* (Fig. 7-6).

The simplest monochromator is a single *glass filter,* although one might question calling it a monochromator, since the band pass of a filter is very wide and the light that passes will include more than one color. Glass filters are made by suspending a coloring agent in molten glass. The thickness of the filter, molded from the mixture, determines how much light will be absorbed. The filter is identified by (1) peak transmittance, (2)

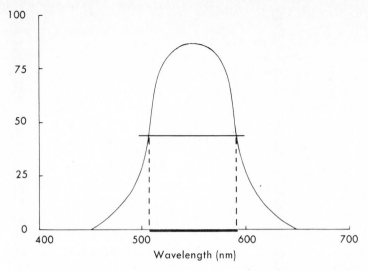

*Fig. 7-6.* Light transmitted through green filter. Heavy line at base indicates band pass.

band pass, and (3) thickness and/or opacity.

A narrower band pass may be obtained by cementing two glass filters of different colors together. Only the wavelengths that are passed in common by both filters will constitute the band pass for this compound filter. For special purposes such a compound filter may be designed to coincide exactly with the emission peak of a mercury lamp to produce true monochromatic light.

Glass filters are used only for transmitting visible and near-visible light. Both UV-absorbing and IR-absorbing, visible light–transmitting filters are available, and near UV–transmitting, visible light–absorbing filters also exist.

For some purposes, filter colorimeters are quite adequate. A good filter colorimeter is sufficiently accurate and quite economical for doing such routine tests as hemoglobin concentration and PSP excretion. Maintenance, calibration, and repair of these instruments are simple and foolproof. One does not need a cannon to kill a fly.

*Interference filters,* made by placing semi-transparent silver films on both sides of a thin transparent layer of magnesium fluoride, will give a narrow band pass. Side bands (harmonics) occur at other wavelengths, however, and may be blocked out by using appropriate glass filters. The band pass of interference filters is determined by the thickness and refractive index of the magnesium fluoride and the angle at which the incident light strikes the filter. This type of filter may have an extremely narrow band pass.

The most widely used true monochromator is composed of an entrance slit, a prism or diffraction grating to disperse the light, and an exit slit to select the band pass (Fig. 7-7).

The *entrance slit* is generally fixed and is designed to limit the collimated light allowed to strike the prism or grating. Reflected light is thus reduced to a minimum. One measure of the quality of a monochromator is the amount of *stray light* it allows to pass. Usually this is expressed in terms of percent of total light. Less than 1% is acceptable for most routine purposes.

When it strikes a *prism,* white light is dispersed to form a spectrum. This occurs because the angle of refraction of light at an interface (such as that between air and a glass prism) varies with the wavelength. Thus, violet is refracted more than red, and the spectrum is formed. The index of refraction determines the spread of the spectrum and the relative width of the color bands. Glass is the

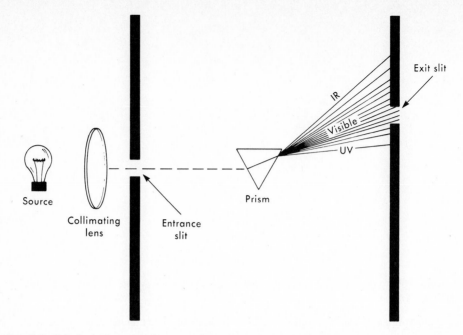

*Fig. 7-7.* Principal elements of a monochromator. Changing the position of the prism causes the spectrum to move up or down on the back wall of the monochromator so that another color passes through the exit slit.

material of choice for visible light; ultraviolet light is absorbed by glass. Quartz and fused silica are preferable for ultraviolet light, but when they are used in the near-IR and IR regions, the color bands produced are too narrow for practical use. The reason for this is apparent in Fig. 7-7. The spectrum is distorted as it is projected at an angle onto the back wall of the monochromator. The red end of the spectrum shows the least distortion; the blue end shows the most. A slit of consistent width placed at the red end and the blue end would produce a significantly different band pass of light.

In past years most high-quality spectrophotometers have used glass or quartz prisms in their monochromators. A very clean spectrum can be produced. The mechanics must be very precise, however. Because high-quality diffraction gratings can now be produced economically, more spectrophotometers of good quality have appeared incorporating diffraction gratings.

*Glass diffraction gratings* are made by cutting tiny furrows into the aluminized face of a perfect, flat piece of crown glass. These furrows are cut at a very precise angle and at a very accurate distance from each other. Cutting is done with a diamond point, and there are usually from 1000 to 50,000 furrows to the inch. Obviously, the engine, as it is called, that cuts these gratings is a very precise machine. Enormous weight prevents any vibrations during the cutting. Original gratings cut in this way take many hours to produce and are very expensive. For this reason they are seldom used in spectrophotometers.

These original glass gratings may be used as *master gratings* in the production of a molded product called a *replica grating*. In the process a parting compound is sprayed on the grating. Onto this a coating of epoxy is applied; and a carrier layer of plastic or glass, called an *optical flat,* is bonded to it. All this is done under vacuum. After

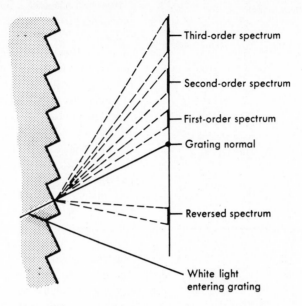

*Fig. 7-8.* Diffraction of light by a grating. Each ascending-order spectrum is more distorted and more diffuse than the preceding.

it is cured, the replica is separated from the master.

As white light strikes the grating, it is diffracted to form several spectra (Fig. 7-8). Each of these is at a different angle from the grating. The brightest of these is called the *first-order spectrum*. It is generally used rather than the more diffuse, higher-order spectra. The angle at which the first-order spectrum is diffracted depends on the angle at which the white light hits the grating and on the blaze angle of the grating. The blaze angle is the angle at which the furrows are cut in the grating (Fig. 7-9). If the grating surface is coated with a layer of silver or aluminum, the spectrum will be reflected instead of passed through the grating. The grating in Fig. 7-9 is the reflectance type.

The spectrum, whether transmitted or reflected, falls onto the wall of the monochromator. A tiny exit slit in this wall allows a small portion of the spectrum to pass through and into the sample to be measured. The particular portion of the spectrum

(wavelength) that passes the slit is determined by the position of the spectrum, and this, in turn, is determined by the relative positions of the light, the grating, and the slit. Some spectrophotometers move the light, whereas others move the grating to select the light that passes through the exit slit.

The *band pass* of the monochromator depends on the width of the slit in relation to the length of the spectrum. A narrow band pass is generally desirable. (The discussion on spectral scanning explains why this is true.) Hence a narrow slit is used. There is a practical limit to the size of the slit, however. For example, one fleck of dust in a very narrow slit may occlude it. Also, the amount of light energy passing a very narrow slit may not be adequate to measure accurately. If the monochromator wall and slit are moved farther from the prism, the spectrum becomes larger and a wider slit may be used. This may not help much, since light intensity decreases as the square of the

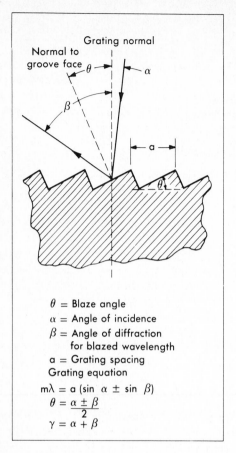

Normal to groove face

Grating normal

$\theta$

$\alpha$

$\beta$

$a$

$\theta$

$\theta$ = Blaze angle
$\alpha$ = Angle of incidence
$\beta$ = Angle of diffraction
     for blazed wavelength
$a$ = Grating spacing
Grating equation

$$m\lambda = a\,(\sin\,\alpha \pm \sin\,\beta)$$
$$\theta = \frac{\alpha \pm \beta}{2}$$
$$\gamma = \alpha + \beta$$

**Fig. 7-9.** Greatly magnified cross section of a diffraction grating. (Courtesy Bausch & Lomb.)

distance traveled (as has been seen earlier), and the light energy of a narrow band pass is still not adequate. It shall be seen later that the best solution to this dilemma is the production of better detectors and amplifiers.

Many of the better monochromators have adjustable slits that allow the operator to determine the band pass. Some slits are adjustable in two directions, allowing adjustment of both the band pass and the total amount of light of those wavelengths which can pass.

In general, grating monochromators are capable of better *resolution* than are those using prisms.

Resolution is best in gratings with the most lines or furrows to the inch. Some stray light in grating monochromators is due to the first- and second-order spectra overlapping and reflecting light of other wavelengths through the slit. Sometimes a double monochromator or a glass filter is used to reduce the stray light. Gratings have the additional advantage of being practical for all wavelengths of light, in contrast to the glass or quartz prisms, which cannot be used in the UV region.

Transmittance gratings lose some light efficiency, since a certain amount of energy is lost in passage through the grating. Narrow–band pass instruments generally use reflectance gratings for this reason, but transmittance gratings allow simpler instrument design.

Replica gratings should never be handled, since fingerprints will seriously damage them. Dust or dirt on their surfaces is also quite deleterious. Laboratory fumes may cause damage to them in time. The condition of the grating can be checked by examining the light entering the sample compartment. If a small piece of white paper is inserted into the sample well, the incident light can be seen. The color should be reasonably monochromatic and clearcut. If the color is streaky or mixed, the grating may be in need of replacement. (*Note:* If the slits are adjustable, open them all the way before making this check.)

*Sample holder.* A few observations concerning *cells* or *cuvettes* used for samples may be pertinent. A square cuvette, which presents a flat surface to the incident light, has less light loss from reflection than does the round cell. This loss is more noticeable in an empty cuvette, since the difference in the index of refraction between air and glass is greater than between glass and a solvent. In routine work this loss is probably not significant, being fairly constant at about 4% for most round cuvettes.

It should be quite obvious that the cuvette must be thoroughly clean and free of fingerprints, etching, and clouding and that the sample and reference cells must be matched for transmittance. It should also be apparent that a longer light path through the sample will allow one to make more accurate readings in very dilute samples. Various types of horizontal cells and spacers are manufactured to provide long light paths for small samples. For routine work a light path of 1 cm has become fairly standard. Most definitions and values are expressed in this term of reference.

Ultraviolet light, as noted earlier, is absorbed strongly by lime glass. For this reason quartz or special-type glass cells must be used to hold the sample in this range.

An obvious but often ignored error is room light entering from the top of the cuvette or elsewhere. A light shield over the cuvette well should be provided and used whenever a reading is being made, otherwise a change in lighting may cause odd and mysterious errors, loss of accuracy, and confusion.

Many types of flow-through and flush-out cuvettes are available. These provide a constant light path and constant absorbance characteristics in addition to the obvious advantages of speed and facility of sample handling. In routine use care must be exercised not to allow them to become cloudy. Cells of this sort should be flushed very thoroughly between types of samples and should not be left in the instrument dry unless they have been rinsed several times with distilled water. Blanks should be run regularly.

Aside from the optical problems of the automatic sample-handling systems, there are often mechanical problems. These devices may suffer from various annoying handicaps that render them awkward for routine use. Totally automated chemistry systems are rapidly taking the place of these semiautomated sample handlers.

It is interesting to note that turbulence, even in a clear, bubble-free solution, will cause an increase in absorbance. This may be a problem in continuous-stream systems (such as the Auto-Analyzer) when the sample system is always in motion.

*Photodetector.* Photo cells, phototubes, photodiodes and other types of detectors are discussed in Chapter 5.

*Readout.* In years past nearly all spectrophotometers used ammeters or galvanometers. Newer digital devices and printers have now almost replaced these, and many instruments relay their electrical output directly to computer circuits where calculations are performed allowing direct reporting of sample concentrations. Readout devices are discussed in Chapter 5.

## Definitions

As stated earlier, a *photometer* is literally an instrument for measuring light intensity, and in the medical laboratory the term is usually used in its generic sense as *any* instrument that measures light. More often than not, however, the person using the term is referring to a filter absorptiometer. In the clinical laboratory a *colorimeter* is always an instrument for measuring the absorption of a colored light by a solution, and the colored light is nearly always produced by simple or compound glass filters. A *spectrophotometer* is an instrument that measures the absorption of monochromatic light, which has been defined by selecting a band from a spectrum produced by a monochromator. General usage of these terms has given them legitimacy in the laboratory, but one should think clearly about what is meant. Absorptiometry is not a commonly used term, but it better describes the functions that have been discussed.

*Flame photometers* measure the emission of an element burned in a flame. *Atomic* absorption photometers measure the light absorbed by certain atoms when excited by heat. *Fluorometers* measure the light, of a specific wavelength, that is emitted by a sample when it is excited by a light of a given energy or wavelength.

In work with absorbance spectrophotometry, there are a number of terms and rules that are commonly used. *Incident light* is the light that falls on the sample. One would like to think that it is pure monochromatic light, but in practice it will contain some *stray light,* of various wavelengths, that has somehow gotten to the sample. Usually the internal surfaces of a monochromator are painted black in an effort to make them *ideal black-body radiators,* or surfaces able to absorb all wavelengths of light, but this is an ideal that is never completely effected. The *transmittance,* designated as *T,* of a sample is the percent of incident light that is transmitted through it. The *percent transmittance,* or %T, of a sample is its transmittance over the transmittance of its solvent alone. *Percent transmission* is a vulgarization of the correct term.

*Absorbance* is a measure of the monochromatic light that has been absorbed by the sample. One would suppose it would be the reciprocal of transmittance but, by general usage, it is expressed as the log to the base 10 of the reciprocal of the transmittance. Absorbance is designated by the capital letter *A.* In laboratories the terms *optical density, OD, absorbancy,* and *extinction* are often used to denote absorbance. All of these terms are ambiguous and should be discouraged.

*Absorptivity* is a proper term and is designated by the small letter *a.* Absorptivity is properly defined as the absorbance of 1 g per liter of a substance, measured in a 1 cm light path at a specified wavelength. There are several other expressions of

absorptivity in common use. For example, $\left\{ \begin{array}{l} 1\% \\ 1 \text{ cm} \\ 520 \end{array} \right.$

would mean that absorbance of a 1% solution in a 1 cm light path at 520 nm. *Molar absorptivity* is the absorptivity of a molar solution in a 1 cm light path at the expressed wavelength. Often the molar absorptivity may be a number (such as 4.6) that could not be read on most spectrophotometers. In practice a dilution of the molar solution is made, and the absorbance value is multiplied by the dilution factor. Molar absorptivity is a convenient expression but not usually practical for direct measurement. In the English literature absorptivity is often called *extinction coefficient.*

*Accuracy* is conformity to an absolute standard or value, whereas *precision* defines the reproducibility of an instrument or method. *Sensitivity* is an expression of the instrument's ability to accurately reflect small changes in a given value. The *reliability* of an instrument means its ability to

constantly satisfy the assumed standards of accuracy, precision, and sensitivity.

## Laws of absorbance

*Beer's law* states that absorbance varies directly with the concentration of the solution in question. This means that if a 1% solution of a substance has an absorbance of 0.1, then a 2% solution should read 0.2 A, and 3% should read 0.3 A. Since most solutions obey Beer's law, it is obvious why absorbance is such a convenient expression. If one has only the %T values, one can plot them against concentrations on semilog paper and obtain a straight line, all points of which should be true. Fig. 7-10 will clarify these values. Mathematically one would say A = 2 log 1/T.

*Lambert's law* simply says that absorbance increases exponentially with increases in the light path. In other words, the absorbance of a given solution in a 2 cm light path will be twice what it would be in a 1 cm light path. Since it is the number of individual molecules of the substance absorbing light that determines absorbance, it makes sense that increasing the concentration of the substance *or* increasing the light path through the solution would have the same effect. It is for this reason that reference is often made to *Beer-Lambert's law,* which implies that the two expressions are saying the same thing.

It is obvious, from Lambert's law, that a small error in the light path through a cuvette may cause a significant error in reading.

When all conditions are ideal, Beer-Lambert's law accurately predicts the absorption of light in a sample. It may not hold true, however, for extremely high or extremely low concentrations. Furthermore, changes in the pH of the sample, temperature change, and interacting substances may cause deviation from linearity. Before calculations are predicated on the linearity of a reaction, the test should actually be set up using several concentrations throughout the expected range. The experimental values should be plotted to ensure that the reaction is indeed linear through the range of anticipated values.

Beer-Lambert's law is simply a way of stating

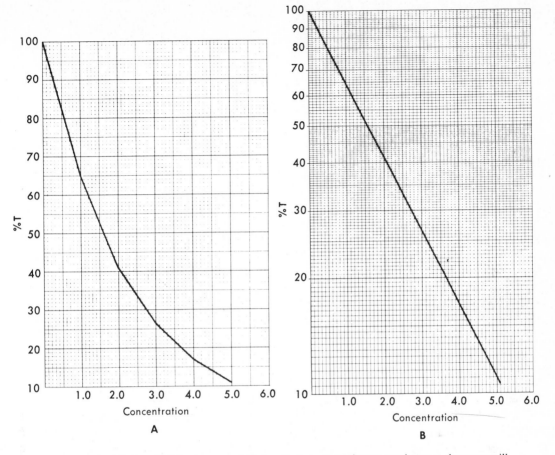

*Fig. 7-10.* Beer's law. If %T values are plotted against concentration on graph paper, the curve will resemble *A*. If semilog paper is used to plot the same information, the curve will be a straight line like *B*. Since absorbance units are log values, plotting them against concentration on ordinary graph paper will give a straight line exactly like *B*.

that each molecule in the solution absorbs a given amount of light. If there are more molecules in the solution, more light will be absorbed. At the same time, if the light path is lengthened, more molecules will be encountered and more light absorbed. If the length of the light path remains constant and the absorbance of a standard and an unknown solution is measured, the following can be said:

$$\frac{\text{Absorbance of unknown}}{\text{Absorbance of standard}} \times \frac{\text{Concentration of standard}}{} = \frac{\text{Concentration of unknown}}{}$$

## Spectral absorbance

It is not surprising that a blue solution transmits blue light almost perfectly. In fact, that is the reason it appears blue. It is harder to say with certainty what colors the solution absorbs best. As mentioned earlier, the human eye sees only the principal component of light—blue in this case—but cannot evaluate what colors are present in lesser amounts. As a matter of fact, it is the absorbance of light at various wavelengths by a compound that provides the most information about its identity.

Let us see how we arrive at this information. If

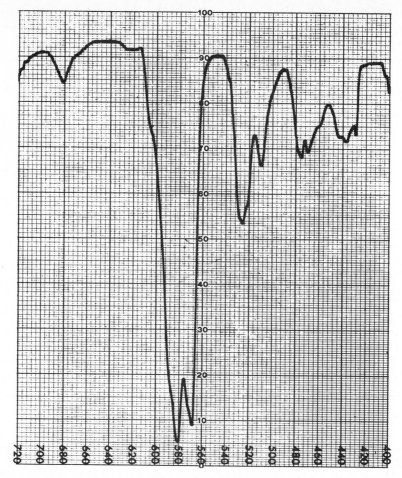

**Fig. 7-11.** Spectral absorbance curve of didymium, using the Beckman DB and the automatic wavelength adjustment option.

one were to prepare a graph, using absorbance on the vertical axis and wavelengths from 400 to 750 nm on the horizontal axis, one could then plot the readings of a solution at each wavelength as one reads it. From this *spectral absorbance curve* it would be seen that the solution transmitted (did not absorb) the color that it appeared to be, as in the preceding example. Some *absorbance maxima,* or peaks where the solution absorbed strongly, would be found. These absorbance maxima are characteristic; indeed, the whole spectral absorbance curve is exactly characteristic of the substance being measured (Fig. 7-11). In toxicology

a substance is often identified by absorbance maxima and their relative heights when compared with each other. The absolute peak height—that is, the absorbance at a given wavelength—depends on the concentration of the substance in the solution. When one sets up a concentration curve (for blood sugar, for example) one is measuring the absorbance peak height at an optimum wavelength, which means at an absorbance maximum or peak.

When one sets up a plot of the spectral absorbance curve, it is necessary to take a number of individual absorbance readings to stake out the

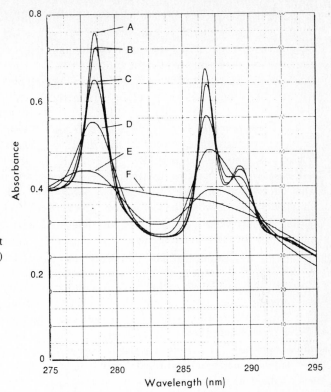

*Fig. 7-12.* Resolution as a function of slit width. (Courtesy Beckman Instruments, Inc.)

Sample: Holmium Oxide Filter
(air reference)

| SCAN | SLIT - mm |
|------|-----------|
| A | 0.15 |
| B | 0.30 |
| C | 0.60 |
| D | 1.20 |
| E | 2.40 |
| F | 2.80 |

curve. If readings were taken at 50 nm intervals only, there would be a very poor curve that might completely miss some of the absorbance peaks. If readings were taken at every 25 nm, there would be a much better curve. If 10 nm intervals were used, it would be even better. It can be said that the peaks are better resolved, or identified, when more points are taken; that is to say that there is better resolution.

As these readings are taken, one is setting the spectrophotometer's monochromator at given points. When the reading is set at 500 nm, light that is nominally 500 nm is being used, but actual-

ly the band pass may have been from 490 to 510 nm. If the band pass had been very wide (50 nm, for example), the *resolution* would have been very poor, and we would not see many peaks. If a 2 nm band pass had been used, the resolution would have been excellent. Thus, resolution depends on band pass (Fig. 7-12).

## Calibration

Unfortunately, no one has ever developed a monochromator that is always true in all circumstances. If small changes are made in the light, the diffraction grating, the slit, etc., the geometry is changed, and the band of color passing through the exit slit may be altered. Hence, when the wavelength dial says light at 520 nm is passing through the slit, there may actually be light at 500 nm instead. It is necessary to have a means of telling whether the monochromator is true or is properly *calibrated*.

It has been pointed out that absorbance maxima or peaks are highly characteristic. The result is that each solution of nickel sulfate, for example, will have a peak at exactly the same wavelength. This information can be used to calibrate monochromators. If absorbance values are checked around this typical absorbance peak, the highest value should be found at the characteristic, defined wavelength. If this does not prove to be the case, the position of the lamp or grating can be adjusted to correct the wavelength setting to correspond to true values.

It is possible to use, as a calibrating standard, almost any substance for which there is a spectral absorbance curve. If a solution is used, there is a risk that there are impurities or that a change in pH has changed the absorbance curve. If a pure crystalline substance is used, this is not a problem; in most cases the crystal will remain unchanged with time and conditions. The rare-earth crystal called *didymium* has a stable crystalline form and also happens to have some sharp characteristic peaks. It is, therefore, a good standard of reference. *Holmium oxide* is another crystalline compound with similarly good characteristics. Fig. 7-11 is a spectral absorbance curve of didymium. Fig. 7-13 shows curves of three commonly used calibrating solutions.

There are also neutral-density filters manufactured specifically for calibrating spectrophotometers. These filters allow a very narrow band of light to pass; this transmittance peak can be used in the same manner as the absorbance peaks of didymium. Also, the U.S. Bureau of Standards sells glass filters that may be used for calibrating.

How an instrument is checked for wavelength calibration depends on the instrument itself and the type of scan it can produce. The first and most obvious means of checking is to identify a very characteristic, sharp absorption peak of a substance and see whether the spectrophotometer actually does show maximum absorption at this point. If methyl orange, for example, has an absorption maximum at 460 nm, one can simply put a sample of methyl orange in a cuvette, turn the wavelength selector knob slowly through the wavelengths from 440 to 480 nm, and observe whether the meter shows maximum absorbance at 460 nm.

This check presupposes, however, that (1) there is only one significant absorption peak in this general area; (2) the instrument has sufficient resolution to discern it as a sharp peak; (3) the absorbance value is on the scale (that is, readable at the concentration used); and (4) if one point of the spectral scan is correct, all others will be. These assumptions are not necessarily true or attainable in all cases. Let us take them, one by one, and examine the problems and their solutions.

*Significant absorption peak.* Many compounds have a great many peaks at close intervals, and it is hard to be sure whether the area of maximum absorbance is actually the wavelength sought. Three precautions may be taken. First, the scan of the substance should be examined to ascertain that the peak to be used is well separated from any other. Second, the color of the light should be consciously noted to verify that it is of the approximate wavelength under consideration. If the wavelength dial reads 650 and the color of light passing through the cuvette is green, the instrument is badly out of calibration, and the meter response is totally irrelevant. Third, the whole spectral scan should be followed to be certain that peaks are in proper relation to each other, in terms of both peak location and peak height.

*Spectrophotometer resolution.* The second problem—whether the spectrophotometer is capable of discerning the peak—can be better visualized if we look again at Fig. 7-12. Notice that the very broad absorbance bands in some areas of the spectrum are not truly peaks; it would be difficult to identify a point of maximum absorbance.

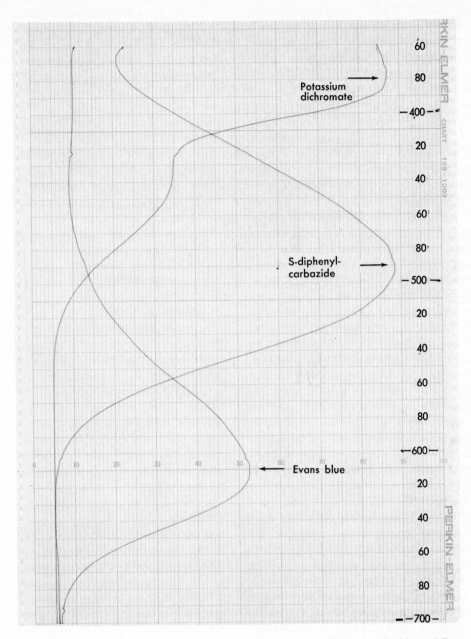

*Fig. 7-13.* Spectral absorbance curves of potassium dichromate, S-diphenyl-carbazide, and Evans blue dye.

This is, of course, true of all scans done at a very wide band pass. With wide–band pass instruments it is probably less important that calibration be absolutely correct, but every effort should be made to achieve the maximum that the system will allow. Calibration of these instruments is done on a somewhat different basis. If the spectral scan of didymium (Fig. 7-11), for example, is examined carefully, it can be seen that there is an abrupt change in absorbance between 580 and 620 nm. This characteristic can be used to calibrate roughly; if enough information is available, even a fairly close calibration can be attained. By turning the wavelength dial with didymium in the light path, it is fairly easy to locate the general area where absorbance drops off precipitously. Exactly what the absorbance reading will be at any one point, of course, depends on such variables as the band pass and grating characteristics. If one is in possession of a didymium scan made on an instrument with the same band pass, grating, and other construction details, it is reasonable to assume that the trace can be duplicated, and the absorbance of the instrument being calibrated will be the same at a test wavelength as that of the sample curve. This rationale is used to establish a calibration point for a broad–band pass instrument, and calibration performed in this way has proved to be quite adequate. This is the rationale of the calibration procedure for the Coleman Junior.

*Readable absorbance value.* The next problem one might encounter in hunting for test absorbance peak would be that it is off scale or that the peak is so small it is of little value for reference. When using a calibrating material in a strange instrument, one may find this is often the case, and if the material is a glass filter, no dilution or concentration of the sample can be done to solve the problem. What one can do if absorbance is too high or too low is change the absorbance by (1) using a brighter light (if the slit can be opened farther), (2) changing the attenuation of the detector by turning the control pots, or (3) using *neutral-density filters*. Neutral-density filters are filters that decrease the total light without selectively decreas-

ing intensity at any given wavelength. Filters of this sort can be purchased in varying thicknesses. With a little experimentation, using neutral-density filters and the standard controls of the instrument, it is normally possible to get a usable scan on the commercially available calibration filters.

*Reliability of readings.* The last problem is that the instrument may not be in calibration at all points throughout the spectrum if only one point has been calibrated. This is a major concern with some spectrophotometers, but only an occasional problem with others, because of the construction of the instrument. It is sound practice to check more than one calibration point occasionally on any instrument. When the instruction manual details it, several points should be checked routinely.

To understand the nature of the problem, let us consider an experiment with a diffraction grating. If a transmittance diffraction grating is held in a beam of light, a spectrum will be formed on a sheet of white paper held in front of the grating. The spectrum will not be directly in front of the path of light striking the grating but will be at an angle. At greater angles to the path of light, other fainter spectra can be seen. The brightest of these spectra is called the *first-order spectrum*. The others are *second-order, third-order,* etc. The first-order spectrum has narrower bands of color and is more uniform in color distribution than are the higher orders. It is the first order that is used in spectrophotometers. Because of the very critical geometry of this system, it is quite difficult to keep the spectrum constant on the sheet of paper without having the light, the collimating lens, the grating, and the paper all held rigidly in position. If a way of holding all these components in position is devised, they can be arranged so that the spectrum is completely flat and all color bands are of essentially the same height and width. If a small window were cut in the paper where the spectrum falls, this would provide a "slit" through which a part of the spectrum could pass. The light that passed would be the "band pass." This arrangement is a monochromator.

If either the light source or the grating is moved

very slightly to the right or left, the spectrum will move, allowing a different band of color to pass. If properly done, the same proportion of the entire spectrum can still pass through the slit, but it will be a different color band. If one end of the white paper is moved a little distance, so that it is no longer parallel to the surface of the grating, one can see the spectrum distorted, with the blue portion very short, narrow, and bright and the red portion wider, longer, and more diffuse. If the movement of the light or the grating is repeated,

one can see the band pass in no longer the same proportion of the spectrum at the two ends of the scale. Also, the movement of the light that shifted the band pass from red to blue now moves it only from red to yellow or green. If one had calibrated on the red part of the spectrum both times, one would have gotten totally erroneous results after moving the paper.

As it happens, the geometry of the monochromator is quite complicated, and the movement of any of these components must be made very care-

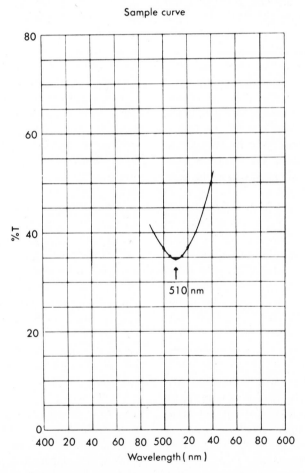

Sample curve

*Fig. 7-14.* Characteristic plot of percent transmittance versus wavelength, using cobalt chloride as a standard with the B & L Spectronic 20. Details of this calibration check are given in the "Spec 20" instruction book. (Courtesy Bausch & Lomb.)

fully if the spectrum is not to be distorted. In some instruments all these relationships are so rigidly positioned that only one element can be moved in one plane. In this case, barring major damage, a one-point calibration is probably adequate in all cases. In other instruments more than one element may be movable, and calibration at several points is advisable.

Several techniques for checking additional points are available, and different filter materials can be purchased or prepared. Didymium is probably the most common of the commercially available filter materials. The principal absorption peak is around 500 nm, and there are four maxima that are usable as calibration points. Didymium glass appears to be light lilac (Fig. 7-11).

Holmium oxide glass is another specially prepared filter. The holmium oxide is mixed into the molten glass and molded to the thickness desired. This filter has about 10 sharp major maxima that can be used. Some of these are in the near ultraviolet, giving it some value for calibration in this area. Holmium oxide glass is light yellow in color.

Cobalt chloride in solution is used as a calibrating agent. A 4.4% solution of $CoCl_2 \cdot 6H_2O$ in 1% hydrochloric acid should show a characteristic peak at about 512 nm (Fig. 7-14). Potassium chromate in a concentration of 4 mg per liter of 0.05 N KOH shows a good absorbance maximum at about 375 nm, and acid potassium dichromate has a significant peak at 350 nm.

It should be apparent that almost any easily reproduced colored solution will have some characteristics that can be used in this way. For example, the green-colored solution of nickel sulfate is often used.

Using any of these possible calibrating materials, it is fairly simple to dial through the length of the spectrum, observing the absorption peaks and comparing them to the available scans or printed values. Correction is then made by adjusting the light or grating according to the manufacturer's instructions.

Another calibration technique, which is excellent, uses a mercury lamp in place of the exciter lamp of the instrument. When mercury is heated, as in the mercury-vapor lamp, it emits a number of characteristic wavelengths. If this light is directed into the monochromator, these emission peaks will pass the slit as the grating is in the proper position and cause the meter needle to move upscale briskly. This calibration method is excellent for checking the entire optical system except, of course, that is does not tell anything about the positioning of the exciter lamp.

### Refinements of the basic colorimeter

Up to this point the *single-beam colorimeters* have been discussed. In these instruments the light from the exciter lamp goes through the sample only and falls on one detector, from which the absorbance of the sample is calculated. This basic instrument has been modified and improved to solve problems and provide additional capabilities. Let us look at these modifications as solutions to problems.

*Problem A.* When a heavy load is placed on an electric power system, lights dim and later brighten. If readings are being made on a photometer at this moment, results will be completely unreliable. If two photocells are positioned at equal distances from the exciter lamp and are attached to the same meter so that they oppose each other, this instability can be cancelled. Photocell no. 1 will drive the meter upscale, and photocell no. 2 will drive it downscale. By the use of variable resistors one can locate the needle at 100% T with the blank in the cuvette well. If the two cells are balanced, a change in light intensity will not cause the needle to move, since both photocells will be affected equally. This is a very simple *dual-beam colorimeter*.

If one wishes to make a *null-balance colorimeter* of this arrangement, one can locate the needle at midscale and, by means of a variable resistor, offset the absorbance of the sample with enough ohms of resistance to bring the needle back to exactly center scale. Ohms of resistance needed to balance the meter will be directly proportional to the absorbance of the sample.

**Problem B.** It is not quite true that the two photocells in a simple dual-beam photometer will balance each other. One beam is passing through a monochromator, and the photodetectors will not respond equally to the white light at the reference cell and the monochromatic light at the sample cell. Two monochromators could be used to solve this problem. If filters were being used, this might be a workable idea, and the cells would balance better.

**Problem C.** Using two grating monochromators to solve Problem B would be quite expensive, and the two monochromators might not be exactly correlated anyway. It is quite easy to insert a *beam splitter* into the light path between the monochromator and the sample so that the light will go to both the sample and the reference detector. Beam splitters may be made in any of several ways. One of the simplest beam splitters is a half-silvered mirror, called a *dichroid mirror*, that allows half the light to pass through to the sample and the rest to be reflected to the reference cell. Other types of splitters are discussed presently.

**Problem D.** Having two detectors can be expensive, and, if phototubes or photomultipliers are used, the wiring detail and power supply become complicated. Also, the two detectors are costly and difficult to balance. One phototube can be used to read both the reference and the sample photocurrent. What one is really doing anyway is reading the net current when the two currents are presented to the meter biased against each other. If one detector output is 40 $\mu$A and the other is 50, there will be a net current of 10 $\mu$A when they oppose each other.

This signal comparison through one detector is accomplished by means of a *photochopper*, which may work in any of several ways. One common light chopper is a mirror that rotates very rapidly. At one moment it directs the light beam *past* the sample, then into a mirror and into the phototube. At the next moment it directs the beam *through* the sample and into the phototube. Now refer to Fig. 7-15. When the beam is going directly to the phototube (position *1*), 50 $\mu$A of current flows.

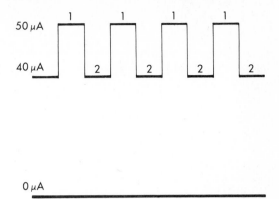

**Fig. 7-15.** Square-wave signal from a phototube receiving "chopped" light, first from a reference cell, then from sample cell.

When the light passes through the sample (position *2*), only 40 $\mu$A of current flows. The output of the phototube is a square-wave current alternating between 40 and 50 $\mu$A. If enough resistance to consume 40 $\mu$A is interposed, the current left varies from 0 to 10 $\mu$A. This can now be rectified to a direct current. (It will not be a 10 $\mu$A direct current but will be proportional to any similarly handled signal, and one assigns it any meter value desired.)

**Problem E.** One has to insert the blank solution in the sample beam, adjust to 100% T, and substitute the sample to be read. With the sophisticated arrangement just described this is no longer necessary. All that is needed now is to provide a sample well for the reference, and one can compare the reference beam, with the blank in it, to the sample beam, with the sample in it. The two can be compared without changing tubes, and a ratio can be established between them. If the output of the detector is fed to a recorder, the system can be called a *ratio-recording photometer*. This system is ideal for following a kinetic reaction in which the sample is changing absorbance as a function of time in response to enzyme activity, heat, or some other force.

**Problem F.** One would like to produce a spectral absorbance curve. This problem is rather easily solved. A drive motor is geared to the diffraction grating to turn it very slowly in the light path so that each color of the spectrum passes through the slit in succession. With the ratio-recording system, one is continuously recording the relationship between the sample and the blank as different wavelengths pass through the sample. This geared motor attachment is called a *wavelength drive*. The recording that is produced is called a *spectral scan* of the sample.

The spectral scan usually identifies a pure substance positively and hence is a very valuable tool. Concentration of the substance can also be calculated from known data, as is explained later.

*Problem G.* The general outline of the spectral scan would look a little like a half-moon, and there is some difficulty in reading peak heights at 400 and 700 nm on the chart. As has been noted earlier, detectors have a spectral response similar to the human eye. At the center of the spectrum the response will be high, but at the ends the response will be considerably lower. This inconvenience can be eliminated by installing a variable slit in the light beam before it reaches the detector. This variable slit is operated by a cam or eccentric wheel whose shape is a function of the shape of the spectral response curve. The cam is turned by and coordinated with the wavelength drive motor so that the slit is widest at the ends of the spectrum and narrowest in the middle. Now the spectral scan will be true, and the absorbance peaks in all wavelengths will be relative. This variable slit controls the intensity of the light but does not change the band pass, since it is regulating the amount of white light before it reaches the monochromator.

*Problem H.* One cannot tell much about the spectral absorbance curve. There are only a couple of large humps that cover half the spectrum. Spectral scans have value only when there is good resolution; that is to say, one must be able to tell specifically what the absorbance at a specific wavelength is, compared with another wavelength 20 nm shorter or longer. To resolve absorbance peaks, the band pass must be short (Fig. 7-12). The relation of band pass to resolution might be illustrated by comparing rides in two cars, of long

and short wheel base, respectively. A very long car evens out bumps and holes in the road, but a short car seems to climb every bump and go to the bottom of every hole. By the same token, the wide band pass levels out all the peaks and valleys of the spectral scan. However, every peak and valley should be seen. Often a very sharp, narrow peak may be the characteristic of a compound that positively identifies it. This would be completely missed if a wide band pass were used.

The peaks of an absorbance curve that show high absorbance are called *absorbance maxima,* and the points of lowest absorbance are the *absorbance minima.* Compounds may be identified in the literature by the exact wavelength of their principal absorbance maxima. Quantitation may be accomplished by comparing the peak height of the unknown with the peak height of a 1-molar solution at a given wavelength.

### Electronic considerations

Obviously, all the optical modifications discussed have created a need for more sophisticated electronics. In the simple single-beam spectrophotometer first discussed, the photocurrent from a photocell was directly measured using an ammeter. When a monochromator is used, light that passes the slit is only a fraction of the total light. With a very narrow slit, very little light is available to activate the photocell.

In double-beam instruments the weak sample photosignal is balanced against the reference photosignal, and the *error signal* (the difference between the two) is very small. Also, a photocell responds too slowly for use with a chopper, so phototubes or photomultiplier tubes are used. This creates the need for a high-quality power supply. The recombination of the two signals after the chopper produces an alternating current, which is usually rectified to a direct current, since alternating current is amplified less easily. This amplified current can be used to activate whatever readout device may be chosen. Other electronic details may be involved, such as the motor that drives the wavelength scanning drive.

Electronic *noise* may appear in the output signal because of the amplification of ripple by the power supply, induction from motors, etc. If one is dealing with a very small electric signal, the noise, when amplified, may be the source of significant error. The rms value of the noise must not be greater than about 2% of the smallest signal one intends to measure. The ratio of the two is called *signal-to-noise ratio*. The use of transistors and other electronic innovations has greatly decreased the noise problem in spectrophotometry.

Most modern spectrophotometers have substituted digital devices, which show absorbance or % T values on a digital display, from the ammeter. To do this the analog signal must be converted to a digital value by an A-to-D converter. Using integrated circuits, this has become very easy to do. It has also become easy, electronically, to convert absorbance values to units of concentration with a log-to-linear converter. These three changes have transformed the appearance of spectrophotometers and have simplified calculations.

Enzyme measurement is so important in the clinical laboratory that many manufacturers have adapted their spectrophotometers to facilitate this performance. These kinetic methods involve measuring the change in absorbance of a substrate as it is exposed to the enzyme. This can be measured most simply by recording the changing absorbance value as a function of time. The recorder tracing can then be translated into enzyme activity units by using appropriate calculations. When a recorder tracing can be examined, the progress of the reaction can be visualized, and the analyst can be assured of its validity. Simply stated without going into the chemistry involved, the reaction must be linear during the period of time selected for calculation. A very simple microprocessor can check the linearity of this absorbance change without producing the record tracing. It is a reasonably simple matter, then, to devise an instrument that takes two or more absorbance readings at precise time intervals and decides if the reaction is proceeding in a linear fashion. If the appropriate factors are provided, a rather simple logic circuit

can then translate the rate of absorbance change into enzyme units. Many manufacturers have produced spectrophotometers equipped in this way.

## Care and operation

In the normal operation of photometric instruments several checks should be made from time to time to ensure accurate, reliable operation. Essentially there are four photometric characteristics that should be monitored.

*Wavelength calibration.* Several methods of calibration have been discussed. Once the instrument is in routine, daily use, some type of wavelength check should be performed each day. Use of a didymium filter or some such standard to check absorbance wavelengths is probably sufficient for routine calibration. These values should be recorded. If there is any significant change, it should be investigated. Most quality instruments will go for long periods of time without need of recalibration, but the routine checking must be done. Whenever lamps are changed or instruments repaired or moved about, the wavelength calibration must be rechecked.

*Linearity.* Each time one prepares a standard curve, one is checking the linearity of the instrument. If the material being used follows Beer's law, the absorbance plotted against concentration should be a straight line. When the plot is not quite linear, one is usually inclined to assume a slight error in measurement and to dismiss it if it does not seem significant. It is wise to watch these deviations carefully to see if there is a tendency for repeated plots to show the same deviation from linearity, which might indicate a lack of linearity of the instrument. Remember that readings below 20% T and over 60% T are inherently somewhat in error, the error being more pronounced at the ends of the scale. Very accurate prepared standards may be purchased; these should be used occasionally as a careful linearity check. These results should be made a matter of permanent record.

*Band width.* Band width is defined as the peak width at 50% T. To check this characteristic properly, a standard *source lamp* (which may be pur-

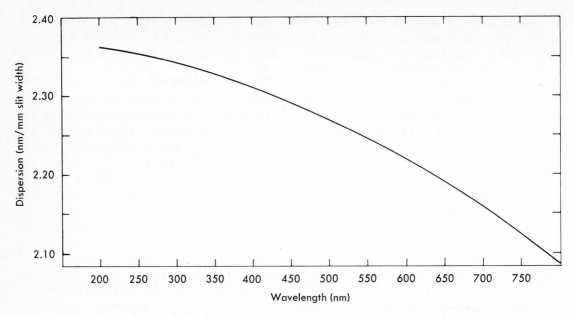

**Fig. 7-16.** Because of distortion of the spectrum, the band pass will be wider at the violet end even though the slit width is constant. (Courtesy Beckman Instruments, Inc.)

chased for use) or a sharp cut-off filter should be available. If a mercury lamp is used, a good isolated peak should be found at 546 nm. Turn the 100% T adjustment knob to set the meter on 100. Then move the wavelength setting toward 700 nm until the meter reads 50% T. Record the wavelength. Now move the wavelength setting toward 400 nm until the meter again reads 50% T. Record this wavelength. The difference between the two recorded wavelengths is the band width. It should correspond fairly closely to the band width claimed by the manufacturer. Remember, however, that in most instruments the spectrum is significantly distorted, so the band width at the red end of the spectrum may be noticeably narrower than at the violet end (Fig. 7-16). There is probably little point in checking this characteristic on fixed-slit spectrophotometers. Instruments with variable slits should be checked occasionally.

*Stray light.* Stray light may be caused by reflection within the instrument, light from the next higher-order spectrum, or room light reaching the detector. Filters can be obtained that almost completely absorb light at a given wavelength. These are called *blocking filters.* Set the wavelength knob at the value of the blocking filter. Zero the instrument in the usual manner, and, with nothing in the cuvette well, set the meter at 100% T. Now insert the blocking filter. Any stray light will cause the meter to move away from zero. Over 2% is generally considered unacceptable. This measurement should be made periodically to ensure proper function of the instrument.

*Common sense checks.* All of the preceding checks are somewhat time consuming, and busy laboratory workers may at times fail to perform them even though they are aware that they should be done. There are many very simple, common sense observations that can be made that show serious troubles. Keeping an eye out for these should become as instinctive as a fisherman checking his boat for leaks.

*Warm-up time.* Turn the instrument on and

set the meter at 100% T. Check for several minutes to see how long it requires to stabilize. Do not use it until the meter stays at zero.

*Fatigue.* If the instrument is left on for some time with the meter on 100% T, does it have a tendency to fade below the initial setting? If the fading is very slow the instrument may be usable, but 100% T should be reset often during use.

*Meter repeatability.* Insert a sample in the cuvette well and set the meter at 50% T. Remove the sample and reinsert it. Check the meter. If the needle does not return to 50% T, the instrument should be serviced by an instrument repairman. Be sure the cuvette is oriented in the well in the same way each time.

*Wavelength repeatability.* With a sample in the well set the meter at 50% T and note the wavelength. Turn the wavelength knob and then bring it back to its exact original wavelength. Does the meter return to 50% T? If not, the instrument should be serviced.

*Grating deterioration.* Insert a slip of white paper into the cuvette well so you can observe the color of light entering the well. Rotate the wavelength knob slowly from 400 to 750 nm. Learn to recognize the approximate colors of various wavelengths. At 555 nm the color should be grass green. At 610 nm it should be yellow-orange. Colors should be sharp and clear. If they are streaky or if more than one color appears at the same time, the grating may be deteriorating or dusty. The instrument should be checked by a competent repairman.

*Low energy.* Place an empty cuvette in the well and set the wavelength at 400 nm. Turn the 100% T set knob fully clockwise. The needle should go past 100% T with ease well before the knob is fully clockwise. Repeat at 700 nm. If the needle reaches 100% T only when the knob is fully rotated clockwise, there is insufficient energy. The exciter lamp may be dirty or going bad, the slit may be dusty, the amplifier (if any) may be weak, or the detector may be defective. Steps should be taken to locate the trouble.

*Room light.* Set the instrument at 100% T us-ing a water blank. Cover the cuvette well completely. If the meter moves, steps should be taken to shield the cuvette when readings are being taken.

*Scratched or defective cuvettes.* Place a water blank in the well and set the meter at 50% T. Rotate the cuvette slowly and watch the needle. If it moves more than 1% T, it should be discarded. Some cuvettes have an index line, and they should be oriented in the well in the same way each time. If this is scrupulously done each time, some latitude might be allowed, but the technician should be alert to this source of error.

*Loose connections.* With the meter set about midscale, thump on the table close to the instrument enough to jar the instrument slightly. Move the power cord and watch for meter response. If the needle moves at all, does it return to its exact position? If not, it should be serviced.

*Defective controls.* Does the on-off switch always work cleanly? Rotate zero and 100% T set knobs slowly. Does the meter respond smoothly and quickly? If the needle moves erratically, the controls should be checked for possible replacement.

Spectrophotometers should be kept clean and dust free. Solution should never be dripped or leaked into the cuvette well. The instrument should not be plugged with extension cords if it can be avoided, and it is best not to share an electric outlet between a spectrophotometer and a piece of heavy equipment such as a motor or heating device. The instrument should be used on a solid counter or bench in a location where it will not be bumped or jostled. At least once each year each instrument should be cleaned and the dust brushed or blown out of its interior. Care should be taken not to damage optical surfaces or disturb alignment.

## Selection of photometric instruments

The introduction of a host of automated devices during the past decade has greatly reduced the use of simple spectrophotometers in the clinical laboratory. There are still many situations in which they are routinely used; it is difficult to imagine a laboratory where there is not a need for some simple colorimetric instruments. Automated colorimetric devices and systems are discussed in some detail in later chapters, but the criteria for the selection of simple colorimeters and spectrophotometers need consideration.

The most important decision to be made is, "Exactly what function is this instrument to serve?" When an employee is being hired, it is of prime importance to have an accurate idea of the job description. By the same token, an instrument should be bought to fill a specific demand. Pathologists and technologists often overestimate the requirement of an instrument and buy something quite sophisticated to do a job that could better be done by a relatively simple device. On the other hand, it is penny-wise to buy an instrument that is inadequate or one that takes valuable time away from important tasks.

Following are some considerations that need defining:

1. Who will operate the instrument?
2. What degree of accuracy is required? Be realistic.
3. How important is a narrow band pass?
4. Is scanning required?
5. What type of tests will be done?
   a. Repetitive tests done rapidly
   b. A few tests done at leisurely pace
   c. Painstaking procedures done in quantity
   d. Research-type activity
6. How important are economic factors?
7. Is ultraviolet light required?
8. Does the instrument need to be a general-purpose tool?
9. What sensitivity is required?

Let us consider these questions in more detail. If one is a busy pathologist who needs a colorimeter to do hemoglobin determinations but who dreams of doing research with untrained helpers, one should not buy a very sophisticated ratio-recording spectrophotometer. It is foolish to buy an expensive or complicated spectrophotometer for most routine, repetitive-type tests. This is espe-

cially true if personnel are not trained in the use of such equipment. The large bulk of hospital and clinical laboratory work can be done adequately on a moderately priced spectrophotometer that is simple to use.

If the instrument is to be used heavily, simplicity and ease of operation are important considerations. Such refinements as variable slits and wavelength scanning may make the instrument more difficult to use and introduce operating error. A digital display or concentration converter may be much more practical. Clinical laboratory errors that cause serious problems are most commonly errors in identification, procedure, or calculation rather than half-percent photometer errors. (This is not meant to discount the importance of accuracy and quality work, of course.)

Obviously, if spectral scanning for accurate quantitation of barbiturates, identification of carboxyhemoglobin and methemoglobin by scan, etc. are to be performed by the instrument, it must be able to scan and be capable of good resolution. In most hospital laboratories one instrument with these capabilities is sufficient.

If routine repetitive tests are to be done, it is wise to get an instrument that is easy to adjust, requires little maintenance, and accepts samples easily. If the load on the instrument is light, more latitude can be allowed for extras. If very careful work is demanded and the load is not heavy, a sophisticated instrument may save much irritation, especially if well-trained personnel are to use it.

In general, price is a minor consideration in buying instruments of this sort. Amortized over the lifetime of the equipment, the difference in cost is negligible if one gets exactly what is needed.

Service is an important consideration. Simple instruments require little service generally and can be repaired by relatively untrained people. The more sophisticated the equipment, the harder it is to get repair parts and service.

Once the instrument is purchased, it should be studied carefully and properly maintained. Service personnel report that the majority of service calls occur because of failure to understand the equipment or failure to take reasonably simple maintenance steps or safety precautions. This situation is usually a result of either an overloaded work schedule or a mania for instant, trouble-free everything. The time required to avoid service pitfalls is usually time well spent, since service personnel are chronically swamped with work and beset by their own problems and repair may be delayed.

### Reading the ''spec'' sheets

Advertising material about an instrument should always include a sheet or section listing the specifications of the instrument in reasonably factual terms. These specifications are designed to set forth in scientifically accurate terms exactly what the equipment has and what it will do. In actual fact, many of these parameters are not quite as amenable to definition as we would like to think. For example, band pass is usually flatly stated in absolute terms even though the band pass generally varies at different points of the spectrum, as previously mentioned. Most reputable manufacturers make a conscientious effort to be reasonably honest but often oversimplify the ''specs'' to make them more understandable.

Many details are mentioned in these specifications, but the following are the most common. In the interest of brevity, only a general idea of each is given here.

*Light source.* As mentioned earlier, tungsten is used in the visible range, and the vapor lamps such as mercury, hydrogen, deuterium, and xenon are used for ultraviolet light. Both types of lamps are used in instruments providing UV capability. When the UV range is desired, the tungsten lamp is turned off, and a power supply for the vapor lamp is turned on. A mirror is then repositioned so the new light source will pass through the entrance slit. Tungsten halide lamps provide more energy in the high UV range. When a quartz envelope is used, the lamps are adequate down to about 320 nm and are often used for enzyme analysis.

*Single beam or double beams.* This distinction has already been adequately explained. It is generally assumed that wavelength scanning is not possible with a single-beam instrument. Gilford Instruments has produced scanning, single-beam instruments, Models 240 and 2400, in which the reference and the sample are moved in and out of the single light beam alternately several times per second. This approach has some advantages and some limitations.

*Monochromator.* Included here may be such items as a glass filter, reflectance grating, transmittance grating, glass prism, quartz prism, and interference wedge. Technical details such as grating rulings per inch, blaze angle, and monochromator configuration are usually listed.

*Detector.* The major element may be identified as a photoemissive cell, phototube, photomultiplier, photodiode, etc. Often more technical explanation—such as catalog number, spectral range, or electrical characteristics—is given.

*Readout options.* Meter, digital display, printer, recorder, or BCD connection (for direct connection to computer) are included.

*Wavelength drive.* When available, the rates of scan provided are listed.

*Sample-handling options.* Automatic or manual sample changers, flow-through cuvettes, cuvette size options, etc. may be listed.

*Definitions.* Several terms are used to define or characterize performance. *Wavelength range* tells the span through which the instrument is warranted to perform satisfactorily. *Band pass* is defined elsewhere and is, of course, a function of *slit width,* which is often stated. At times variable slits or multiple slits with different widths are available. *Resolution* is primarily a function of band pass but may be listed separately. *Stray light* is the portion of the total incident light that is not of the wavelength indicated by the monochromator. In grating instruments much of this comes from higher-order spectra overlapping the first order (unless eliminated by appropriate filters). Reflected light also adds some stray light. This is normally less than 1% and on better instruments generally approaches 0.1%. *Baseline drift* results primarily from variations in the brilliance of the light source, sensitivity of the detector, and instability of the amplifier. *Noise* or *short-term stability* is a measure of the fluctuations in readings taken over a short time period. This is usually expressed as absorbance units variation per 15-minute period. *Drift* or *long-term stability* is essentially the same measurement but made over the period of an hour. *Wavelength calibration* should indicate the accuracy with which the wavelength scale reading may vary from actual wavelength when the instrument is in proper calibration. *Sensitivity* indicates the amount of light to which the instrument is accurately sensitive. This is indicated, in general terms, by the readout scale.

Most general laboratory spectrophotometers have scales that read from 0 to 1 A. If a higher sensitivity is indicated, the scale may go to 2 A or even to 3 A, suggesting that the instrument can read the very small amount of light that would be transmitted at this point of the scale. Sometimes an additional stage of signal amplification is added to provide greater sensitivity, and a separate scale may be used in this case. *Photometric accuracy* is a composite of several factors such as *meter accuracy* and *detector linearity*. *Photometric reproducibility* tells how closely repetitive readings will duplicate each other. Linearity tells how faithfully Beer-Lambert's law would be enunciated with an ideal solution.

As mentioned earlier, there is a tendency to provide many extra features such as temperature-controlled cuvette wells, timing mechanisms, and microprocessors to time sequences and to calculate results. Each of these features may also be described in the ''spec'' sheets and performance specifications set forth.

## Some common photometric instruments

In the past few years automated computer-assisted chemistry analyzers have largely supplanted colorimeters and spectrophotometers in medical laboratories. For those occasional tests that have not yet been automated, the older spectrophotometers have been kept, since the purchase of a new, high-performance instrument is not warranted. In the following pages several of these older instruments are presented because they are still in occasional use.

About 40 years ago, Beckman Instruments, Inc. introduced the Model DU Spectrophotometer, which was a single-beam instrument with a quartz prism monochromator. At that time it was probably the best instrument of its kind, and it was many years before a spectrophotometer with better resolution was produced. When they came, the newer instruments were mostly dual-beam, wavelength scanning, recording instruments with an array of timers, sippers, samplers, and other attachments.

With the introduction of integrated circuits and microprocessors, spectrophotometers have undergone a radical change. It has become fairly easy to design instruments that monitor their own performances, cycle through entire sequences, and perform a variety of calculations. There is a trend back to single-beam instruments, since computer circuits can store reference data and compensate at all times. These newer instruments are more compact, faster, and more accurate, and they can provide many time-saving conveniences. A few of these newer instruments are also presented here even though they are not widely used.

*Leitz Photometric Colorimeter (E. Leitz, Inc.).* This is one of the most economical general purpose colorimeters on the market. It has stood the test of time with relatively little change in design. A transformer and capacitors provide and stabilize the 6 V current that the exciter lamp requires. This power supply is well insulated and rugged and almost never fails. It compensates fairly well for normal line voltage fluctuations but is inadequate to compensate for heavy surges and drops.

This instrument is typical of glass filter colorimeters. Having been on the market for about 40 years, this colorimeter has had many modifications and improvements added. It is simple, easy to understand, fool-proof, and reliable. Like all glass filter instruments, it has a wide band pass and is severely limited in many characteristics but adequate for some situations.

*Coleman Junior Spectrophotometer (Coleman Instruments Division, Perkin-Elmer Corp.).* The Coleman, Perkin-Elmer, Hitachi group has produced more spectrophotometers for the medical laboratory than any other manufacturer. In past years the Coleman Junior Model 6 has been the most common spectrophotometer in the clinical laboratory. Since there are still many of these instruments in use and since it is a good example of this type of instrument, let us consider it in some detail. This instrument has stood the test of time well. Its power supply is usually an external 6 V constant-voltage transformer, although an electronic power supply is available. The electronic supply is capable of handling greater fluctuations in line voltage, but it is relatively expensive and bulky and has had its share of electrical problems.

Light from the exciter lamp passes through a collimating lens to strike the transmittance-type diffraction grating, which is immediately behind the lens. The spectrum created is thrown onto the front wall of the black chamber located between the grating and the sample compartment. A small slit allows a 35 nm band of light to pass through the sample and onto the photocell. Changing the position of the exciter lamp (by turning the wavelength knob) shifts the spectrum to the right or left, causing a different color band to pass through the slit.

The photoelectric current, produced when light strikes the photocell, activates the galvanometer. One side of the circuit goes directly to the base of the galvanometer while the other side is passed, in series, through the two variable resistors marked "coarse" and "fine." These potentiometers modify the photocurrent so the galvanometer can be set on 100% T.

The galvanometer lamp is focused on the galvanometer mirror through a collimating lens with a hairline that is mounted in a tubular mounting close to this lamp. The mirror reflects this image onto a second mirror at the rear of the instrument, from which it is again reflected onto the scale panel. All these components and relationships can be seen on the schematic diagram in Fig. 7-17. The basic design remained unchanged for about 25 years until the advent of the Coleman Junior II.

*Micro-Sample Spectrophotometer 300-N (Gilford Instrument Laboratories, Inc.).* This instrument was introduced several years ago and has gradually gained good acceptance in most areas (Fig. 7-18). It is one of the first popular spectrophotometer designed primarily for microsamples. A 500-microliter ($\mu$l) sample allows a 1 cm light path. The spectral range is from 340 to 700 nm, with a band pass of 8 nm. A linear, digital voltmeter is used for the readout, allowing absorbance values from 0 to 2 to be read to 0.001 A. Concentration can also be read directly, of course. Adjustment of the 0 A end of the scale is made by varying the intensity of the lamp. Lamp temperature is kept quite low so that lamp failure is unusual. Samples are drawn through a measuring cell by a vacuum pump outside the instrument.

This instrument has been coupled with samplers, microprocessors, and printers to produce small automated chemistry analyzer systems. This model and its newer versions have functioned well and have been popular.

*Beckman Models DB and DB-G Spectrophotometers (Beckman Instruments, Inc.).* These instruments are dual-beam and ratio-recording spectrophotometers capable of wavelength scanning (Fig. 7-19). When equipped with an external power supply for the hydrogen lamp, they will cover the range from around 200 to 800 nm. They are capable of very high resolution for spectral scanning.

Fig. 7-20 shows the details of the electrooptical system. There are two exciter lamps—one an ordinary tungsten lamp, the other a hydrogen lamp for UV work (Fig. 7-20). The instrument's power supply provides a carefully modulated 6 V to the tungsten lamp. The UV power supply, external to the instrument, furnishes a higher voltage for

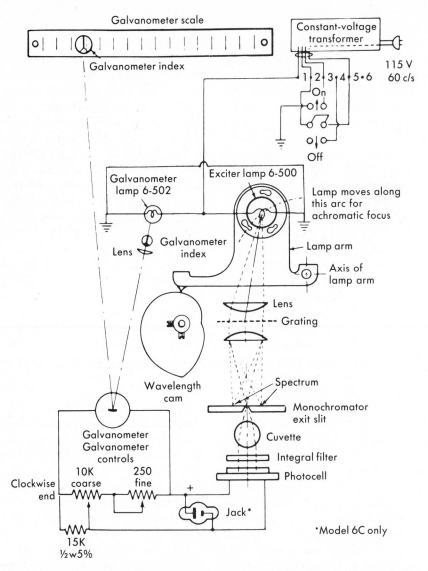

*Fig. 7-17.* Schematic diagram of Coleman Junior Spectrophotometer. (Courtesy Coleman Instruments Division, Perkin-Elmer Corp.)

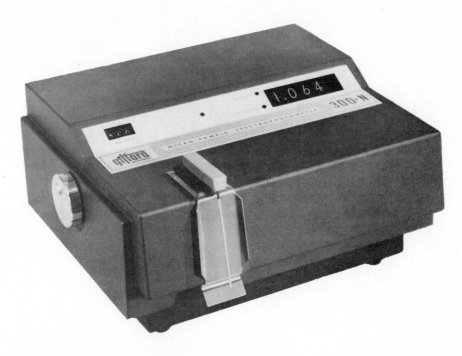

*Fig. 7-18.* Gilford Micro-Sample Spectrophotometer 300-N. (Courtesy Gilford Instrument Laboratories, Inc.)

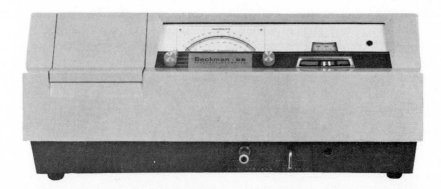

*Fig. 7-19.* Beckman Model DB Spectrophotometer. (Courtesy Beckman Instruments, Inc.)

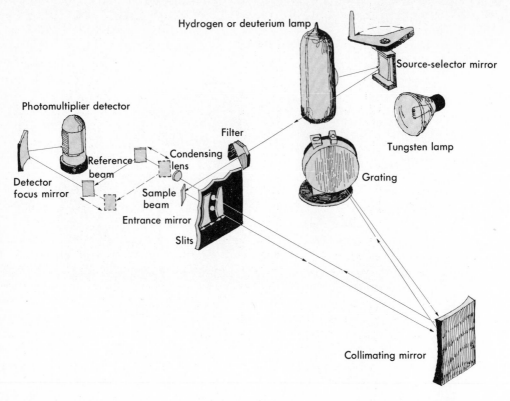

*Fig. 7-20.* Electrooptical system of the Beckman Model DB. (Courtesy Beckman Instruments, Inc.)

firing and maintaining the hydrogen lamp. A mirror can be moved to the right or left to direct the beam from either lamp into the monochromator. Model DB has a prism monochromator, but the newer DB-G uses a reflectance grating of high quality with a stray-light filter. The grating monochromator is rotated by means of a cam that can be mechanically driven through its entire wavelength span at either of two speeds. As the cam changes the position of the grating monochromator in relation to the light, different areas of the spectrum are continuously presented to the slit; hence the term *spectral scanning*.

The band pass of light through the exit slit is directed to a mirror attached to a vibrating reed. At one instant the light is reflected by the mirror through the reference solution (blank), and

at the next, the beam is reflected through the sample. At the other end of the vibrating assembly another mirror catches the transmitted light, first from the reference, then from the sample, and directs it to the phototube. This process causes the phototube to produce a square-wave alternating current, the high side of which is the reference photocurrent and the low side, the sample photocurrent. This new current is now amplified and presented to the meter and to a recorder (if so equipped). If such a record is made at a single wavelength, the optical changes of the sample may be recorded. If the recorder is running while the cam is rotating the monochromator, a spectral scan will be drawn, describing the absorbance of the sample at each wavelength of the spectrum. The narrower the band pass and the slower the scan speed, the better the resolution displayed in the spectral scan.

As mentioned earlier, detectors have a peak area of sensitivity, and sensitivity falls off toward both ends of the spectrum. Since this is true of the phototube of the DB Spectrophotometer, some compensatory mechanism needs to be made to take care of the greatly diminished output of the phototube in the violet and red areas. This is done by adjustable slits that open to accept more light at the high and low wavelengths. The slit adjustment is operated by the same motor that drives the wavelength cam, the opening being exactly proportional to the sensitivity of the phototube at any given wavelength.

The DB Spectrophotometer fills a definite need in the clinical laboratory. It is able to read the absorbance of a compound accurately and with fine resolution. It can monitor a chemical change in a solution by recording the change in absorbance. When plotted as a function of time, a rate of change that is especially useful in enzymology is established. This instrument can also do spectral scans and thus establish the identity and concentration of a substance in solution. All this capability has been provided in the instrument at a reasonable price and in good quality.

This is not to say that there are no problems with the Beckman DB Spectrophotometer or that it has no competition. The early models had many problems with components, and many people were discouraged with them before a workable system was developed. There have been problems with the automatic shutter assemblies, which have occasionally failed to operate correctly. Wear of the shutter parts has caused some problems. In the DB the small circuit board at the left rear of the instrument has generated too much heat, and the 6973-6AK5 vacuum tube on this board has had to be replaced often. Unfortunately, this replacement cannot be made without removal of the instrument cover, which is awkward and time-consuming.

The vibrating reeds are controlled by a neon chopper located directly below the sample well. The chop speed of approximately 35 c/s is determined by an oscillator on the main power board. The rate of chop may be controlled by a pot located at the right end of the instrument and accessible through a hole in the cover. Variation in the rate of chop may cause serious meter instability when components fail or change values.

The DB-G is a newer instrument in which many of the troublesome features of the DB have been eliminated. The use of transistors has eliminated many problems of tube aging and failure, and redesigned circuitry has solved the overheating that was chronic on the amplifier board. A redesigned optical system incorporating an excellent reflectance diffraction grating and filter has improved the very good resolution to 0.5 nm, which is more than adequate for any routine medical laboratory work. Stray light is under 0.1% at 220 nm. Wavelength accuracy, which was a little erratic at times with the DB, is markedly improved.

The cell compartment is designed to allow its temperature to be accurately controlled. A water jacket surrounding the cells is fitted with ports so that hoses can be attached and water from a thermostated bath can be circulated through. This feature is essential for enzyme work, in which temperature is critical, and it is most useful for many other procedures.

Any piece of equipment as sophisticated as the DB and the DB-G is almost certain to have some mechanical and electronic problems if heavily used. These instruments are not exceptions, but the number and type of problems experienced with the model DB have not been excessive, and its capabilities have far outweighed its shortcomings.

***Beckman Models 34 and 35 UV/Vis Spectrophotometers (Beckman Instruments, Inc.).*** These instruments are dual-beam, scanning, and recording spectrophotometers. They are adaptable for scanning gels by suppressing the reference beam. Both models have an operating range of 190 to 700 nm but the model 34 can accommodate the ultraviolet portion of the spectrum only when an ultraviolet accessory is added. The monochromator uses a single filter grating with 1200 lines per mil-

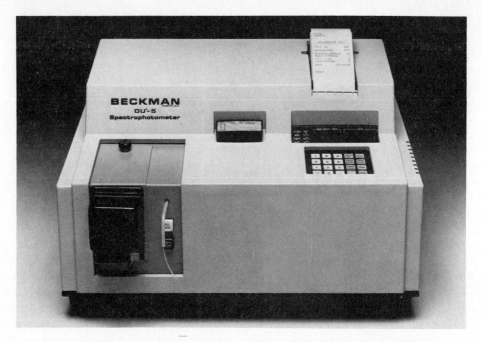

**Fig. 7-21.** Model DU-5 Spectrophotometer. (Courtesy Beckman Instruments, Inc.)

limeter, blazed at 250 nm. The principle difference between the two models is in band pass. The Model 34 has a fixed 0.8 nm slit, which allows a 2 nm band pass, whereas the Model 35 has variable slits with a normal and a wide program, which allows from 0.125 to 5 nm band width. The photometric range for both instruments is from 0.0 to 3 A with an accuracy of 0.5%. Scanning speeds can be set in six steps, from 1 to 250 nm per minute. If the absorptivity of a compound is known, the K-factor (1/absorptivity) can be entered into the digital display, and concentrations will be directly calculated, saving the time of preparing and reading calibrating standards.

Either of these models can be used for kinetic measurements, spectral scanning, chromatography gel scanning, or rapid and point analyses. Both instruments are straightforward, high-quality spectrophotometers without computer capabilities.

***Beckman Model DU-5 Spectrophotometer (Beckman Instruments, Inc.).*** This is one of the newer single-channel computer-directed instru-

ments mentioned earlier (Fig. 7-21). A silicone photodiode is used as the detector, giving a wavelength range from 260 to 1100 nm. Subassemblies are used, which can be easily removed and replaced, saving downtime for repair.

The most interesting feature of the instrument is the microcomputer, which can store three programs and accept five others from the "Memory-Pac Module." Wavelength can be changed, and as high as five different wavelength readings made sequentially with a program. Concentrations can be calculated from the reading of a standard, or a factor can be entered through the keyboard and concentrations calculated. Zeroing is done automatically, and blank subtraction is carried out. The printer can be programmed to report results and all critical data. When kinetic testing is done, linear regression is calculated from 1-second sequential readings.

By using calibration solutions and a computer self-check program, wavelength accuracy, stray light, repeatability, linearity, and accuracy can all be easily monitored.

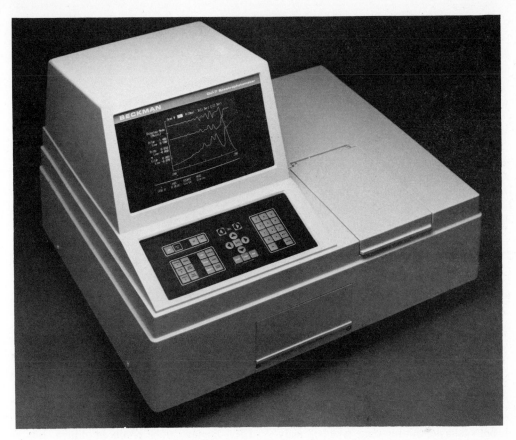

*Fig. 7-22.* Model DU-7 Spectrophotometer. (Courtesy Beckman Instruments, Inc.)

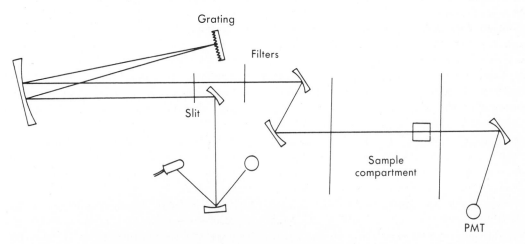

*Fig. 7-23.* Optical diagram of the Beckman Model DU-7. (Courtesy Beckman Instruments, Inc.)

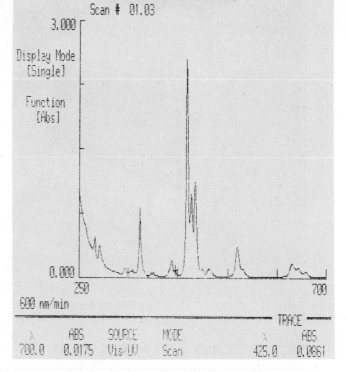

**Fig. 7-24.** Didymium scan made with the DU-7 Spectrophotometer. (Courtesy Beckman Instruments, Inc.)

All this is contained in a case that is only 20 × 16 × 12 inches. Since there is no recorder, scanning is not available, but for some types of analyses this spectrophotometer would be quick, convenient, and accurate.

**Beckman Model DU-7 Spectrophotometer (Beckman Instruments, Inc.).** This is an example of a highly sophisticated computer-directed instrument (Fig. 7-22 and 7-23). The specifications for the spectrophotometer portion are not a great deal different from those discussed. The wavelength range is from 190 to 800 nm. The standard model scans at 120, 300, and 600 nm per minute. Slits at 2, 1, and 0.5 nm must be changed manually. The computer capability of this instrument is, however, considerably more than those previously reviewed. There is a CRT display that is used to provide printed messages concerning parameters setup and display spectral curves, as well as first and second derivative curves and other data. Abscissa and ordinate axes can be expanded for closer study; sequential and related curves can

be overlaid; and data can be stored for later retrieval and display. With the video copier, any CRT display can be produced in hard copy within about 40 seconds (Fig. 7-24).

This sort of instrument lends itself to research activity more than routine analysis, and it would most likely find utility in medical laboratories only in developmental or research areas.

### Other light-measuring devices

Although conventional photometry is the chief concern in this chapter, there are other techniques dealing with the measurement of light that should be mentioned.

*Turbimetry.* There are some situations in which one wishes to measure the turbidity or cloudiness of a solution. The suspension or emulsion to be tested is often white or nearly colorless. The white light (or a specific wavelength may be used) that is absorbed or dispersed by the material in suspension can be measured. For clinical applications an ordinary filter photometer or spectropho-

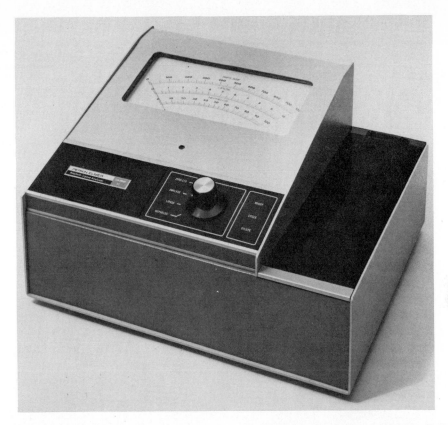

*Fig. 7-25.* Amylase-Lipase Analyzer, Model 91. (Courtesy Coleman Instruments Division, Perkin-Elmer Corp.)

tometer such as has been described is used for this purpose. A curve can be prepared using appropriate standards.

*Nephelometry.* Particles in solution may also be measured by nephelometry. A nephelometer measures the light that is reflected by the particles in suspension rather than the light absorbed. The sensing photodetector is placed at an angle of at least 30 degrees from the path of incident light so that transmitted light does not strike it, and only light that is scattered or deflected by the particles is sensed. The instrument is standardized using a curve prepared with test materials appropriate to the analysis being performed. The nephelometric principle is used in a few clinical instruments that are rather widely used in medical laboratories. A few of these are presented here.

*Amylase-Lipase Analyzer, Model 91 (Coleman Instruments Division, Perkin-Elmer Corp.).* When amylase is incubated with a buffered suspension of amylopectin, the turbid solution becomes more clear as the amylopectin is broken down into smaller fragments. In the case of lipase, olive oil emulsion is cleared as the droplets of oil are converted to fatty acid. This reduction in turbidity can be measured and the change related to units of the enzyme. The nephelometer, similar to the one just described, is equipped with an 8-inch meter that is calibrated in units of amylase, lipase, and nephelos. Since the company provides the standardized substrates for the enzymes, it is possible to accurately predict the change that one unit of enzyme will produce on this substrate in a given period of time. The instrument is automatically

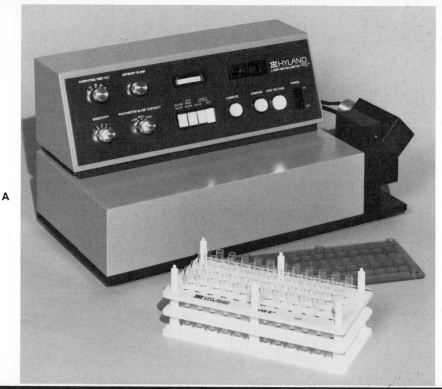

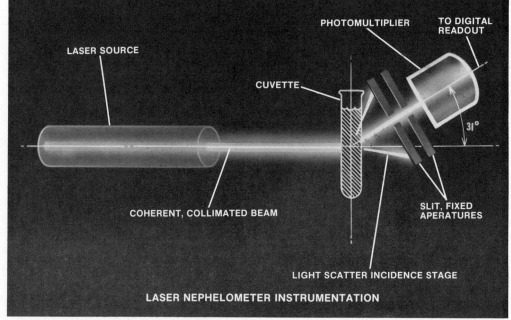

LASER NEPHELOMETER INSTRUMENTATION

*Fig. 7-26. A,* Laser-Nephelometer-Hyland Model PDQ. *B,* Path of laser beam through the sample, showing deflection of light path by particulate matter in solution. *C,* Basic measurement concept of the electronic componentry in the Laser-Nephelometer PDQ is graphically depicted. (*Percent relative light scatter.) (Courtesy Hyland Laboratories.)

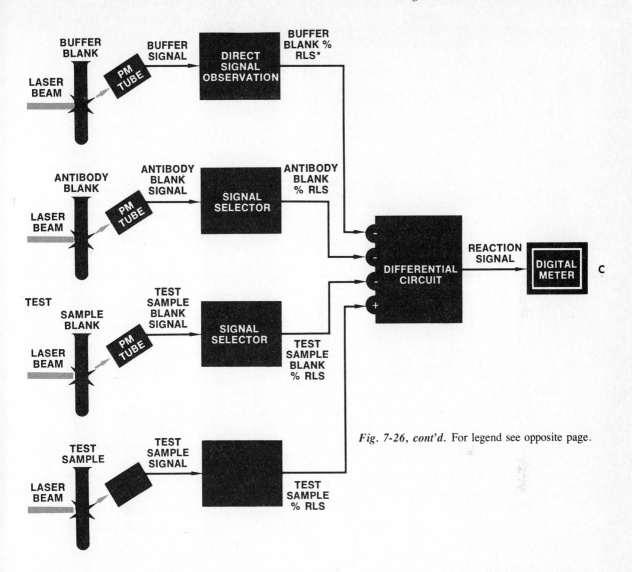

*Fig. 7-26, cont'd.* For legend see opposite page.

zeroed at the start of a cycle, and a built-in timer arrests the meter at the completion of the cycle. Premeasured substrate is maintained at 37° C in the dry well at the right side of the temperature-controlled cuvette well. The selector buttons labeled amylase, lipase standard, and nephelos control the timing sequence. Lipase is measured at 6 minutes and amylase at 2 minutes 15 seconds. Turbimetry standards are provided for checking the accuracy of the instrument.

Since standard manual methods for measuring these enzymes are time consuming and subject to considerable possible error, this instrument has been enthusiastically received. The user is totally dependent on the company to provide accurately prepared buffer. Aside from a very few obviously bad lots, this has not been a significant problem, and the instrument has performed well. It is simple in design and, if properly treated, should require very little maintenance or repair (Fig. 7-25).

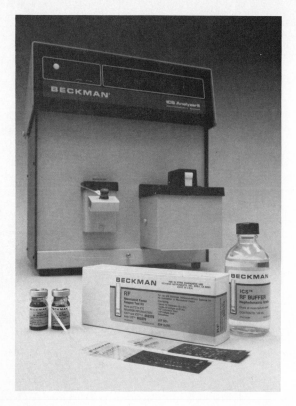

*Fig. 7-27.* The Beckman ICS Analyzer II showing a typical reagent kit. (Courtesy Beckman Instruments, Inc.)

*Laser-Nephelometer-Hyland Model PDQ (Hyland Laboratories).* This instrument works in much the same way as those just mentioned except for the rather important difference in light source (Fig. 7-26, *A*). Whereas the instruments previously discussed use light from an incandescent lamp, this instrument uses a helium/neon laser to produce a coherent, intense, collimated beam of light that can be used with much greater precision. The instrument is primarily used to measure light scatter in immunoprecipitin tests. Prior to the introduction of this instrument, the immunoglobulins were separated and estimated using immunoelectrophoresis, which is an exacting and rather expensive technique requiring considerable time. Turbimetry and ordinary nephelometry are not sensitive enough to accurately measure these protein fractions. This system can give IgA, IgM, IgG, and human complement C′₃ values in about one hour. Since other instruments using

lasers are presented, it is appropriate to discuss laser technology briefly here.

The term *laser* is an acronym for *l*ight *a*mplification by *s*timulated *e*mission of *r*adiation. In the case of the instrument just discussed, a helium/neon laser is used. These gases are contained in a glass plasma tube that has a reflective mirror at one end and a partially reflective mirror at the other. When the electrode contained in the plasma tube is electrically charged, helium atoms are raised to a high energy state. By collision energy is transferred to the neon atoms. This happens because the excited states of the two species of atoms share a common energy level. As interaction between atoms occurs, the light energy produced is amplified, and photons produced bounce back and forth between the two end mirrors, stimulating increasing numbers of atoms. By this process a very intense beam of light of precisely defined wavelength is generated. In order for this light to

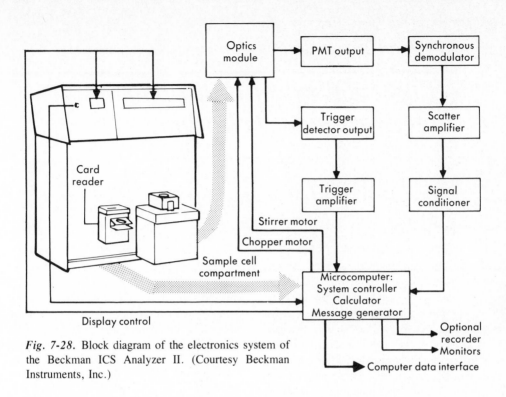

*Fig. 7-28.* Block diagram of the electronics system of the Beckman ICS Analyzer II. (Courtesy Beckman Instruments, Inc.)

bounce back and forth between the two mirrors, light waves must be exactly parallel; hence the light is very monochromatic, organized, and collimated. Obviously light that is so specifically defined is ideal for light-measuring techniques. Fig. 7-26, *B,* is a diagrammatic presentation of the laser source and its light path through the Hyland PDQ Nephelometer.

*Beckman ICS Analyzer II (Beckman Instruments, Inc.).* This is a sophisticated system built around a rate nephelometer (Fig. 7-27). Its principal use is the quantitation of specific proteins and therapeutic drugs by immunochemistry. It measures the rate at which turbidity occurs following the combination of an antigen with its specific antibody. A quartz iodide lamp is the light source, and the scattered light is measured by a photomultiplier tube.

The system furnished by Beckman includes a fixed ratio diluter and a fixed volume dispenser for pipetting the calibrator sera, patient samples, diluent, and antibody. The test is performed in a cell that contains buffer and a magnetic mixing bar. A one-point calibration is calculated by the microcomputer using data from a machine-readable mylar calibrator card, which is supplied with each test kit. The microcomputer provides the operator with instructions, discrepancies, and test results through an alpha-numeric display. Computation is also, of course, performed by the computer. Some self-testing, such as internal voltage measurement, can be performed using the display. Fig. 7-28 is a simplified block diagram of the electronics system.

Beckman has recently introduced a fully automated system that combines all steps for over 15 different assays into one test instrument that is capable of 40 to 60 assays per hour.

# CHAPTER 8

# Light emission and absorption measurement (photometry)

### Emission flame photometry

When a metallic salt is burned in a flame, colors are produced. These colors are at very specific wavelengths that are characteristic of the ion being burned. The heat energy, which the ion absorbs, drives one or more electrons out of their usual orbital positions. As the ion cools, the absorbed energy is released in the form of light, the electrons returning to their normal positions (ground state). Any particular ion may have more than one electron that is excited. The heat energy absorbed and the light emitted on cooling are characteristic of the particular electron orbit involved, as well as the ionic species. For this reason each metal, when heated, has its own emission spectrum, showing emission at various characteristic wavelengths. The number of emission bands may increase as the temperature of the flame is increased and more stable electrons in the ion are excited. If the temperature becomes high enough, the electrons may be thrown so far out of their orbits that the ion is destroyed and the electrons do not return to their proper positions with the characteristic emission of light. Electrons thrown out of position assume characteristic new orbits until they return to ground state. They may return to normal by dropping to one or more intermediate new orbital positions before finally returning to ground. These partial energy releases cause the emission of light at other characteristic wavelengths.

Further confusing the picture is the fact that there are generally many different ionic species in a flame when a solution is burned; these ions may be present as free ions or parts of atoms, molecules, aggregates, or particles. Various areas of the flame will have different temperatures, and the introduction of water into the flame has a cooling effect. All these facts point up the difficulties involved in practical flame photometry. It is extremely important that conditions be duplicated exactly in all details and that standards be run if the results of flame photometry analyses are to be accurate.

The flame photometer is a device for burning solutions to be analyzed and measuring the wavelength and intensity of their emissions. The design of the instrument is not complicated, but the details of construction must be quite precise. There are two major parts involved. The *atomizer-burner* assembly must introduce a constant amount of solution into the flame, which must burn at a constant temperature. The *colorimeter* portion of the instrument must measure the color and intensity of the light emitted by the flame. Since one is normally concerned with one element at a time, an interference filter for the wavelength of the brightest emission peak of the selected element is placed between the flame and the detector so that only this characteristic wavelength passes. There is then only the problem of reading the intensity of the light and comparing it with the intensity of a standard to establish the concentration of the element in the solution being burned.

The design of the atomizer-burner has been the

subject of a great deal of engineering research. A fuel gas such as propane, methane, or butane is brought together with an oxidizing agent such as oxygen or compressed air and burned to produce a flame of predictable heat. The choice of gases and the mixture of fuel and oxidant determine the temperature. The solution to be burned is pulled into the flame by *Venturi action* as the gases rush by the tip of a capillary tube whose other end is immersed in the test solution.

There are two general types of atomizer-burners in use. The first, called a *total-consumption burner,* draws the solution directly into the base of a small flame, where most of it is vaporized and burned (Fig. 8-1). The second, called a *premix burner,* is designed in such a way that the gases rushing past the tip of the capillary nebulize the sample and spray it in a fine mist into a closed chamber beneath the flame (Fig. 8-2). The larger droplets fall to the floor of the chamber, and only the very fine droplets are carried upward into the flame by the flow of gas.

The total-consumption burner is a much simpler design. Concentric tubes around the capillary sweep the gases upward past the capillary tip and carry the droplets of fluid into the flame. Other factors being equal, it should be possible to work with lower concentrations in this sort of system, but there are several rather serious disadvantages. The large droplets of water that are not dispersed cool the flame considerably. This is particularly bad, since small changes in viscosity, surface tension, and pressure may alter the size of the droplets and vary the flame temperature at any moment. Also, a larger amount of solid material passes through the burner, and the part that is not burned tends to fall back to dry and cake around the burner orifice, causing further problems. The flame, because of the large droplets, has an uneven turbulent quality that causes erratic meter readings. For these reasons most of the newer flame photometers on the market are of the premix atomizer-burner design with an atomizer chamber.

It should be apparent that the fuel content of the gas and the pressure and composition of the

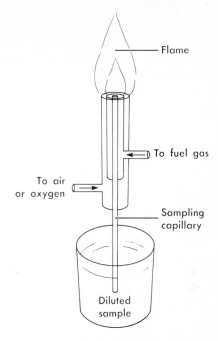

**Fig. 8-1.** Cross section of total-consumption burner.

gas mixture are critical. Both gases should be accurately and consistently metered, and all gas lines and the burner should be clear and unobstructed. Moisture in compressed air, when such air is used, can be a serious problem, and a moisture trap and filter should be used. Where piped gas is used, care should be taken that the gas be relatively clean and consistent as to fuel content.

The total pressure of the gas mixture will determine the flame height, and it is important that the right portion of the flame be in front of the detector. In the base of the flame, where it is hottest, the element absorbs heat energy. As the element rises, it moves into the cooler part, where it gives off its light energy; it is in this area that the emission should be monitored.

Some instruments operate at a temperature that is barely adequate to achieve the desired emission. In most instruments fewer than 5% of the ions passing through the flame are energized. If the temperature falls slightly because of changes in gas

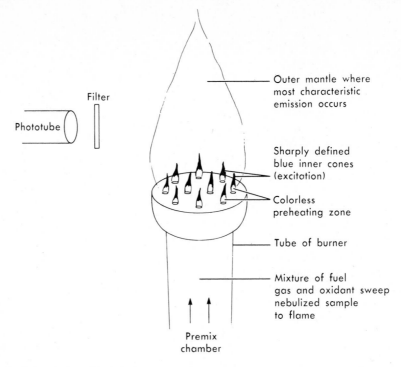

Filter

Phototube

Outer mantle where
most characteristic
emission occurs

Sharply defined
blue inner cones
(excitation)

Colorless
preheating zone

Tube of burner

Mixture of fuel
gas and oxidant sweep
nebulized sample
to flame

Premix
chamber

*Fig. 8-2.* Cross section of premix burner and flame, showing where detector should be relative to flame.

pressure, fuel content, or water in the flame, the accuracy of the instrument may be seriously impaired. If this happens, there will be insufficient energy to activate the photometer properly, and, when a precalibrated scale panel is used, it becomes impossible to set the high and low ends of the scale using the high and low standards.

The photometer part of the instrument must be designed to detect and measure a very small light signal. The light intensity of a flame is much less than that of an exciter lamp. Also, an interference filter with a very narrow band pass is generally used to isolate the specific energy peak (wavelength) that is characteristic of the element being measured. Hence the light reaching the detector is very weak. For this reason a phototube or photomultiplier is generally used, and the output is amplified considerably before it is presented to the readout device.

Because of the many variables involved it is expedient to use an internal standard whenever possible. An internal standard contains a known concentration of an element with an emission peak appreciably different from the unknown so that the two can be readily differentiated. The internal standard is mixed with the test solution. A separate filter and photodetection system is provided. When the test solution with the standard is burned, the two photosignals are compared electronically (Fig. 8-3). Since the standard and test are affected similarly, variation in aspiration rate, atomization, or amplification will virtually be eliminated. To some extent, the effect of variation in flame temperature is also cancelled. Since the optimum emission temperature for the internal standard and the element being tested may not be quite the same, a disproportionate percentage of the two ionic species may be excited. In the case

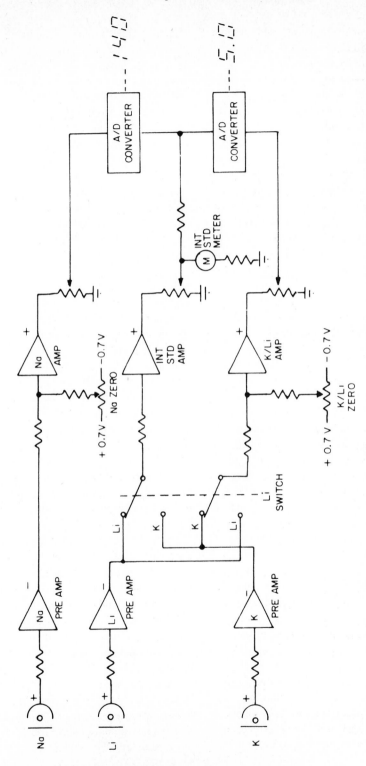

*Fig. 8-3.* Block diagram showing the Lithium Photosignal as a reference for both sodium and potassium. (Courtesy Instrumentation Laboratory, Inc.)

of sodium and potassium compared with lithium as a standard, this variation is minimal.

Calcium presents a special problem in that there are a number of emission maxima at wavelengths that overlap those of sodium. Since sodium is present in body tissues in concentrations up to 40 times that of calcium, the interference is very hard to completely eliminate. The problem is further complicated by the low percent ionization at low temperatures and the differences in the emission spectra at higher temperatures. An entirely adequate system for doing serum calcium determinations by emission flame photometry without previous chemical separation has not been developed.

For many years serum calcium determinations were done by flame photometry, and normal standards were routinely found to read correctly, but many analysts complained that high or low values were not correct. Explanations were contrived, yet careful work revealed that the complaints were justified. Both sodium and protein seem to have contributed considerably to the error. These interferences could be eliminated by preparing a washed calcium oxalate precipitate of the calcium and redissolving in the solution to be aspirated. This procedure is rather pointless, however, since the calcium oxalate could as easily be titrated.

*Quality control.* Several quality control steps should be taken when one is using a flame photometer. As with any instrument, there should be a careful inspection of the flame photometer and its operating characteristics before tests are made. The moisture trap on the air line should be free of water. Adequate fuel and oxidant (air or oxygen) pressures should be ensured. If a small propane tank is used, there will probably not be a gauge to indicate pressure, but a "no fuel" indicator light is usually provided. When a compressor is used to provide compressed air, the gauge should be regularly checked.

The height and form of the flame should be checked from time to time. With no fluid being aspirated, the flame should be pale blue, and the cones of flame from each orifice should be distinct. The flame should be steady and should burn rather quietly. When the lithium internal standard is as-

pirated without a sample, the flame should assume a characteristic pink-red color, and the brightest part of the flame should be at the level of the light lenses.

Most modern flame photometers have a meter that indicates lithium response. This meter should be centered on the scale. If the meter cannot be brought to center-scale, the aspirator tube should be checked to ensure that it is not partially blocked by clots or dried material. The aspiration rate should be checked occasionally by measuring the time required to draw up 1 ml of water. The operator's manual will specify what this rate should be. Adjustment can be made by raising or lowering the sampling capillary tube.

At least two calibrating standards should always be used. Response is adjusted to one standard. A higher or lower standard is then introduced. If it does not read correctly without further adjustment, the instrument must be repaired or adjusted before specimens are tested. The cause of the problem may be a flame that is too cool because of improper gas mixture, or the slope adjustment may be incorrect. The slope should be adjusted by a qualified repairman.

The instrument should always be flushed with water after use, and the flame should burn clean and blue before it is turned off. The atomizer chamber should be cleaned occasionally. If any cleaning agent is used, this should be thoroughly rinsed away with distilled water before the chamber is reassembled.

Some newer flame photometers are self-standardizing. Even when this is the case, reference sera (controls) must be run with each batch of tests to verify calibrations.

If samples are diluted manually, the accuracy and precision of the dilutor or pipettor should be verified occasionally. The reproducibility of automatic dilutors can be checked by replicate testing of a standard.

### Emission flame photometers in common use
*IL Model 143 Flame Photometer (Instrumentation Laboratory, Inc.).* The IL Model 143 was the first instrument in general use to employ an internal standard. For several years it was the most

common flame photometer in hospital laboratories. Most of the flame photometers used today are of the same basic design. Some Model 143 Flame Photometers are still functioning well in daily use. Both Instrumentation Laboratory, Inc. and other manufacturers have introduced newer models with automatic sampling capability, self-standardization, and electronic readout, but nearly all of these use a basic design very similar to the Model 143. For this reason the Model 143 is considered in detail.

The IL Model 143 was designed specifically for performing sodium and potassium determinations on serum and urine. It is a sophisticated instrument, well designed, with relatively few problems when used and maintained as recommended. Sodium and potassium values are recorded simultaneously within about 5 seconds on digital readout devices.

A plastic atomizer chamber attaches under the burner housing on this instrument. Compressed air entering the chamber through a small jet draws up the sample through a capillary and nebulizes it. The stream of air and propane sweeps the smaller droplets up into an open burner, where several small cones of flame burn and coalesce into a larger flame where emission occurs. The emission is monitored by three phototubes with interference filters for sodium, potassium, and lithium. The photosignal from each of these tubes is amplified. The sodium signal is then related to the lithium signal, and the difference is amplified and used to drive a sodium digital readout. The potassium signal is also related to the lithium signal, and this difference is amplified and used to drive a potassium digital readout. Meanwhile a portion of the lithium signal is fed to an edge meter, which serves to monitor the lithium concentration. Obviously, the lithium signal will be inadequate or unsteady if the flame is too high or low or if aspiration is poor. The electronics involved are all solid state and of high quality, giving negligible problems. Each function is on a separate circuit board to make checking and replacement easy.

In addition to the circuits just mentioned, several convenience and safety checks and controls have been added. There is an automatic igniter that throws a high-voltage spark across the top of the burner when the machine is switched on. When the flame lights, a small indicator light, activated by a photocell close to the burner, indicates that the flame is on. If there is no gas pressure, a small pressure switch in the gas line closes a circuit to light a "no gas" indicator. A "no air" indicator works in the same way. If there is no air, a proportional mixing valve makes it impossible for the gas to flow, thus preventing a possible gas fire. When the machine is off, a solenoid valve closes the gas supply. Of course, for safety, the gas should be turned off at the tank also.

The propane gas comes in a small tank of the size used for hand welding torches. This tank is acceptable for use inside buildings without difficulty under almost all fire codes. Exchange of these tanks can be performed quickly and easily without tools. Only a filtered grade of propane such as that sold by the company should be used with this instrument. Propane is a "dirty" gas normally, and industrial grades have debris that quickly clogs the built-in filter and causes considerable trouble. Even with the special propane provided, the filter gets quite dirty after a couple of years of use. A preheater, which is an aid to combustion, is provided on the air line. The valve first used on the propane tank is somewhat fragile and should neither be forced closed nor be opened more than about a half-turn. Later models have supplied a much better gas valve that is somewhat sturdier.

Most of the operational problems with this instrument are the result of inadequate or irregular aspiration and clogging of the capillary of the aspirator. The ideal flow rate is slightly less than that required to get maximum deflection of the lithium meter. If the lithium meter is unsteady, the capillary may be partially occluded and should be cleaned or replaced. The newer models have an easily replaced capillary. Each time the capillary is replaced, however, the aspiration rate must be readjusted; this can be time consuming.

Moisture in the air lines is a serious problem

with this instrument. Compressor air may contain considerable moisture, and unless a moisture trap and filter are provided, difficulty will almost certainly follow. The moisture trap should be drained daily if any moisture is accumulating. The filter should be changed every 4 to 6 weeks. If air from piped compressed air lines is used, it should be dehumidified and filtered before it comes to the instrument. Piped air lines in moist climates can accumulate quantities of water, which must not reach the instrument.

The automatic striker on the IL Flame Photometer was one of the first built into this type of instrument. It is a real convenience and has been hailed as a most welcome innovation. Like most new ideas, it has had to go through a few design changes before problems were eliminated. The earliest models had a wire about 1 inch long positioned close to the flame. A high-voltage spark jumped from it to the metal burner and ignited

the gas. The wire corroded badly and also got bent away from the flame area so that it would sometimes fail to ignite the gas. The next change was to have only a small unprotected tip of metal protruding from a ceramic insulator fixed firmly in place. This was a considerable improvement, but when corrosion of the igniter tip and buildup of material on the striker and burner occurred, the burner would fail to light, and the higher-voltage current would short-circuit out through the buildup on the striker and burner. If the burner and striker surfaces were carefully cleaned, the instrument would work well again. A new striker housed in plastic is now in use. It has a replaceable electrode that can be discarded when it corrodes. It is easy to change and seems to work extremely well.

When the burner fails to light and air and gas are both available, the striker is usually the problem. One can easily check whether adequate current is getting to the striker. If the banana plug

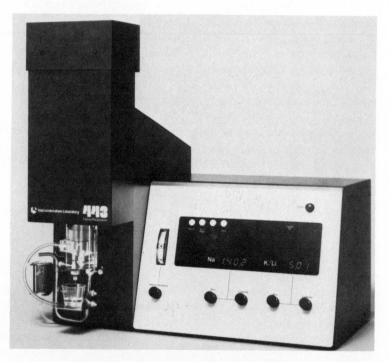

*Fig. 8-4.* IL Model 443 Flame Photometer. (Courtesy Instrumentation Laboratory, Inc.)

in the top of the Tesla coil (large black coil behind the flame compartment) is removed and the switch is turned on, a stream of sparks can be seen to jump from the plug to its receptacle. Absence of a spark indicates an electronic problem in the power amplifier. (Exercise care in making this check because you are dealing with very high voltage.)

Just inside the case, below the burner, is a small valve that controls the flow of gas to the burner. Behind this valve is a proportioning valve that maintains a constant proportion of gas and air. Thus, although they enter the atomizer by separate lines, both propane and air are adjusted by turning the one gas-control valve. This setting is rather critical to good instrument performance, and, once the proper flame height is set, the valve should not be readjusted. If the setting is far off, the instrument is hard to light.

Early models had no dilutor, and it was necessary to make a lithium dilution manually. A peristalic-type dilutor was developed later that could be added to the Model 143. This first dilutor had a number of problems, but on later IL flame photometers it was improved and built into the instrument. The newer dilutors have been largely trouble free.

Several newer, more automated flame photometers have been added to the IL series (Fig. 8-4). All have been essentially trouble free and accurate and have found wide acceptance.

*FLM2 and FLM3 Flame Photometers (Radiometer).* These instruments are from a Danish firm (Fig. 8-5). The FLM3, which is the newer model, is now being manufactured in the United States. Both instruments are basically similar to the IL flame photometers described earlier. The principal

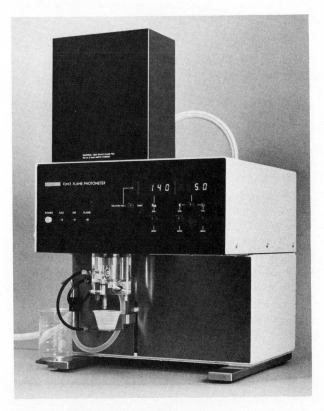

*Fig. 8-5.* FLM3 Flame Photometer. (Courtesy Radiometer.)

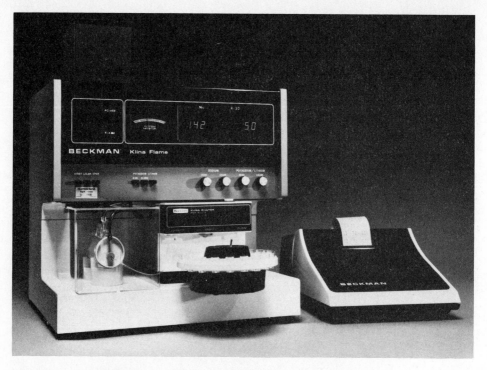

*Fig. 8-6.* Beckman Klina Flame System with automatic sampling carousel and printer. (Courtesy Beckman Instruments, Inc.)

differences are in the placement of controls and indicators and in the electronics, The Model FLM3 has a new, convenient air-pressure regulator that contains an air filter and settling bowl that traps any water in the air supply and automatically drains it off whenever the air pressure is cut off. This model should respond in approximately 3 seconds and stabilize at about 6 seconds. When stabilized, the indicator lamp lights, and the answer stays on the digital display until the sample is lowered from the capillary. No dilutor or automated handling device has been offered for these instruments. Radiometer instruments use high-quality components and are carefully manufactured. They are distributed in the United States through The London Co.

*Klina Flame System (Beckman Instruments, Inc.).* Beckman has had rather bad luck with clinical flame photometers in the past, but this unit seems very promising indeed and reports on it are good (Fig. 8-6).

There is an automatic ignition system, and in case of malfunction an automatic shutdown functions. The premix atomizer chamber is in the front, where it can be easily removed for cleaning. Dilution is performed automatically within the sampler-atomizer portion. A measured sample of serum and an aliquot of diluent are swirled together in a small cup from which the dilution is drawn into the atomizer. A vibrator aids mixing, and the chamber is rinsed between samples. Three different dilution ratios may be selected with the flip of a switch.

There is a capability built in that allows one to switch over to reading sodium and lithium (rather than sodium and potassium). When lithium is used as an internal standard, it is monitored and adjusted electronically. If the aspiration rate is

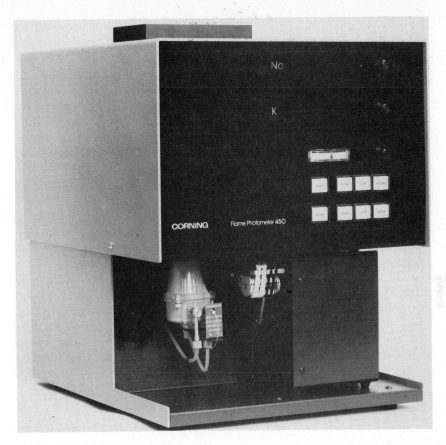

*Fig. 8-7.* Model 450 Flame Photometer. (Courtesy Corning Scientific Instruments.)

incorrect or if certain other malfunctions occur, a system monitor reports the fact, thus reducing erroneous readings.

This system uses photomultiplier tubes, rather than phototubes, which makes possible a considerable improvement in precision and a reduction in background noise. Readout is by Nixie tubes, but a printer is available, and BCD output is provided for computer connection.

If the Klina Flame System works as well as early reports seem to indicate, it should find wide acceptance in those laboratories that are not automating electrolyte procedures.

*Models 430 and 450 (Corning Scientific Instruments).* These instruments are basically very sim-

ilar in design to those already discussed (Fig. 8-7). The atomizer chamber has a somewhat different appearance but operates like the other two. The dilutor is also similar. Controls and displays are arranged in a slightly different pattern but serve nearly identical functions. The Model 450 provides an automatic scale expansion for reading urine samples, which is activated by the press of a button. A button for activating a printer may be added.

## Atomic absorption photometry

In *emission flame photometry,* which has been discussed, a very specific amount of energy, in the form of heat, is absorbed by an atom. This energy causes certain valence electrons to move to new orbital positions more distant from the nucleus. The atom is *excited,* or in a higher energy state. Since this is an unstable state, the extra energy is given up in a very short time as the atom moves to a cooler part of the flame. This energy is released as light, and the wavelength (energy level) is the precise energy involved in the electron transition.

In *atomic absorption* the process is essentially reversed. If one can dissociate the atom in question from its chemical bonds, one finds that an un-ionized, unexcited atom will absorb light of a specific wavelength, that is to say, of a certain energy level. This is the exact energy required, in emission flame photometry, to excite the atom by moving certain valence electrons to new, defined orbital positions. In other words, the un-ionized atom will absorb light of the wavelength that it would emit if emission flame photometry were used.

The best way found, until now, to cause the atom to dissociate from its chemical bonds is to heat it in a flame. When heated, some of the atoms emit, but it is estimated that only about 1.5% do so, and all of them will absorb light energy. Thus, the error is small and reasonably constant and can be compensated. The energy band that is absorbed is very narrow—in the order of 0.0001 nm—and at exactly the wavelength that would be emitted if the atom were excited. Since the disassociated atom will absorb exactly the wavelength (energy) that an excited atom of the same element emits, it is most convenient to produce the energy band by heating the element.

These very fine emission lines are produced in the atomic absorption photometer by a *hollow cathode lamp.* This is a neon or argon lamp with a cathode composed of the metal in question. The lamp will emit only the spectrum of the gas plus that of the heated metal. If this light is directed into the flame containing the metal, the atoms of the metal in question will absorb the emission from the metal in the hollow cathode lamp. Absorption will follow Beer's law so that there is a logarithmic

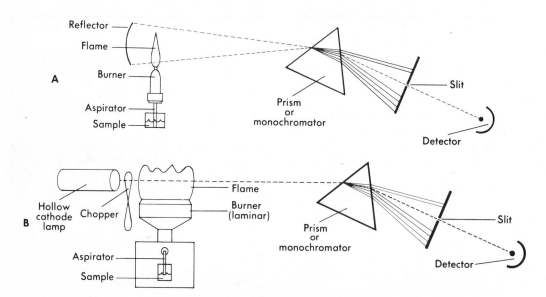

*Fig. 8-8.* Atomic absorption technique. *A,* Emission flame photometer measures light emitted by the flame. *B,* Atomic absorption photometer measures absorption of light from the hollow cathode by the flame. (Courtesy Beckman Instruments, Inc.)

relationship between absorption and concentration of element in the light path, just as in spectrophotometry.

For this arrangement to work accurately, it is imperative that a very narrow emission peak of the hollow cathode lamp be measured and that all extraneous light be rejected. To accomplish this a very good monochromator with a very narrow band pass is necessary.

Fig. 8-8 compares emission flame photometry with atomic absorption.

The atomic absorption (AA) flame photometer, then, in its simplest form, consists of a hollow cathode lamp, an atomizer-burner, a monochromator, a detector, and a readout. It is similar to a spectrophotometer. The hollow cathode lamp acts

as the exciter lamp, and the flame acts as the cuvette. Fig. 8-9 may facilitate visualization of the principle.

In actual practice most AA photometers include many additions, refinements, and details that are not described in this rather oversimplified summary. Let us consider some of these further.

A hollow cathode lamp is made for virtually every metallic element. Westinghouse and Perkin-Elmer, together, make almost all the hollow cathode lamps on the market. Until recently the life of one of these lamps was about 100 hours of burning time. Since there was a rather long warm-up time for lamps of many elements, the actual use time was shorter. Recently lamps have been produced with a much longer life, and in some cases

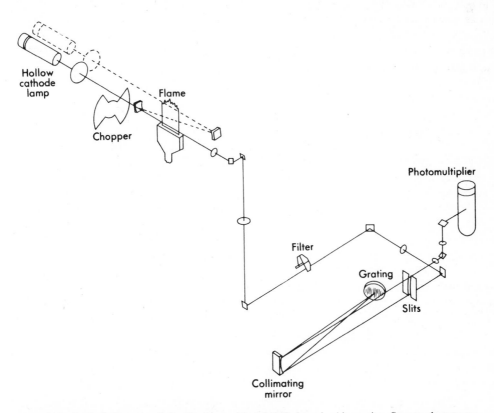

*Fig. 8-9.* Optical diagram of the Beckman Model 440 Atomic Absorption Spectrophotometer. It is a single-beam instrument with triple- and single-pass optics. (Courtesy Beckman Instruments, Inc.)

the warm-up time has been reduced. These lamps are rather expensive. More than one element has been inserted in one cathode in some cases so that one lamp can be used for two or more elements. This practice saves somewhat on initial cost; however, the lamp life is still the same. Also the multielement lamps may have interference between the elements.

The importance of lamp warm-up time has been somewhat controversial. The spectral emission of the lamps of certain elements fluctuates considerably during the first few minutes after the lamps are ignited. With some elements this instability has lasted for 30 to 45 minutes. In an effort to obviate the need for a long warm-up time, some companies have produced a double-beam instrument that works very much like a double-beam spectrophotometer. The emission from the hollow cathode lamp is directed to a beam splitter, which by one means or another routes half the light around the flame. Regardless of the variations of the cathode lamp output, the reference beam and the beam passing through the flame are now comparable. This modification is, in general, inclined to improve the stability of the instrument (Fig. 8-8).

At least one company (Instrumentation Laboratory, Inc.) believes that this does not go far enough and that the double beam does not monitor variations in flame characteristics. It has inserted an internal standard (usually lithium) and has provided an additional hollow cathode lamp to continuously monitor the flame as the tests are performed.

Perkin-Elmer has a deuterium background corrector, which does essentially the same thing. Rather than use an additional hollow cathode lamp, such as lithium, this company uses a deuterium lamp with a broad band emission. Monitoring the deuterium lamp output gives the necessary corrective information.

As the flame burns the sample, a few atoms of the element to be tested are excited and give off light of the same wavelength as the hollow cathode lamp. Also, some stray light from the room and the burner may coincide with the cathode lamp emission. To eliminate these sources of error, the beam from the hollow cathode lamp is chopped, and only the chopped light reaching the detector is measured. As has been seen earlier, this is fairly easy to do. In the double-beam instruments, the chop may be the alternative viewing of the reference and sample beams.

Burner design has been the subject of much study during the past few years. Since absorbance varies directly with the optical path through the flame, it has seemed expedient to use a ''curtain'' or''fishtail'' flame, with the hollow cathode beam passing through the length of the flame. Some instruments have the facility to turn the flame at an angle to shorten the path if this becomes desirable. The burner designed to give a curtain of flame is called a *laminar-flow burner*. Some burners have three slots in the head, which give the curtain of flame more width. A higher-temperature, nitrous oxide burner is made for those refractory elements that will not atomize at lower flame temperatures.

It is important that the monochromator of the AA photometer be of very high quality, since the emission bands that are being measured are very narrow. A band pass of about 0.2 nm is, on occasion, required for good resolution.

Atomic absorption is primarily used, in clinical laboratories, to measure trace metals of medical significance and to detect and quantitate metallic poisons. Zinc seems to be involved in the healing process, growth, appetite, and sexual drive. Copper is involved in porphyrin metabolism and is a constituent or activator of various enzymes. Many other metals such as cobalt, molybdenum, selenium, lithium, and tin are known or thought to be important to health—in very small amounts. Arsenic, lead, thallium, beryllium, and many other metals are poisonous, even in very small amounts. Increasing use of many of these in industry makes accidental poisoning more common.

Until recently many of these metals were very difficult to detect, and routine analyses of body fluids and tissues were seldom routinely checked.

Food and water supplies could not possibly be monitored by the tedious chemical methods available. With the development of the atomic absorption spectrophotometer these analyses can be done quickly, economically, and quite accurately. This has allowed us to learn much more about these elements and this, in turn, has stimulated a heavy demand for many analyses. With the present emphasis on the environment, many more tests of this sort are being requested on industrial wastes and on water, air, and foods.

Although the use of these tests has become much more common, the measurement of atomic absorption is still restricted, in most cases, to the larger laboratories and hospitals or to specialized laboratories.

Several companies now have instruments that seem practical for clinical work. Some of these are presented here. The list is not exhaustive, and only a cursory evaluation of each is made. Selection of a system such as an atomic absorption spectrophotometer involves many technical details and parameters, and space does not allow adequate consideration here. The serious student or prospective buyer should study carefully the claims for each, read all available literature on each, and talk with someone who has had experience with the instruments, if possible.

*Atomic absorption spectrophotometers in common use.* There are probably more Perkin-Elmer atomic absorption spectrophotometers in use in clinical laboratories than any other. This company has produced instruments for study of atomic absorption since 1960. Perkin-Elmer scientists have published much material and conducted many fine workshops and training programs that have advanced the use of these instruments. There are two principal models in wide clinical use.

*Perkin-Elmer's Models 290B and 303 (Perkin-Elmer Corp.).* The 290B is a single-beam instrument designed with a readout in linear concentration units. The monochromator covers the range from 200 to 700 nm, using a grating ruled at 1800 lines/mm. Resolution of 0.2 nm is possible, and a choice of 0.2, 0.7, or 2 nm band pass is available.

Since some hollow cathode lamps require some warm-up time before their output is stable, a three-lamp warm-up supply accessory is available to save time. Where a large number of analyses are to be done on one element, the Model 290B is an excellent instrument. A scale expansion of $4.5\times$ is built into the instrument, which can be increased to $18\times$ by using an external 10 mV recorder.

Their Model 303 is a double-beam instrument. In this case the chopper is a rotating mirror that alternately directs the reference and the sample beam into the detector. The ratio is then read electrically. This process helps to offset drift in hollow cathode lamp output and detector sensitivity. Lamp warm-up time can be virtually eliminated. With the Model 303 it is possible to use the deuterium background corrector, which emits a broad emission. Background in the flame absorbs both the deuterium and hollow cathode emission, whereas the element of interest absorbs only the hollow cathode's narrow band of emission, providing a basis for correcting for background effect. It is also possible to use the digital concentration readout accessory with the Model 303 to provide readout in units of concentration. See Fig. 8-10 and compare the light paths of Model 290B and Model 303.

The Model 303 is a sensitive, stable, and versatile instrument that is generally considered to be the leader among atomic absorption spectrophotometers in clinical use. This is not to say, of course, that competing companies do not have some extremely fine instruments and excellent points to make for their own developments and modifications. A wide choice of burners and other accessories is available.

*IL Model 453 Atomic Absorption–Emission Spectrophotometer (Instrumentation Laboratory, Inc.).* This instrument is by far the most sophisticated of those discussed here (Fig. 8-11). It is, in effect, a double double-beam instrument; that is to say, the beams from two hollow cathode lamps are passing through the flame simultaneously, each with its own reference beam around the flame. The second cathode element may be used as an

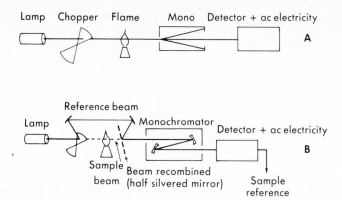

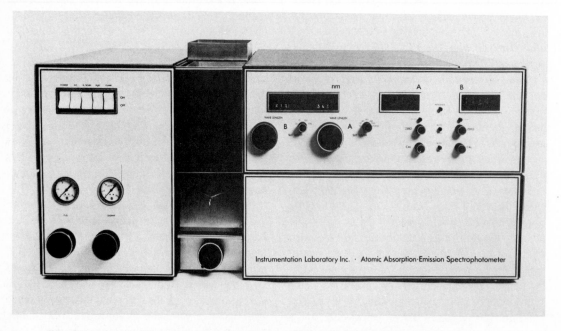

**Fig. 8-10.** Comparison of optical paths in single-beam and double-beam atomic absorption spectrophotometers. *A*, Single-beam ac system: in this sytem, light from the hollow cathode lamp is chopped, either mechanically or electronically, to differentiate it from unchopped light emission. The monochromator is tuned to select the resonance line of the element being determined. The chopped lamplight causes an alternating current flow in the photomultiplier detector—hence the name "ac system." The Model 290B uses this system. *B*, Double-beam ac system: in the Model 303, the chopper is a rotating sector mirror that divides the light from the hollow cathode lamp into two beams. The electronic output appears as the ratio of the sample and reference beams. The effects of changes in lamp emission and detector sensitivity are thereby eliminated. Compared to the single-beam system, double-beam gives better precision and detection limits. (Courtesy Perkin-Elmer Corp.)

**Fig. 8-11.** Atomic Absorption–Emission Spectrophotometer, Model 453. (Courtesy Instrumentation Laboratory, Inc.)

internal standard, or there is the option of performing tests for two elements simultaneously. This instrument also can be used as an emission-flame photometer. It is equipped with an automatic ignition as well as a number of monitoring functions.

There is a digital concentration readout, and scale expansion is possible. An ingenious correction circuit that permits linearization of nonlinear signals by means of a single adjustment is provided. Since atomic absorption is such a dynamic process, one should check standards carefully at frequent intervals, however.

A great deal of thought has been given to safety in the design of this IL instrument. In addition to the automatic remote control of flame ignition and extinction, fail-safe devices that take over in certain circumstances have been built in. If air or gas pressure drops, all valves are immediately and automatically closed. If the flame becomes irregular or if it "lifts off" the burner, the fail-safe comes into play. If the wrong burner for the gas mixture being employed is installed, the ignition system is neutralized and cannot function.

Conversion to nitrous oxide may be effected by a control on the front panel, and, when the nitrous oxide flame is extinguished, air is injected into the system to prevent excessive soot formation and flashback explosions. If such a flashback does occur, a diaphragm ruptures gently away from the operator.

Another attractive feature of this unit that seems excellent is the built-in circuit-testing feature. Using the controls on one panel, one can electrically check 20 different points without extensively dismantling the instrument.

The electronics are all solid state and superbly designed. The optical system seems very good. The band pass, of the Ebert-type (grating) monochromator, is 0.6 Å. Design of the gas-handling system, the fail-safe features, and the safety features appear to be excellent.

Many features that are provided as extra, optional accessories on other atomic absorbance units are built into this one. The digital readout, linearizer, electronic integrator, and built-in circuit testing might be considered as extras. The price of the unit is comparable to the competitive units with these accessories.

An intriguing additional feature is a motorized wavelength scanning drive that permits scanning of the hollow cathode lamp's emission or the emission of the flame itself. This spectral scan may be recorded, of course.

The IL atomic absorption spectrophotometers have now established themselves as serious challengers and have had wide acceptance. Early arguments that the unit is overengineered have apparently, at least, been overstated, since its performance record seems good. There is possibly something to be said for the loss of sensitivity involved in the many optical surfaces of lenses, mirrors, and beam splitters. This loss seems to have been largely offset by good electronics.

The Model 453 has recently been superseded by the Model 351, which is modular in design, allowing for the addition or deletion of some modules to suit the user's need.

*Model 603 Atomic Absorption Spectrophotometer (Perkin-Elmer Corp.).* This sophisticated, double-beam instrument was introduced during 1976. One of the more interesting features is the microprocessor, which controls many of the instrument's functions. There are two memory devices. One is the *ROM* (read only memory) and contains the necessary software to instruct the unit in its operation. It is hard wired and cannot be changed or dumped. The second unit is the *RAM* (random access memory) into which the operator may insert concentrations of standards and times. Various function keys are provided on two keyboards and are labeled in English (not machine language).

The microprocessor makes possible an automatic calibration routine. The operator instructs the instrument concerning the concentration of the standard, lights the machine, presses zero, aspirates sample no. 1, pushes standard no. 1 button, aspirates no. 2, pushes standard no. 2 button, and repeats with no 3. The curve is recorded in the instrument's memory and is available until cleared. Curve correction is automatically performed.

The microprocessor also prevents some types of mistakes. Calibration standards will not be accepted out of sequence. If the system is changed to a new element, all calibration information is erased. When switching between modes, however, the calibration information stays in the system. Out of range calibrations are shown by an OVER CAL. indicator light. Indicator lights also show what function is in progress at any time.

The optical system is double beam, with the sample beam passing through the flame and the reference behind it. As stated earlier, this provides protection against variations in power and light intensity. Lamps may be used immediately after ignition, even though they may not stabilize for some time. A deuterium background correction (discussed earlier) is provided.

A variety of burners are available for various gases and both air and nitrous oxide. The flame is shielded from the operator for safety and comfort. Safety interlocks are provided on the burners to avoid ignition when the proper burner is not in place.

An optional gas control is available that programs the gases to come on in the right order and ignition to occur at the proper interval. Changeover to nitrous oxide with a compensating change in acetylene flow can be accomplished by pushing a button.

This system is representative of the new generation of atomic absorption spectrophotometers and, indeed, says a great deal about the state of the art in instrumentation in general.

# CHAPTER 9

# *Fluorescence and fluorometry*

## *Phenomenon of fluorescence*

When some types of molecules are exposed to light or other electromagnetic radiation, they absorb this energy and then reemit it as light of another wavelength. The radiant energy displaces certain electrons from their customary orbital positions and moves them into characteristic new positions farther from the nucleus. In its natural condition the molecule is said to be in the *ground state*. When the electrons have absorbed energy in the above manner, the molecule is said to be in an *excited state*, or a *higher-energy state*. Such electrons usually occur in balanced pairs. When one of the pair of electrons is raised to its first characteristic excited state, it is said to be in a *first singlet*, or $S_1$, stage. If the electron absorbs still more energy, causing it to move into a more distant orbit, it may be placed in an $S_2$, $S_3$, $S_4$, etc. stage. A typical, highly reproducible amount of energy is required to place the electron in a particular orbit.

It has been noted that the wavelength or color of light determines its radiant energy. A specific color or wavelength of light will characteristically excite a molecule to a specific singlet stage by displacing an electron from its normal position.

At the same time other wavelengths of light, with different energy levels, from the same source may be displacing other electrons of the same molecule to new characteristic positions.

Excited molecules do not stay in this state very long. Within microseconds or even nanoseconds the displaced electron returns to its normal position, with the release of the absorbed energy. In

the process, however, a little energy is lost, and the *emitted* energy (light) is of a lower order (longer wavelength) than that of the *exciting* energy. Hence a molecule may absorb violet light and then emit red light. The energy that is "lost" in this process can probably be accounted for by vibration and by collisions (Fig. 9-1).

This process is called *fluorescence*. The ability of a molecule to absorb light of a given wavelength and reemit it at another, characteristic wavelength is such a specific and characteristic phenomenon that it can be used as a certain method of identifying a particular compound. Also the amount of light that will be reemitted is a linear function of the concentration of the compound. These circumstances make *fluorometry* a very specific and sensitive testing procedure.

If energy is not released until a few milliseconds after excitation of the molecule, the process is called *phosphorescence*. The luminous dial of your watch provides an example of phosphorescence. For clarity it is usually called phosphorescence when a lapse of $10^{-4}$ second occurs before the light is reemitted; much longer time lapses are, of course, very common.

When the electron is raised to the second or third singlet stage, it can lose its absorbed energy in two or more steps, thereby emitting more than one characteristic wavelength of light energy. Considering the possibility of electrons in different orbital positions, each reemitting a characteristic wavelength of light, and further considering the possibility that some may lose their energy in several stages, one might predict that the

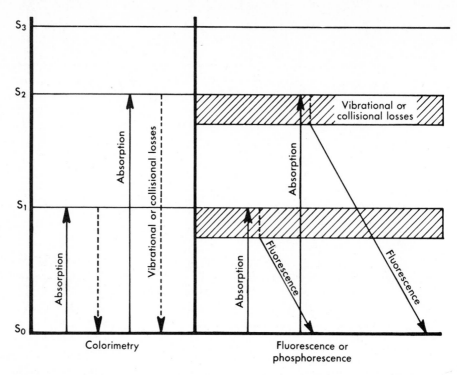

**Fig. 9-1.** Diagrammatic representation of the absorption and reemission of energy in fluorescence or phosphorescence compared with the same process in normally nonfluorescing compounds.

fluorescent light emitted by a compound could contain a considerable number of characteristic emission peaks. This is, indeed, the case, and it is possible to identify a compound, in many cases, by the emission spectrum of that compound. If one wishes to quantitate a compound by fluorescence, however, one selects a specific characteristic wavelength *(an emission maximum)* at which the intensity of light emission relative to suitable standards is measured.

Since some energy is always lost in the process of absorption and reemission and since the reemitted energy is generally visible light, it stands to reason that the exciting energy might often be in the UV or near-UV region, where wavelengths are shorter and energy levels higher. The light source used to provide this energy in a fluorometer may be a *hydrogen lamp,* a *mercury arc,* a *xenon lamp,* or another similar emission source.

These sources require relative high voltage to fire, and a high-voltage transformer is always a necessary part of a fluorometer. Fluorescent lighting such as that used in the home emits some energy in the near UV range and can be used in special situations.

It is interesting to note that the phenomenon of fluorescence is not limited to the UV and visible range. Some molecules may absorb energy from x-rays and reemit in the soft–x-ray or far-UV range. Since it is more difficult to detect and resolve radiation of such short wavelengths, this region has never been used in routine analysis.

### Fluorometry

A very simple fluorometer would have a configuration similar to that in Fig. 9-2. The power supply would need to be sufficiently stable to provide a constant voltage to the exciter lamp. The

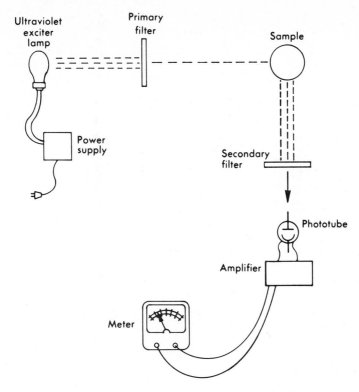

*Fig. 9-2.* Typical configuration of a simple fluorometer.

exciter lamp would have to have adequate emission at the specific wavelengths needed for whatever analyses were contemplated. The primary filter would provide the wavelength that would excite the solution under examination. The resolution required of the instrument would dictate the sort of monochromator to be used.

Since the entire sample in a fluorometer is saturated with light, the light does not have to be collimated into a sharply defined path through the sample. Therefore, small blemishes and scratches on the cuvettes are of relatively less consequence as a source of error. If the material being tested is fluorescent, the entire content of the tube emits light and becomes, in effect, a light source, the brilliance of which is measured with the detector. The detector is usually placed at a 90-degree angle to the beam of the exciting light so that only emitted (not transmitted) light is measured.

The secondary filter defines the specific emission peak that is to be used for analysis. Again, the quality of resolution required will dictate whether a filter or a more sophisticated monochromator is used.

A phototube or photomultiplier is usually used as a detector in fluorometers, since the total emitted light may possibly be much weaker than in photometry. Fig. 9-3 shows the optical path of a typical fluorometer.

As mentioned earlier, ultraviolet light is absorbed by ordinary glass, and the amount of this absorption is quite significant at the shorter wavelengths. Quartz or a special type of glass is used in the optics of better fluorometers, and, in some cases, the use of quartz or Infrasil cuvettes may be advantageous or necessary. Front-surfaced mirrors are also generally used, since the ultraviolet light traveling through the glass to a reflective

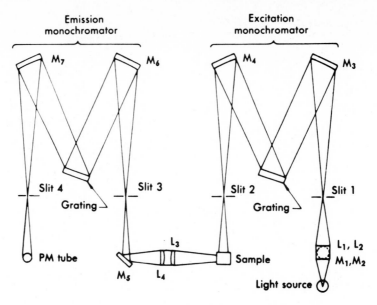

*Fig. 9-3.* Optical path of the SPF 125 Spectrofluorometer. (Courtesy American Instrument Co., Inc.)

coating and being reflected back through the glass again would lose much of its energy.

The time required for fluorescent emission to occur after excitation may vary somewhat between orbital electron positions and between molecular species. This delay is usually in microseconds and is not significant when readings are taken reasonably soon after the specimen is exposed to light. If the specimen remains in the light path for a considerable time, however, this may result in a gradually increasing emission. A shutter is often supplied between the light source and the sample. The shutter is left closed until the reading is to be made, to prevent the sort of error just described.

As a general rule, the intensity of fluorescence is proportional to the concentration. When dealing with an unknown, one should plot a curve using known standards. In some cases a phenomenon known as ''quenching'' occurs, in which the fluorescence actually decreases as the concentration of fluorophores exceeds an optimal value.

Fluorescent procedures should be followed exactly, since small changes in chemistry may make significant changes in fluorescence. Some fluoresc-

ing compounds are so sensitive to changes in pH that their emission can be used as a sensitive measure of pH change. In fact, there are several excellent fluorescent indicators for use in acid-base titrations.

It is interesting to note that the excitation wavelengths (those that excite a molecule and cause it to fluoresce) are the same as those at which the molecule will absorb light. The emission wavelengths are generally somewhat higher, but there may not be much resemblance between the total *excitation spectrum* and the emission spectrum. The term *quantum efficiency* is used to express the ratio of emitted light to absorbed light.

Fluorometry is a more specific means of measurement than absorptiometry. If one measures the light absorption of a solution at a given wavelength, one is measuring absorption by the material in question plus any other that might be present. In fluorometry, however, one deals only with the substance that absorbs at the specific wavelength *and* emits light at a second characteristic wavelength.

Fluorometry is extremely sensitive. It is esti-

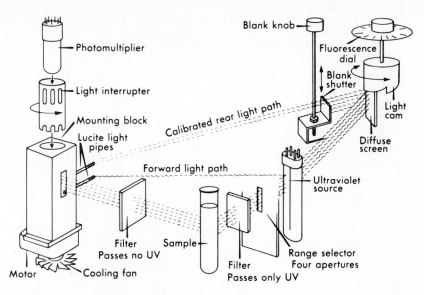

*Fig. 9-4.* Optical path of the Turner Model 111 Fluorometer. (Courtesy G.K. Turner Associates.)

mated that it can detect materials in a concentration of 1 in 10 billion. This is about a thousand times the sensitivity of absorptiometry. The material must naturally fluoresce or be made to fluoresce by some tagging technique, of course. This tagging technique can be accomplished with many materials, but it is often as easy and more expedient to detect and quantitate a substance by some other technique. Fluorescence for many substances, however, is the obvious technique of choice.

In the past several years, classical fluorescence chemistry has been largely replaced by better conventional methods and by automated systems using other principles. A new application of fluorescence has developed, however. Antibodies can be produced to many substances such as therapeutic drugs, hormones, and protein fractions. These antibodies can then be tagged with fluorescent material, which can be easily detected in specially designed fluorometers. Fluorescence immunoassay may become an important method of detecting and measuring many substances that have previously been analytical problems. The Syva Ad-

vance System is one of the best instruments of this sort.

### Fluorometers in common use

*Turner Model 111 (G.K. Turner Associates).* This instrument has become the standard for instruments in this category. Fig. 9-4 shows the optical configuration of its system. Light from the UV source strikes the sample, causing fluorescence that impinges upon the photomultiplier. At the same time, light from the UV source is reflected from a diffuse screen and is reflected to the photomultiplier. A light interrupter (chopper) causes the photomultiplier to sense the fluorescent light from the sample at one instant and the reflected light from the diffuse screen the next. The forward light path, shown on the optical schematic, is a very small light signal that falls on the photomultiplier to produce a constant dark current to operate the servomechanism even when nonfluorescent blanks are used. The consequent photocurrent is an alternating current (square-wave) that can be amplified. This error signal is then fed back to a light cam that by a sort of servomechanism automatically adjusts the reflected light until the

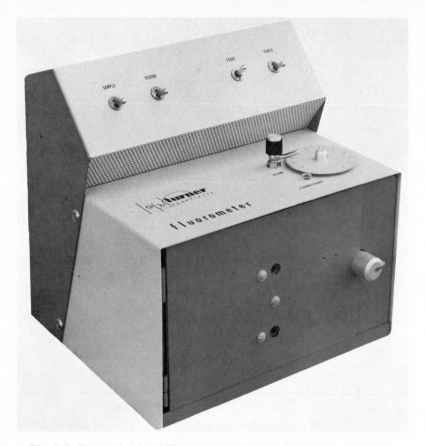

*Fig. 9-5.* Turner Model 111 Fluorometer. (Courtesy G.K. Turner Associates.)

two light signals (sample and reference) are equal. The correction that has been made is indicated on the fluorescence dial. This correction is a linear function of fluorescence so the concentration of the sample may be accurately ascertained.

This sort of dual-beam arrangement, which Turner calls an *optical bridge,* eliminates the effect of variations in line voltage, light source, and detector sensitivity. As noted earlier, cuvette variations and light collimation are of minimal importance in fluorescence measurement; therefore, the system has less chance for error than one would suppose.

As has been noted, glass absorbs ultraviolet light rather strongly at lower wavelengths, so front-surfaced optics are used. The filters are glass.

The secondary filters will not be in the UV range, and the fact that the primary filter absorbs some ultraviolet light is not too significant, since this absorbance is constant for any particular filter.

A flow-through cuvette door is available, making possible the use of this instrument with the AutoAnalyzer for fluorescent methods. Also, special doors are available for scanning fluorescence of filter paper strips.

The electronics of this instrument are fairly complicated, and major repair should not be attempted by anyone but a factory-trained repairman. In use the Turner has had relatively few repair problems and has proved to be a very sensitive and reliable instrument.

G.K. Turner Associates has probably done more

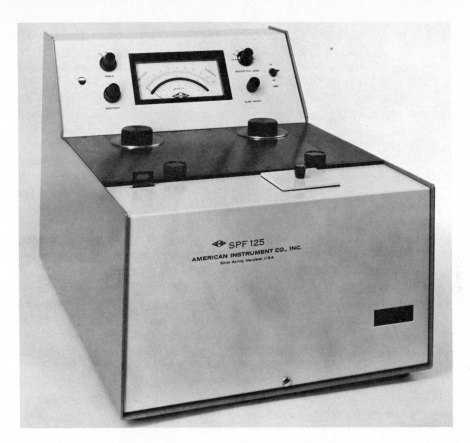

*Fig. 9-6.* SPF 125 Spectrofluorometer. (Courtesy American Instrument Co., Inc.)

to advance the field of fluorescence measurement than has anyone else, both by its monumental design innovations and by its research and publication of fluorescence methods for clinical determinations. The company maintains an outstanding bibliography and reference service, which it has generously made available to Turner users and nonusers alike. The popular Turner Model 111 is shown in Fig. 9-5.

*Spectrophotofluorometer (American Instrument Co., Inc.).* This is a sophisticated and rather expensive instrument with more capability than the filter fluorometers discussed. In place of primary and secondary filters, this instrument uses grating monochromators.

A high-intensity xenon arc lamp is used. There is some danger from the buildup of ozone around the lamp, caused by ionization of oxygen. Ozone is normally considered healthful, but if present in excessive quantities, it may have deleterious effects. Such a buildup occurs only when the instrument is used continuously in quarters that are not well vented. Flushing the area around the lamp with nitrogen or ventilating the area is adequate protection. A high-voltage dc power supply, required to fire the xenon lamp, is housed in a separate cabinet.

Several excitation and emission exit slits are provided to determine the band passes used. These slits are manually substituted in the instrument.

The high-quality monochromators are motor driven to provide automatic scanning. An X-Y plotter is available to correlate wavelength with emission regardless of scan speed or interruptions in the scan.

A photomultiplier tube is used as a detector. Even though this is a single-beam instrument, it has very good stability because of the high-quality electronic components employed in power supplies and amplifier circuits.

The output of the photomultiplier is amplified in the Fluoro-Microphotometer, which is housed in a separate case. This unit consists of amplifying and control circuits, chopper, amplifier, and a 6-inch ammeter. It is used with the recorder and oscillograph, which may be attached, a total of five separate units are involved in the Aminco Spectrophotofluorometer system, and at least 6 feet of bench space is required. It is an excellent research instrument with high resolution, good accuracy, and fine sensitivity but seems to be expensive and cumbersome for routine clinical use.

*SPF 125 Spectrofluorometer (American Instrument Co., Inc.).* In response to the obvious need for a smaller, more economical, and handier instrument, the American Instrument Company has introduced the SPF 125, which incorporates many of the features of the Spectrophotofluorometer in a

much smaller unit and at a considerably lower price (Fig. 9-6). The instrument is all solid state (except for the detector, of course), and all components are housed in a single cabinet $15 \times 22$ inches deep (front to back) and 14 inches high. The X-Y plotter or printout accessories are not included in this cabinet but may be attached easily.

Resolution of the instrument is 1.5 nm, and sensitivity is very high. A larger thermostated cell compartment is available. Temperature control of the sample is important, since fluorescence, in general, increases with temperature; the heat buildup in this kind of instrument can be appreciable. Manual scanning is available if desired.

The fixed, substitutable slits are 0.1, 0.2, 0.5, 1, 2, and 4 nm. These are mounted on a turret operated by selector knobs on the front panel.

The SPF 125 appears to be a great improvement over the excellent, but awkward, older Spectrophotofluorometer, which it is designed to replace. A flow cell and debubbler, as well as a strip scanner, are available, as are a number of other accessories. This instrument seems to be well adapted to clinical laboratory use and is of research quality.

# CHAPTER 10

# Electrochemistry and ion-selective measurement

## General review of potentiometric measurement

The activity of a wide variety of ions plays essential roles in our physiological well being. Thus, measurement of specific ions is an important diagnostic procedure performed in the clinical chemistry laboratory. Analysis of ionic activity is accomplished through the measurement of a potential. Potentials can and do develop as a result of chemical reactions. This phenomenon is known as *electrochemical activity*. Use of electrochemical reactions in determining activity of ions was first applied to pH measurement, and later the application expanded to include a variety of electrolytes. After a general review of potentiometric measurement, pH, $Po_2$, $Pco_2$, and other ion-specific measurements are presented.

Nearly all conductors of electricity are either metals or electrolytes. The carrier of current will be either electrons or ions. When current passes from metal to electrolyte or from electrolyte to metal, the type of carrier usually suddenly changes, and certain interesting phenomena occur.

Whenever there is an interface between a metal and the ions of that metal in a solution, an electric potential is produced. This potential is called the *electrode potential* of that metal. Nonmetallic elements such as hydrogen also have electrode potentials. It is impossible to assign a specific value to each substance because the absolute value depends on such factors as concentration and temperature, but each is assigned a *relative* electrode

potential using hydrogen as 0.0. Thus, calcium has an electrode potential of $-2.87$, and mercury has $+0.789$ V.

An electrode potential is also produced when different concentrations of an ion are separated by a membrane that is semipermeable to that ion.

To measure an electrode potential, another voltage source (such as another metal/solution interface) is needed against which the first can be measured. Each such electrode arrangement is called a *half-cell*. In such a measuring system, one of these half-cells, or electrodes, is set up in such a way that the potential will be absolute. This electrode is then called a *reference electrode*. It is possible to measure the potential difference between these two electrodes and calculate the concentration of ions in the solution of the first (measuring) electrode (Fig. 10-1).

To clarify this concept, let us look at a specific measuring system. If a silver wire is immersed in a solution of silver chloride, ionization of the silver metal occurs with the formation of silver ions ($Ag^+$) and electrons. An electric potential now exists between the wire and the solution.

If one uses two half-cells, each with a silver wire or foil immersed in a different silver solution, and connects the two solutions through a meter, one can detect a difference in potential between them (Fig. 10-2). Since the potential of each solution depends on the concentration of silver ions in it, the concentration of ions in one solution can be predicted if the value for the other one and the

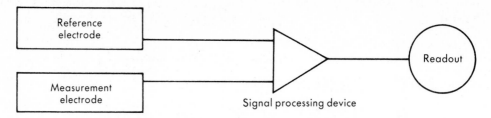

**Fig. 10-1.** Basic functional units of electrode system.

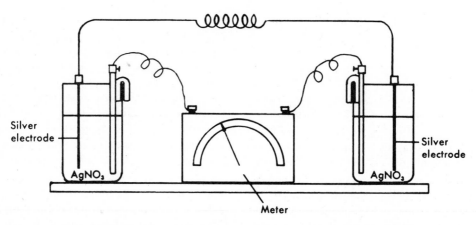

**Fig. 10-2.** Two silver half-cells connected through a meter. If one knows the potential difference and the concentration of silver nitrate in one beaker, one can calculate the other.

difference in potential between them are known. A temperature difference between the two would affect the relationship, however, and there are other minor technical factors involved. In practice one can set up such a system and, by calibrating it against known standards, arrive at a very workable measuring system.

In this process, it is not necessary that the two half-cells contain the same materials as long as two similar potentials are produced. In fact, it is possible to devise a reference electrode that will give a very precise and reproducible potential. Using a reference electrode with a highly reliable potential, it is possible to calibrate the system with known standards and measure the concentration of the ion in question on a precalibrated scale.

Potentiometric methods are based on the quantitative relationship between the potential of a cell as given by the following distribution of potential:

$$E_{cell} = E_{reference} + E_{indicator} + E_{junction}$$

Since the reference and junction potentials are constant, the indicator potential can be determined. The potential of the indicator (measuring electrode) can then be related to concentration.

Electrode systems used in the clinical laboratory have precalibrated readout devices that give results in concentration units. The cell potential is related to concentration through the Nernst equation:

$$E = E° + \frac{2.303 \, RT}{nF} \, \log \frac{[ox]}{[red]}$$

E = Potential of an electrode
E° = Standard electrode potential
R = Molar gas constant (8.314 joules)/(moles) (°K)
T = Absolute temperature (°K) (273° + °C = °K)
n = Number of electrons transferred in the electrode reaction
F = Faraday's constant (96,500 coulombs/equivalent weight)
[ ] = Concentration of oxidized and reduced forms

To simplify this equation, the voltage developed between the reference and measuring electrodes will be:

$$E = KT \log (C_1/C_2)$$

$$K = \text{Constant} \left( \frac{R}{nF} \right)$$

$(C_1/C_2)$ = If either $C_1$ or $C_2$ is known, the concentration of the unknown can be calculated from the measurement of the potential developed

In summary, the potential of a reference electrode is a known constant potential. An indicator electrode is sensitive to the concentration of a specific component of the solution being analyzed. The potential due to the species being measured is obtained by finding the difference between the reference and measuring potentials. By using the Nernst relationship, concentration is calculated. Different types of reference and indicator electrodes are described.

## Reference electrodes

Electrodes that generate a constant potential to be used as a reference include the standard hydrogen electrode, the saturated calomel electrode, and the silver-silver chloride electrode.

*Standard hydrogen electrode.* The standard hydrogen electrode is the international standard but is seldom used for routine work, since more convenient types with reliable calibration buffers are available. These hydrogen electrodes are produced by coating a platinum electrode with platinum black—finely divided particles of platinum. Hydrogen gas is then bubbled around the coated platinum. Although this type of electrode is quite accurate, it is unstable and very awkward to use.

It is still the absolute standard of hydrogen electrodes but is not used routinely on any instruments.

*Saturated calomel electrode.* The saturated calomel electrode is a widely used reference electrode. Its function is based on the reversible reaction:

$$Hg_2Cl_2 + 2e^- \rightleftharpoons 2Hg + 2Cl^-$$

The calomel electrodes contain a nonattackable element, such as platinum, in contact with mercury, mercurous chloride (calomel), and a neutral solution of potassium chloride of known concentration and saturated with calomel. The saturated calomel electrode in which the solution is saturated with potassium chloride (4.2M), is commonly used because it is easy to prepare and maintain. For accurate work the 0.1M or 1.0M electrodes are preferred because they reach their equilibrium potentials more quickly and their potentials depend less on temperature than do the saturated type. Calomel electrodes become unstable at temperatures above 80° C and should be replaced with silver-silver electrodes.

To make an electrical connection between the electrode and the sample solution, some means must be provided that will itself produce a negligible potential and be reproducible. This can be done by means of a salt bridge. The potentials are called *liquid-liquid junction potentials*. A saturated potassium chloride salt bridge is commonly used, since it provides the advantages presented in the following explanation.

Refer to Fig. 10-3, a conceptual diagram of an enlarged section of a liquid-liquid junction. Consider the $A^+$ ions and the $B^-$ ions. Initially there are none of these in the sample solution, but there is a large concentration of them in the salt bridge. These ions, following the laws of thermodynamics, will diffuse from the region of greater concentration to the region of lower concentration. Since the $A^+$ ions are smaller, they will diffuse more quickly than the larger $B^-$ ions, and the result will be that a small positive-negative charge difference (or potential) is established. The same

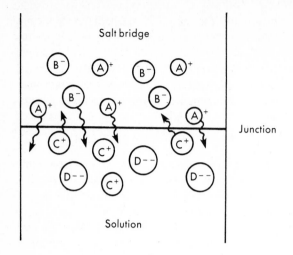

Salt bridge

Junction

Solution

*Fig. 10-3.* Liquid-liquid junction.

process can happen with the $C^+$ and $D^{--}$ ions in the sample diffusing into the salt bridge. The cumulative result, which is the liquid-liquid junction potential, can amount to 20 to 30 mV. This is a large value when one is measuring electrode potentials to a few tenths of a millivolt.

If the hydrated positive ion and the negative ion were the same size, they would diffuse at the same rate, and no potential would be established. Because potassium ions and chloride ions have about the same mobility, potassium chloride is a good compound for use as a salt bridge. This similarity in mobility of the ions results in reducing the junction potential considerably, from the standpoint of the electrode. There is no such choice of ions in the sample solution and no control of this kind to reduce the diffusion of ions from the sample. This diffusion is controlled by having a saturated potassium chloride solution. This results in many ions diffusing from the salt bridge against which the sample ions must diffuse. Diffusion of ions from the sample to the junction is thus reduced so that the junction potential is 1 mV or less. One can then measure fractions of millivolts more accurately.

If the salt concentration around the electrode is different from the salt bridge concentration, an-

other liquid-liquid junction potential is established. For this reason the salt solution in a calomel electrode is usually saturated.

***Silver-silver chloride electrode.*** The silver-silver chloride electrode is a very reproducible electrode. Its operation is based on the reversible reaction:

$$AgCl + e^- \rightleftharpoons Ag + Cl^-$$

The electrode is prepared by electroplating a layer of silver on a platinum wire and then converting the surface silver to silver chloride by electrolysis in hydrochloric acid. The solution surrounding the electrode should be saturated with potassium chloride and silver chloride.

### Indicator electrodes

The term *ion-selective electrode* (ISE) is increasingly used to describe the technology used in instruments for measurement of ions. Evolution of ISEs has resulted in numerous useful electrodes for this application. The ion-selective electrode unit simply consists of a membrane separating a reference solution and reference electrode from a solution to be analyzed. The complexity of ISE design is in the membrane formulation, which determines its ionic selectivity. Several types of ion-selective indicator electrodes are described.

***Glass electrode.*** The glass electrode is a commonly used electrode for measurement of pH. With certain kinds of glass, an electrical potential can develop across a thin film of the glass when solutions of different hydrogen ion concentrations are on opposite sides of the film. A glass electrode consists of a small bulb of special glass and contains on the inside a solution of known hydrogen ion concentration (for example, 0.1N HCl) and an internal reference electrode, usually calomel or silver-silver chloride. The special composition of hydrated glass containing $Na_2O$, $CaO$, $SiO_2$, and perhaps small amounts of other ions makes possible the ion-exchange reaction of hydrogen at the surface of the glass. As a hydrogen ion combines with an oxygen ion within the lattice on the outer glass surface, a hydrogen ion leaves a binding site on the opposite surface. This combined activity on the glass surface maintains the electrical neutrality of the glass while establishing a hydrogen equilibrium and thus producing a potential. Because of the high resistance of the glass, electronic amplification is necessary for measurement of the potential.

When the glass measuring electrode and the calomel electrode are immersed in a solution containing hydrogen ions, the small potential difference between these two half-cells is measured on a very sensitive meter. When the instrument is calibrated against standards and adjusted for temperature effect, the concentration can be read very accurately. A very sophisticated, stable, and sensitive measuring train is of course required. This combination of parts is a *pH meter*.

The pH meter is designed to measure the *effective concentration* of hydrogen ions in a solution. In general terms three parameters are involved in the effective concentration. The first of these is the *actual molar concentration* of hydrogen. The second is the *dissociation constant* of the acid, or the pKa. The third is the *temperature*.

The *pH* is defined as the negative log of the hydrogen ion activity. Water at $25°$ C has 0.0000007 mole of hydrogen per liter. This may be expressed as approximately $10^{-7}$; that is to say, the log of the hydrogen ion concentration is $-7$, and the negative log would be 7. Therefore, the pH of water at $25°$ C is 7. An acid would have a higher concentration of hydrogen ions (as, for example, 0.08 mole per liter), which would represent a pH of about 2. A strong alkali solution such as sodium hydroxide would have a higher concentration of hydroxyl ions and a lower concentration of hydrogen ions. Such a solution might easily have 0.0000000000006 mole per liter of free hydrogen ions and would be said to have a pH of 13. The stronger the acid, the lower is the pH. One may also refer to the pOH or the negative log of the hydroxyl ion concentration. The sum of the pH and the pOH is always 14. Very strong acid solutions, such as some pure acids that are highly ionized,

may have a pH of $-1$. The pOH of such a solution is 15.

*Buffer solutions* have the ability of maintaining their pH when acid or base is added. Buffers are usually made up of weak acids and their conjugated base. The excess hydrogen ions are rendered inactive as they become part of the conjugated base radical and hence un-ionized and inactive.

Buffers have three properties of primary significance. First is their buffer value, which is indicated by the Greek letter *beta* and is also called the *Van Slyke buffer value*. The buffer value indicates the resistance of a buffer to pH change, on the addition of acid or base, and is defined as the amount of completely dissociated acid or base in gram equivalent per liter necessary to cause one unit of pH change. The second property of interest is the dilution value of the buffer, which is defined as the pH change of the buffer on dilution with an equal quantity of pure water. The third property is the temperature stability or the magnitude of change in pH with a change in temperature. Obviously all these values vary with the pH under consideration. In selecting a buffer, the pKa of the buffer system should be close to the pH desired; this means that the pH should be close to the flat portion of the buffer titration curve.

This brief review of pH and buffers may be of some help in the discussion of the mechanics of pH by meters.

Since the early twentieth century, various workers have reported that a difference in electric potential could be measured between two solutions of different pH separated by a thin glass membrane. All the measuring devices available, however, had such a high internal resistance that the amplitude of the current produced could not be measured. Around 1930 an amplifier system was devised that allowed the pH meter, as it is known now, to develop.

When a calomel reference electrode is used, the potential produced by hydrogen ions is quite constant, amounting to 59.15 mV per pH unit when measured at $25°$ C. As previously mentioned, temperature has considerable effect, Each degree of temperature increase raises the cell's output by about 0.2 mV.

For convenience both the glass measuring electrode and the reference electrode are sometimes built into a single glass housing and called a *combination electrode*. Combination electrodes are convenient to handle and can be used where a very small amount of fluid sample is available. No significant accuracy is lost.

It is immediately apparent that there are a number of interfaces in this total pH-measuring chain. One must assume that the potential at each of these interfaces is constant in all situations when one is making measurements.

To measure the flow of electrons between the two half-cells, a rather sophisticated electrometer had to be devised.

If a difference in potential of 59.15 mV represents one pH unit, one must then have a device that can measure a voltage change of 1.2 mV to indicate a change of 0.02 pH unit. When the many imponderables, such as the various junctions in our measuring train, the temperature effect on each of these, and variables in electrical components, are considered, one becomes aware of how complicated this process is.

Resistance of this circuit is between 50,000 and 200,000,000 $\Omega$. The tiny potential discussed is extremely hard to measure. For this reason a device similar to a vacuum tube voltmeter is used. Because of the high resistance of the electrode system, a circuit that will measure very high impedance is required.

When very alkaline solutions were tested with glass electrodes, it was found that pH measurements were strongly affected by the presence of sodium and some other alkali ions. By changing the composition of the glass, this kind of error could be minimized. At the same time it was found that glass electrodes could be developed which, under proper conditions, could actually measure sodium ion concentration. We shall return to this idea presently. When measuring very high pH values, some small sodium correction may be necessary. This correction is usually stated by the manufacturer.

One of the first pH meters developed for laboratory use was the Beckman Model G. A few of these instruments are still in use. The meter was housed in a wooden case with an access door in the front of the cabinet to hold the electrodes. Reproducibility was not outstanding, and sensitivity was not particularly high, but the meter was a pioneering, workable system.

A "battery" was used as a voltage reference for the Model G, a galvanometer was null balanced by a slide wire as the reference, and the amplified unknown currents were compared. The resistance imposed by the slide wire, to null the two currents, was indicative of the pH, and calibration was established by use of standards. A resistance was introduced to compensate for temperature; and a zero adjust was provided.

Although this sort of system might be considered somewhat primitive today, it was a landmark accomplishment at the time it was introduced. The system is still quite adequate if high accuracy is not needed.

Modern pH meters are, of course, quite different instruments. Electrode design has progressed to the point that nearly any type of configuration for any sort of use can be obtained. Tiny electrodes can be inserted into veins, and rugged electrodes are made for pushing deep into underground sewer lines. Very small, trouble-free combination electrodes are available for routine laboratory measurements in nearly any sort of container or condition. We shall presently look at the anaerobic, temperature-controlled pH electrode used for blood pH measurement.

Electronic amplifiers have also been miniaturized and made more rugged and reliable so that tough, accurate systems can be made quite small and convenient. Ammeters have largely given way to electronic digital displays such as LEDs, and measurement to three decimal places is common.

***Liquid ion–selective electrode.*** Liquid ion–selective electrodes have been developed that use liquid ion-exchange resins or electroactive substances for electrode membranes. The liquid electroactive substances are allowed to fill the pores of a porous membrane by capillary action or are bound by other forces, such as electrostatic action, in a membrane. The external and internal solutions then develop potentials on the surfaces of the electroactive substances in the membrane in much the same way that the glass membrane in a glass electrode does. The choice of electroactive substance is an important factor in determination of the ionic selectivity of the electrode. Neutral ion-carriers such as nonactin or valinomycin are used in ISEs for $K^+$, $Ba^{++}$, $Na^+$, $Ca^{++}$, and $NH_4^+$. $Ca^{++}$- and $Mg^{++}$-sensitive ISEs use phosphoric acid esters. $NO_3^-$, $Cl^-$, and other anion determinations are obtained with ISEs using membranes with electroactive substances of substituted arsonium, phosphonium, and ammonium salts.

*Precipitate-impregnated membrane electrode.* Once the ion-exchange mechanism of the glass electrode was established, electrochemists started to investigate ion-exchange membranes with the hope of devising an anion-sensitive electrode. In this type of electrode, a slightly soluble salt containing the anion to be measured is immobilized in a silicone rubber matrix. For example, an electrode that is to be chloride sensitive would be constructed by forming a silicone rubber membrane that contains about 50% weight-to-weight silver chloride and silicone rubber. The silver chloride particles are generally about 5 to 10 $\mu$m in diameter, and are in actual physical contact throughout the silicone rubber. Such an electrode functions because of the selective permeability of the membrane. This type of electrode can be used for measurement of anions such as chloride, bromide, and iodide.

*Solid-state electrode.* The solid-state electrode is a second type of anion-sensitive electrode, which functions on the same principle as the precipitate-impregnated electrode. The active membrane portion of the solid-state electrode consists of an inorganic single crystal doped with a rare earth. For example, the solid-state fluoride electrode has a crystalline lanthanum fluoride membrane that has been doped with europium (II) to lower its electrical resistance and facilitate ionic charge transport. This type electrode has been commercially produced for $Br^-$, $Cd^{++}$, $Cl^-$,

$Cu^{++}$, $CN^-$, $F^-$, $I^-$, $Pb^{++}$, $Ag^+$, $S^{--}$, $Na^+$, and $SCN^-$ ion measurements.

A membrane produced by Beckman appears to be solid but is not solid state. It is lipid in structure. The true solid membranes are crystallographic in structure, whereas the firm lipid structure is due to close spatial orientation of molecules. Lipids provide a medium in which electrostatic forces function. An ISE for $K^+$ consists of diphenyl ether, valinomycin, lecithin, and Nujol, and an $NH_4^+$-sensitive electrode is prepared with bromodiphyl, nonactin, lecithin, and Nujol.

*Oxygen-sensing electrode.* The anode and cathode are separated from the sample by a gas-permeable membrane, polyethylene. A small potential between the anode and cathode causes an oxidation-reduction reaction with the oxygen diffusing through the membrane. A current is generated proportionately to the partial pressure of oxygen in the sample. Since oxygen diffuses instantaneously, sensor response is fast.

*$PCO_2$-sensing electrode.* A standard glass pH electrode has been modified to measure the concentration of carbon dioxide in aqueous solution. The electrode is placed in contact with the solution being analyzed for carbon dioxide content. Carbon dioxide can pass through the Teflon membrane because Teflon is highly permeable to the gas. After a period of a few seconds, the solution on the inside of the Teflon membrane is at equilibrium with the solution on the outside. The solution on the inside of the Teflon membrane contains sodium bicarbonate. Thus, the carbon dioxide concentration has a large effect on the concentration of hydrogen ions in solution. Hydrogen ions can easily permeate a cellophane membrane that separates the reaction chamber from the glass electrode. The hydrogen ions are then detected by the glass electrode. In this way the carbon dioxide concentration effects the pH, and the pH can then be measured directly.

Blood pH and the partial pressures of oxygen and carbon dioxide have become significant parameters in diagnosis and treatment. Many advances in the diagnosis and treatment of acidosis, electrolyte imbalance, emphysema, and cardio-

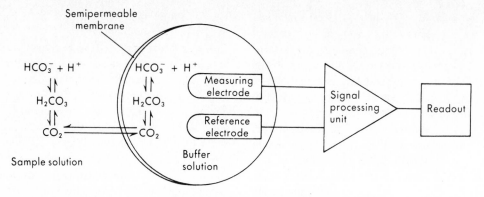

*Fig. 10-4.* Principle of $P_{CO_2}$ electrode system.

vascular disease have been possible because of the improvement in instrumentation in this general area.

Reference is sometimes made to pH, $P_{O_2}$, and $P_{CO_2}$ as if they were comparable terms of measurement. The term *pH* has been discussed earlier, and you will remember that it relates to the effective concentration (*puissance* or "force" in French) of hydrogen ions. The capital P of $P_{CO_2}$ and $P_{O_2}$ does not denote effective concentration but partial pressure.

*Partial pressure* simply refers to the part of the total gas pressure (atmospheric pressure, for example) that is contributed by the gas under consideration. To calculate the partial pressure of a known gas concentration, take the following steps:

1. Determine ambient barometric pressure in millimeters of mercury (mm Hg).
2. Subtract the vapor pressure of water at the temperature of measurement. At 37° C this is 47 mm.
3. Multiply the remainder by the percentage or decimal fraction of the gas under consideration. The product will be the partial pressure (P).

The technique of measuring pH has been previously discussed. Measurement of $P_{CO_2}$ is accomplished in the same manner, but the details of the electrode require some explanation (Fig. 10-4). The blood sample is separated from a combination pH electrode system by a membrane.

Carbon dioxide can pass through this membrane from the blood sample into an electrolyte solution, which perfuses the sensing tip of the electrode. As the carbon dioxide is absorbed by the electrolyte, carbonic acid is formed, altering the pH. This pH change is a linear function of the carbon dioxide content of the blood, and it can obviously be measured by the electronics of the pH meter on an appropriate scale. This arrangement may be called a *Severinghaus electrode* (Fig. 10-5). The electrolyte solution perfusing its tip makes contact with both measuring and reference electrode elements. The carbon dioxide electrode in various systems may differ in physical arrangement from the electrode pictured in Fig. 10-5 but will function in the same way.

Measurement of the partial pressure of oxygen requires a somewhat different approach. The $P_{O_2}$ electrode works on a polarographic principle.

The fact that nearly all conductors are metallic or electrolytic in nature was mentioned earlier. When electricity passes from a metal to a solution of electrolyte or vice versa, the type of carrier changes abruptly, and either an oxidation or a reduction takes place. In the case of oxygen in solution, oxygen is reduced with the release of electrons, and the current increases as a direct function of the electrons released. Hence the change in current is an analog of the oxygen concentration in the solution.

This electrode consists of a platinum cathode

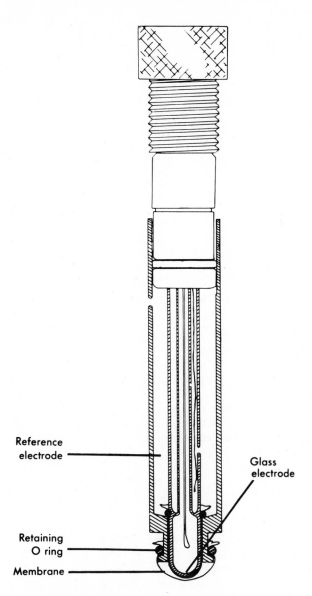

Reference electrode

Glass electrode

Retaining O ring

Membrane

*Fig. 10-5.* Diagram of a Severinghaus $P_{CO_2}$ electrode. (Courtesy Instrumentation Laboratory, Inc.)

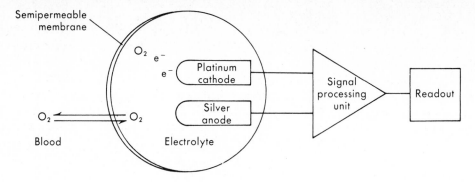

*Fig. 10-6.* Principle of Po$_2$ electrode system.

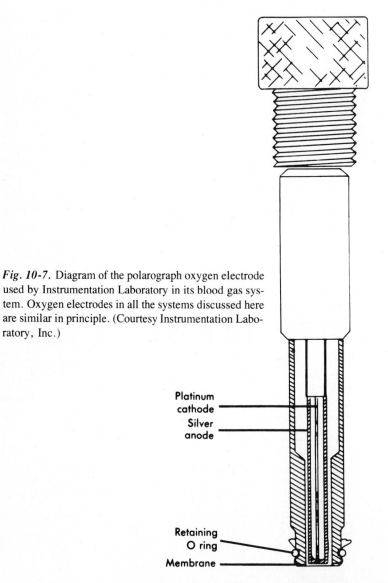

*Fig. 10-7.* Diagram of the polarograph oxygen electrode used by Instrumentation Laboratory in its blood gas system. Oxygen electrodes in all the systems discussed here are similar in principle. (Courtesy Instrumentation Laboratory, Inc.)

with a tubular silver anode around it. The two are insulated from each other and make contact only through a drop of electrolyte at the electrode's tip. A gas-permeable membrane holds this drop at the tip of the electrode and separates it from the blood to be measured. Oxygen in the blood diffuses across the membrane into the electrolyte, where it is reduced and measured (Fig. 10-6).

Measurement of the gain or loss of electrons in a chemical reaction, by electrical means as previously described, is called *polarography*. Polarographic apparatus is widely used in analytical chemistry but has seldom been employed in clinical laboratory methods until recently. The very tiny change in current sensed by the $Po_2$ electrode is amplified and measured by a sensitive electrometer against a reference current provided by a reference cell or Zener source. The pH meter's ammeter can be used for actually reading this signal on an appropriate scale. A polarographic electrode is the usual means of measuring $Po_2$ in the systems described here. A cut-away view of a $Po_2$ electrode is shown in Fig. 10-7.

*Enzyme electrode.* Enzyme electrodes have been developed to extend the application of ISEs to the measurement of nonionic compounds. In enzyme ISEs an intermediary reaction is used to generate ions that can be directly related to the concentration of the compounds of interest. Enzymes are perfectly suited to catalyze the production of ions from a compound such as glucose or blood urea nitrogen. Enzyme electrodes have been used specifically for glucose and BUN analysis; therefore, these two applications are described.

Generally, an enzyme electrode is made by polymerizing a gelatinous membrane of immobilized enzyme directly over an ISE. A specific glucose enzyme electrode is made by polymerizing a gelatinous membrane of immobilized glucose oxidase over a polarographic oxygen electrode. When the enzyme electrode is in contact with a glucose-containing solution, the glucose and oxygen diffuse into the immobilized glucose oxidase layer. Oxygen diffuses through a plastic membrane to the oxygen electrode where it is detected. The polarographic electrode is used to measure the oxygen consumed when glucose oxidase reacts with glucose in the sample solution. Therefore, decrease in the amount of oxygen detected by the oxygen electrode is related to an increase in the amount of glucose present. This type electrode can also be used to detect the rate of reduction of oxygen rather than the absolute reduction and to relate it to glucose concentration.

In another approach to glucose analysis, glucose oxidase acting on the glucose produces hydrogen peroxide, which is measured by a polarographic electrode. It is the level of peroxide production, rather than the reaction rate, that is proportional to glucose concentration.

An enzyme electrode can be used for the determination of urea. The electrode consists of a membrane containing immobilized urease over a $NH_4^+$-selective glass electrode. The urea in the sample diffuses into the enzyme-containing membrane where it is hydrolyzed to $NH_4^+$. $NH_4^+$ is measured by the glass electrode and is related directly to urea concentration.

*Microelectrodes.* Efforts are being directed to miniaturize electrodes to accommodate measurement with small amounts of solution. A creative design for a microelectrode is the combination of ISEs with transistors. In one approach an ion-selective membrane is placed over the gate of a MOSFET (metal oxide–semiconductor field effect transistor). Such a microelectrode has been constructed with a MOSFET using a $K^+$-selective membrane. When the electrode is in contact with the test solution, $K^+$ activity at the gate results in a current drain that can be monitored and related directly to $K^+$ concentration. Initially, poor stability of the measured signal limited the use of this microelectrode, but the advantages of small size and direct electronic handling of the signal are incentive enough to rectify this problem. Microelectrodes will become popular with improved designs that give the performance required for quantitative analysis.

## Thermal conductivity detection

Thermal conductivity detection is used for analysis of carbon dioxide in an instrument that is designated Model E 100 (Ericsen Instruments). This ingenious instrument is designed to detect only carbon dioxide by using an analytical principle not previously discussed in this chapter. When an electric current is passed through a resistance wire, some electrical energy is lost as heat energy, and thus the temperature of the wire increases. As the wire gets hotter, resistance, in turn, increases. The heat produced is radiated into the air or surrounding gas and dissipates at a rate determined by the composition of the gas. Thus, heat would dissipate more quickly in carbon dioxide than in helium, for example. As the heat dissipates, the temperature, and hence the resistance, of the wire decreases. A *thermal conductivity (TC) detector* is a measuring device set up to sense the resistance change that occurs when the gas surrounding the resistance element changes. In most configurations the sensor is one arm of a Wheatstone bridge, which is a configuration of four resistors set up to very accurately measure resistance.

In the Carbon Dioxide Analyzer, carbon dioxide is displaced from the serum sample using lactic acid. The released gas is then forced from the reaction chamber by fluid displacement into the sensing chamber. Here the displaced carbon dioxide serves to change the relative percentage of carbon dioxide in room air, and this is sensed by the thermal conductivity detector.

The instrument is semiautomated. A sample is injected into the reaction chamber and the cover closed. The start button is depressed, initiating a mixing sequence. Reagent fills the chamber, forcing the carbon dioxide into the TC detector. The electronic circuit converts the sensed change in resistance to millimols per liter, and the result is displayed. Recycling the instrument flushes the sample and prepares the instrument for a new sample. A 100 $\mu$l sample is required, and the test cycle requires less than a minute.

## Coulometric titration

Several chloride titrators have been produced that work on the coulometric principle. If a carefully controlled current is passed between two silver electrodes in an ionic solution, silver ions will be released by ionization at one electrode. If chloride ions are in the solution, these will combine with the released silver ions to produce insoluble silver chloride. The chloride titrator makes use of this idea. A silver-detecting electrode and reference half-cell are included in the system to sense the excess of free silver ions when the chloride is used up. When silver is detected, the current to the silver-releasing electrode is discontinued. If the amperage of the ionizing current and the time it was flowing are known, the coulombs that passed can be calculated. Faraday's law states that the ionization produced when an electric current is passed from a metal into an electrolyte depends only on the coulombs passing through the current. Hence one can calculate the ions of silver released by ionization, which will exactly equal the ions of chloride that were present in the solution.

## Electrolyte system

Flame photometry, as has been seen, presents a number of problems, and the maintenance of flame photometers provides many operational headaches and safety hazards. A search for safer, more accurate, and less cumbersome ways of determining sodium and potassium has led many companies to examine electrochemical methods. Since chloride and carbon dioxide determinations are nearly always ordered along with sodium and potassium, several companies have sought methods of combining all four tests into one instrument. Methods other than electrochemistry are used in some electrolyte systems.

An example of an electrolyte system currently available is the IL 508/504. The IL System 508 is a microprocessor-controlled multichannel electrolyte and chemical analyzer. It has a central console, an electrolytes section (to the right of console), a chemistry section (to the left), and a counter work space. System 504 consists of the above, with electrolyte or chemistry section only.

Sample cups in racks of 10 are placed in the sample tray where the racks are fed forward to a sampling position. Computer-controlled mechanisms then distribute the sample, add diluent and reagents, and deliver the mixtures to measuring transducers. Tests are run at a rate of 100 per hour.

A keyboard, in conjunction with the CRT screen, allows two-way communication between the operator and the minicomputer. Patient identification along with the lists of tests for that sample are keyed-in by the operator. Tests are carried out automatically after instructions for an entire batch of samples have been keyed-in.

The sodium/potassium module utilizes ion-selective electrodes. The sodium determination employs a sodium glass electrode in conjunction with a reference electrode. For potassium an elec-trode with a neutral carrier membrane, valino-mycin, is used in conjunction with a reference electrode. The chloride is determined colorimet-rically at 525 nm, measuring the absorbance of the ferric thiocyanate complex resulting from a mercuric thiocyanate reaction.

The $TCO_2$ module incorporates a unique application of traditional manometric procedures (Van Slyke or Natelson), patent pending. Sample and mild lactic acid are mixed in a controlled-volume syringe. Released carbon dioxide adds pressure to the gas phase of the syringe contents. This added pressure is directly measured by a pressure transducer.

Calibrations for each channel are performed automatically or can be called up via the keyboard. The calibration fluids are internal. Quality control can be carried out by running standards as samples.

# CHAPTER 11

# Separation techniques

## General principle

Early in the twentieth century a Russian botanist by the name of Tswett worked at separating plant pigments and devised a system very similar to the paper chromatography that is in use today. Since he worked primarily with colored solutions, he suggested the name *chromatography* and the term has persisted even though many of the separations commonly done today have nothing to do with color.

Chromatographic separation is accomplished by subjecting a mixture of components to two opposing forces. One of these forces tends to move particles in one direction while the other tends to restrain this movement or oppose it. Let us consider *ascending-paper chromatography*, for example. If a sheet of filter paper is suspended above a dish containing phenol so that the lower edge of the paper is in the solution, the paper will act as a wick, and the phenol will gradually rise in the paper by capillary action. If a mixture of two components is placed on the paper slightly above the fluid level in the dish, the flow of phenol will have a tendency to wash the components upward while the texture of the paper tends to restrain them. The result is that the smaller molecules are washed along fairly easily while the larger molecules are held back. Over a period of time a definite separation occurs.

Components that have been separated in this manner can be identified with fair certainty by their $R_F$ values, or the distance each has traveled relative to the moving front of the solvent used. In complex mixtures the $R_F$ values of all the substances in the mixture are compared.

*Thin-layer chromatography* is a varient of chromatography that has made a large contribution to separation techniques during the past few years. A gel preparation is applied to a glass plate or film and allowed to dry. This very thin gel layer is used as the support medium for the separation of unknown materials. The technique is a valuable one, and there is a great deal of literature available on the subject. It is, however, outside the general scope of this book.

## Electrophoresis

The technique of electrophoresis is similar in many ways to chromatography. In electrophoresis the *impelling force* is an *electric potential* that tends to move electrically charged particles toward the negative or the positive pole, depending on their electric charge. The difference in $R_F$ value of various components depends principally on the difference in their electric charge and on their size. The *retarding force* is frictional and is influenced by the porosity and general architecture of the absorbent material.

In electrophoresis a phenomenon known as *electroosmosis* occurs. When an electric current is conducted through a capillary filled with fluid, there is a tendency for the fluid to be displaced toward one of the electrodes. Other factors being equal, the larger the current imposed, the larger will be the flow of liquid toward the electrode. Porous material might be thought of as a collection of capillaries of various diameters, and the phenomenon of electroosmosis occurs in them also. This force may act to either impel or retard the migration of a material being separated, depending on the direction of the electroosmotic current relative to the direction of migration. It is a factor that has considerable influence in this type of separation.

Electrophoresis is especially practical for the separation of macromolecular substances such as proteins and lipids, although it is applicable to many other substances as well. In routine clinical testing the various protein substances in human serum are separated and quantitated, enzymes are separated and identified, and various hemoglobin fractions are identified. The isolation and quantitation of lipoproteins is also of practical value.

Enzymes such as lactic acid dehydrogenase and creatinine phosphokinase are composed of protein molecules. Various fractions (isoenzymes) of these enzymes can be identified with organic functions within the body. These fractions vary in molecular size and electric charge and can be separated by electrophoresis. One of the important uses of electrophoresis in recent times has been the fractionation and quantitation of various isoenzymes. This technique is of special value in differentiating coronary disease from various other conditions that can cause an elevation of enzymes.

*Immunoelectrophoresis* has become an important diagnostic tool. In this variation, serum proteins are separated by electrophoresis. Specific antisera are spotted near to various zones in the gelatinous matrix, and the interactions of antisera and protein are observed. In this way specific protein fractions can be identified and roughly quantitated. The antisera may be placed in slits or small wells in the gel at a position and distance that have proved to be most advantageous. The technique is not difficult to perform, but the reading and evaluation are technically complex and beyond the scope of our discussion. The diagnostic information that can be obtained can be of considerable diagnostic importance.

The principal equipment for electrophoretic separation consists of a cell, in which the migration and separation occur, and a power supply that provides the electric charge to impel the particles to be separated.

*Power supply.* Typically the power supply must be able to convert line voltage into the required 100 to 500 V of direct current and provide 100 mA or so, depending on the system. The current must be nearly ripple free, and random variations of more than 0.1% would be quite undesirable. Control of the voltage produced is usually by a potentiometer, and meters are used to indicate the voltage and measure the amperage. Many economical and adequate power supplies for this application are commercially available. The quality of the separation obtained depends on the quality of the current provided. Newer power supplies are all solid state, trouble free, and convenient.

Some of the more common problems with power supplies have been transformer failure, short-circuited capacitors, and resistors that have either short-circuited or opened. When a transformer fails, it usually short-circuits and overheats, with considerable smoke and odor. When the voltmeter needle vibrates rapidly, it may be that a capacitor has short-circuited. However, a capacitor may short-circuit without such a manifestation. Faulty resistors can sometimes be located by visual inspection. Potentiometers often become defective and cease to provide smooth control of voltage. Switches are always subject to failure. As with all electronic equipment, moisture is quite detrimental. Electronic components have improved to the point that component failure of this sort is no longer a very important problem, however.

*Cell.* There are many types of electrophoresis cells in use. Several requirements dictate their general design. The paper or membrane must conduct the current from one end to the other without contacting any conductor, which would shunt the current elsewhere or dissipate it. The membrane must be moist at all times, but fluid must not be allowed to pool or flow through it. The electrodes should not directly contact the membrane or be too close to it, since breakdown products from the electrodes might contaminate the material being separated. Temperature should be relatively constant. Vibration and other physical disturbance should be minimal. If heat is generated in appreciable amounts, some system of cooling must be effected. The best arrangement from a theoretical point of view is to have the membrane horizontal so that there is no gravitational effect on the liquid in it. Some cells have a flat surface on which the membrane can lie.

Originally filter paper was the principal absorbent or support medium in general use. There was some tendency for components, notably proteins, to adhere to the fibers and produce the effect known as tailing, in which the separation is not clear-cut and some of the component lags behind the trailing edge of its zone. Also, variation in the pore size of the paper does not permit the sharpness of separation that might be desired.

Various types of gelatinous films, membranes, and cellular acetate strips are now used in place of paper. These provide much more uniform migration and sharper and faster separation. Migration times and distances can be drastically reduced and sharp, readable zones produced. These media readily absorb contaminants from the fingers and other surfaces; they should always be handled with forceps, and care should be taken to avoid contamination. Wetting of the membrane should be done carefully to avoid entrapment of bubbles of air in the fine porous structure. When these precautions are taken, very sharp zones can be obtained, and tailing is almost nonexistent. Frequently materials that would have migrated as a single zone on filter paper strips can be separated on cellulose acetate. The migration time that would have required 15 hours now takes 30 minutes. Membranes in use include *polyacrylamides, polyacetates, cellulose nitrate,* and *agarose film.*

The solvent used in the electrophoresis cell is of considerable importance. Changes in the pH of the system affect the mobility of charged particles by altering the actual electric charge. Ionic strength affects the electroosmotic current through the paper or membrane. Substances such as the *glycols* are added at times to reduce evaporation from the strips, especially when high voltages are used and there is evolution of considerable heat. *Urea* and other substances have been added to suppress formation of various complexes of the solute and the support material. Other materials have been added to reduce the amount of solvent that can be absorbed into the support material, in an effort to minimize the effect of electroosmosis.

In most cases the materials that are separated cannot be seen on the electrophoresis strips. The most common means of recognition and quantitation use stained strips. Techniques for staining will vary with the material in question and the choice of stain. Usually the protein materials are fixed by immersion in methyl alcohol. After the staining is performed, the strips are washed several times and dried. A typical electrophoresis routine for serum protein on cellulose acetate, as recommended by Beckman, is reproduced in Fig. 11-1, along with an explanation of the steps involved.

## Densitometers

Densitometers are instruments designed to read the density, or concentration, of material deposited along the electrophoresis strip. A densitometer is very similar to a colorimeter except that light is passing through the electrophoresis strip instead of through a cuvette or test tube.

Most densitometers are essentially double-beam recording colorimeters. The sample beam is focused to a pinpoint of light that scans the migrated material as the strip is fed through the densitometer. As in double-beam spectrophotometry, the reference beam scans an area of the strip where no material is deposited, and the reference detectors pass their respective signals to amplifiers. The difference between the amplified reference and sample signal is used to drive a recorder, which draws a tracing. This tracing represents the quantity of material deposited along the membrane during its migration.

Appropriate colored filters are used to enhance the absorbance of light by the dyed material on

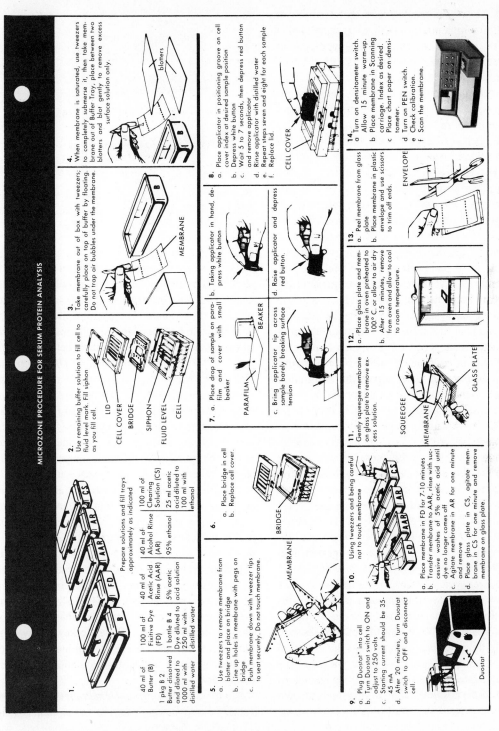

*Fig. 11-1.* Typical electrophoresis technique, showing sampling, separation, staining, and quantitation. Essentially all systems in common use are similar in these details. (Courtesy Beckman Instruments, Inc.)

the strip. Most densitometers have the capability of adjusting the light beam to scan a larger or smaller area. Modern densitometers often use photodiodes or phototransistors as detectors.

Early densitometers used a mechanical integrator to calculate the area under each peak of the recording. Electronic integrators are now used. The amplitude and duration of the current that drives the pen can be used to calculate the amount of material deposited in each zone along the membrane. The change in current at the end of each peak can also be used to sense the "valley" between recorded peaks so that each zone of deposited material can be separately measured. By relating the measurement of each zone to the total for the strip, the densitometer can report the percent of the total that each zone represents.

Some newer densitometers are designed to detect and measure the material on electrophoresis strips using fluorescence or reflectance photometry, as well as the more conventional transmittance just described.

***ACD-15 Automatic Computing Densitometer (Gelman Instrument Co.).*** This instrument has a solid-state voltage regulator that supplies power to a tungsten exciter lamp. This light is focused on the entrance slit of the grating monochromator. A wavelength span from 475 to 700 nm is available. Monochromatic light leaving the exit slit is in a 0.5 × 3 mm beam that passes through the membrane and falls on a silicone phototransistor, which measures the transmitted light energy.

The signal from the phototransistor is electronically adjusted to compensate for the light absorbed by the clear membrane (automatic zeroing) and is then fed to a log converter, which effectively converts the electrical information to units of concentration in conformity to Beer's law. This information is then presented to the recorder, where a heated stylus traces the pattern. Simultaneously the instrument can process the electrical signal through an A-to-D converter and print out the percentage each peak (fraction) represents of the total. If the absolute value of the total is entered into the instrument keyboard by the operator, the absolute value of each peak is calculated.

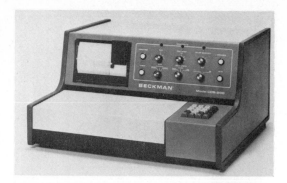

**Fig. 11-2.** Model CDS-200 Clinical Densitometer. (Courtesy Clinical Instruments Division, Beckman Instruments, Inc.)

The system is designed to accommodate nearly any kind of media, including cellulose acetate, agars, starches, paper, and gels. A scan is completed in 15 seconds. The operator may define the peak areas to be considered, or the instrument will automatically sense the separation between peaks.

***CDS-200 Clinical Densitometer (Beckman Instruments, Inc.).*** This is typical of newer densitometers (Fig. 11-2). It is designed for reading most electrophoresis strips by transmittance densitometry, certain other separations by fluorescence, and thin-layer chromatography plates by reflectance photometry. A tungsten lamp is used as a source. There are four interference filters at 520, 550, 570, and 600 nm. Two slits are provided. A photodiode is used for transmittance measurement, but for reflectance and fluorescence a photomultiplier tube is the detector.

A small microprocessor performs simple calculations such as reducing concentrations to percentages and calculating area under a curve. A keyboard allows entry of patient and sample data, date, time, or other information that can be expressed in seven digits. Separate keys allow suppression of extraneous peaks, eliminate unwanted delimiting marks, and allow calculation of area under a curve.

***Model 750 Scanning Densitometer/Fluorometer/TLC (Corning Scientific Instruments)*** (Fig. 11-3). The Corning line of densitometers was

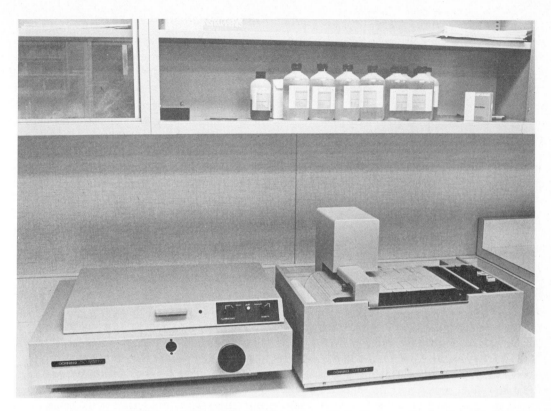

**Fig. 11-3.** Model 750 Scanning Densitometer/Fluorometer/TLC. (Courtesy Corning Scientific Instruments.)

previously designed and manufactured by the Clifford Instrument Co. Since acquiring the Clifford Co., Corning has done much design work on these basically good instruments. The Model 750 can employ transmission, reflectance, fluorescence, or fluorescence quenching and can accept almost any type of electrophoresis or thin-layer chromatography media. The grating monochromator can provide a wavelength range of 400 to 700 nm. White light and light at 356 nm or 254 nm is also available. A variety of exit slits is available, ranging from 0.2 mm wide to 10 mm high.

*Auto Scanner Flur-Vis (Helena Laboratories).* This instrument also provides fluorescent capabilities. In place of a monochromator, however, a series of optical filters is provided. Many of the automatic features of the previously discussed instruments are lacking on this model. The price is accordingly lower, and the operator has both the control of and the responsibility for many functions. The operator's manual is carefully and clearly presented.

*TG 2980 Scanning Densitometer (Transidyne General Corp.).* This very sophisticated instrument provides transmission and fluorescence modes. The monochromator provides a wavelength range of 350 to 750 nm and a variety of exit slits. A nine-stage photomultiplier is used as a detector, and an 8 nm band width is provided. Six different protocols are programmed into the instrument and made available by push button. Wavelength, gain, mode, scan speed, and slit can all be preselected and actuated with one control.

Transidyne General manufactures a number of models, including some that are sold under other companies' labels. This instrument is of unusually high quality and design, providing almost every capability that most hospital laboratories are likely to need.

• • •

All systems discussed provide a full line of power supplies, cells, single- and multiple-sample applicators, and reagents. There are also many other companies providing electrophoresis equipment. Basically these systems are very similar in capabilities and approach, and those presented seem to be an adequate representation of the field.

*Antigen Crossover Electrophoresis System (Hyland, Division of Travenol Laboratories, Inc.).* This is a small, special-purpose electrophoresis system designed specifically for the detection of hepatitis-associated antigen (HAA). The patient's serum is placed in one well of a negatively charged gel plate. The antibody to HAA is placed in another well. Under the influence of the current, the antibody is displaced toward the cathode while the antigen, if any, moves toward the anode. A distinct zone of precipitation can be observed in positive cases after 30 to 45 minutes.

A number of companies manufacture small, special-purpose units of this sort.

*Quality control of electrophoresis equipment.* Certain steps should be taken to ensure proper functioning of electrophoresis equipment. Cells should be properly cleaned. Power cords, switches, and electrical controls should be checked for wear or damage. Voltage applied to cells should be regularly checked. Reagents must be correctly prepared and labeled and properly stored. Membranes should be properly stored and handled to avoid deterioration or contamination. Controls must be included with each run and results compared with their assay values. If tracings do not show clear separation into sharp zones free of trailing or background, the run should be rejected.

## Gas chromatography

Gas chromatography is similar to column chromatography in many respects. In the simplest sort of system the material to be separated is in the form of a gas, and the substrate is porous material that is able to mechanically retard the advance of larger molecules in the material. The impelling force, pushing the sample forward, is flow of an inert gas through the column.

Although the basic idea of gas chromatography is quite simple, the devices that are in use may be complicated and may vary considerably in all details. The basic ingredients of a gas chromatograph are (1) a *carrier gas system* to carry the sample forward, (2) a *column* packed with some sort of material to selectively impede the forward movement of the sample, and (3) some means of sensing and measuring the sample as it passes a point in the system.

Many of the samples to be analyzed are in a liquid state. These may be volatilized by raising the temperature. In order to accomplish this, the column may be housed in an *oven* whose temperature can be accurately controlled. The signal from most types of detectors is too small to measure conveniently without some amplification; therefore an *electrometer,* with some type of measuring device, is required. Let us consider these parts of the gas chromatograph in detail.

*Carrier gas system.* Any inert gas may be used to carry the sample forward. Technical considerations may determine which gas will be used. Helium is probably the most widely used, although nitrogen is somewhat cheaper. Other gases in common use are argon and hydrogen. The flow of the gas must be extremely consistent because any change in rate will vary the $R_F$ values of the materials being separated and cause unstable and unreliable results. The flow of gas acts as a background value to the detectors, and a constant baseline cannot be achieved if there is any fluctuation in the carrier gas. When the flow rate is increased, the material moves forward faster, and the $R_F$ value, measured in seconds or minutes, is shortened. When the flow rate is too high, the migration becomes ragged, and the sample is presented to a detector as a less compact bolus, during a longer period. Thus, the corresponding recorder peak is lower, wider, and less sharply defined. Usually a combination of at least two valves is used to control the carrier gas flow. A fairly common arrangement uses a two-stage regulator on the tank of gas and one or more needle valves. It is extremely important that the gas be very dry. It is usually passed through a filter of desiccant or a molecular sieve to remove moisture and other contaminants. On some systems several feet of stainless steel capillary tubing, before the column, serve as a resistance to reduce pressure and stabilize the flow rate. Metal and glass are generally used throughout, since rubber may be a source of contamination. Also, since helium is a very small molecule, it tends to pass through the walls of ordinary rubber tubing.

*Column.* Column technology has become an exact and complicated science. Only the principal considerations are discussed here. The column may be made of stainless steel or glass and may vary considerably in length and diameter. A column of $1/8$-inch diameter is most widely used. However, when the system is to separate large quantities of material for commercial use or further study, a larger column may be desirable. Also a capillary column, which contains no packing material but a coating on the walls of the tube, may be used.

Materials with similar $R_F$ values may require a long migration before they separate adequately, whereas easily separated materials may require only a short time. Most columns in routine clinical use are more than 18 inches and less than 10 feet in length.

The columns are generally packed with a porous material to help retard the progress of the sample. This material is called the *solid phase, stationary phase,* or *column support.* Crushed fire brick, diatomaceous earth, and molecular sieve are examples of commonly used solid-phase materials. There are many others. The size of the particles of material is spoken of as the *mesh.* Granular material that is 40 to 50 mesh will pass through a screen that has 40 wires per inch but will not pass through one with 50 wires to the inch. For various situations solid-phase packing of 60 to 120 mesh may be used. The smaller the particles, the more tightly the material will pack and the slower will be the passage of gas through it; also, the more will be the retarding action on the migrating sample.

The material used as a solid phase is commonly coated with a viscous liquid to help retard the progress of the sample. This material must be stable at high temperatures, and must be effective in the differential partitioning of the sample components. It must be a good solvent for the sample components and must not react with them or with the solid phase. Various glycols, silicone oils, and paraffin oils have been employed.

After the solid material is coated with the liquid phase, the column must be conditioned by heating and flushing with inert gas. Excess liquid phase and various impurities are driven off, and the system is gradually stabilized. At high temperatures the column may continue to "bleed" or lose some volatilized liquid phase.

Columns are formed in U shapes or coils so that they will fit easily into ovens of workable dimensions. The ends are attached to the carrier gas supply and to the detector by means of threaded Swagelok fittings or some similar easily connected device. Different analyses require columns of different length and composition, and it is desirable to be able to change them easily, even when they are hot.

The oven into which the columns are installed is designed to control the temperature within very narrow limits. Most modern systems include controls that enable the oven to heat up to a preset temperature quickly, to maintain that temperature very exactly, and to cool back to room temperature with a minimum of lost time. They are also programmed so that increases in temperature can be performed at a regular, even rate that can be controlled. A regular and even increase of 1 degree per minute or 20 degrees per minute can be attained with ease and accuracy. This aids in the differentiation of compounds that volatilize at different temperatures.

There is usually a separate temperature control for the point in the system where the sample is injected into the column. This *injection port* is usually maintained at a slightly higher temperature than the column so the material will be driven into the column immediately and not remain at the point of injection. There is also a separate temperature control for the area around the detector. This temperature is also maintained a little higher than that of the column to prevent the material from redistilling at the detector. The temperature at these points may be monitored by a system having a thermistor probe in each location, a switching arrangement, and a single meter.

*Detector.* There are many types of detectors used with gas chromatography. The simplest of these is the *thermal conductivity cell*—a type often referred to as a TC detector. A hot wire conducts electricity at a rate dependent upon its temperature. Heat is dissipated at a rate that depends on the type and concentration of gas passing the wire. The resulting change of temperature of the wire determines its resistance and hence the flow of electricity through it. Two such *hot-wire detectors* may be used in conjunction. One of these monitors the stream of inert gas prior to injection of the sample, and the other monitors the effluent from the column. The difference in resistance between the two wires is then amplified and used to drive a recorder, meter, or digital readout. Many instruments actually use two hot-wire cells located before the column and two located after the column. This serves to average the signals in each case, minimizing errors caused by slight variations in gas pressure and hot wire temperature. A thermistor may be used in place of the hot wire. The thermistor works on the same principle as the hot wire. A semiconductor material that conducts much more readily at high temperatures than at low is enclosed in a small glass capsule and installed in the flow lines.

A second type of sensing mechanism is the *ionization detector*. As the material being separated is swept out of the end of the column by the carrier gas, it is burned in a small but very hot hydrogen flame. The resulting breakup of molecular structures produces ion pairs. An electric field of high potential is set up in the area of the flame. The ion pairs contribute to the current in the field, and the increase is measured by a highly sensitive electrometer. For this system to function, the current passing across the detector must be very constant when at baseline. Gases must be dry, and the flow rate must be extremely steady. Impurities from the column must be minimal. Since the ionization current is very small, even slight variations in these factors can cause severe problems.

Since many of these conditions are hard to control with adequate precision, two columns, each with its own detector, are sometimes used. The second column and detector act as a reference system against the sample side. Hence the two must be parallel in every detail. The columns are the same length and contain the same packing. They pass through the same heating oven in proximity, and the injection-port heaters and detector heaters are at the same temperature. As the column temperature is raised, there is a tendency for the liquid phase to volatilize or bleed, causing some ionization at the flame. If dual columns and detectors are used, this bleed is compensated and the net effect is negligible.

Ionization detectors are most efficient for the detection of compounds with many electrons that are easily displaced. Organic compounds rich in carbon are easily detected, and the hydrogen-flame detector is best suited for these.

Another type of detector occasionally used is the *cross-sectional ionization detector*. The sample is ionized in a small cross-sectional area of the column by a stream of beta radiation from an isotope. The amount of ionization occurring is measured by a sensitive electrometer in the same manner as with the hydrogen flame.

The *argon detector* is a two-stage mechanism. A radioactive material ionizes argon gas molecules, which then collide with the molecules of

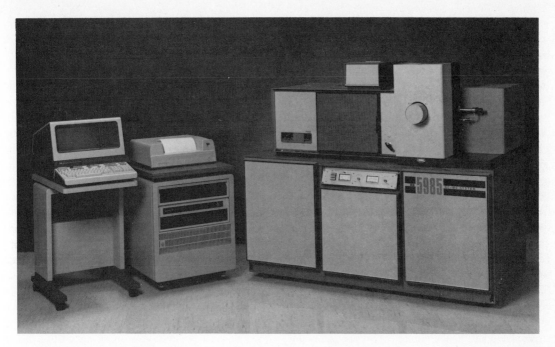

***Fig. 11-4.*** A gas chromatograph is often coupled with a mass spectrograph as in the Hewlett-Packard 5985 GC/MS system shown. (Courtesy Hewlett-Packard Co.)

the sample to be measured, causing ionization.

In the *electron-capture detector* the process is more or less reversed. Certain halogenated gases, peroxides, and metal organic compounds are able to capture and bind free or loosely bound electrons. As the sample reaches the end of the column, it is bombarded by beta radiation. The free electrons are captured by the electron-binding gas, thus decreasing the current flow.

There are several other types of detectors available for specific analytical problems. The hot-wire and hydrogen-flame detectors just discussed are the most common systems in medical applications.

It is possible, in the case of the hot-wire detector, to reclaim the entire sample fraction in its naturally occurring state. Various gas traps are provided to collect these fractions as they leave the detector and are flushed out of the column. In the case of the hydrogen-flame detector, a *stream splitter,* which allows a portion of the sample to pass into the flame while the rest goes on to the fraction collector, may be provided.

The fractions that are separated by the gas chromatograph may be fed directly into a mass spectrometer where the mass-to-charge ratio is determined (Fig. 11-4). By using these data along with the $R_F$ value and quantitation data provided by the gas chromatograph, a computer can quickly identify and quantitate all components of the sample. A discussion of mass spectrometry follows.

Gas chromatography is not widely used in the clinical laboratory at the present time; however, it is the method of choice for the analysis of several drugs of abuse and for the quantitation of some therapeutic drugs and steroids. The metabolites of bacteria, particularly the anaerobes, can be identified as an aid to rapid identification. The specialized gas chromatographs for this purpose are discussed later. An instrument was recently developed for the quantitation of carbon dioxide in serum by gas chromatography, and other applications are under development. This interesting technique may, in time, become more important.

## Mass spectrometry

*History*. The first mass spectrometric work was done in England by J.J. Thompson (discoverer of the electron) in 1912 and by F.W. Aston in 1919. Thompson demonstrated the existence of the isotope neon-22, which was the first step in the identification of stable isotopes. In 1940, mass spectrometers were commercially available. At that time the primary application was the quantitative analysis of hydrocarbon mixture constituents in the petroleum industry. Not until 1960 was mass spectrometry recognized for its capabilities in the identification and structural analysis of organic compounds. Mass spectrometers are not usually found in hospital clinical laboratories. These complex expensive instruments require expert operation and maintenance. However, mass spectrometry is being used in laboratories of specialized interests for clinical applications such as identification of dangerous drugs and detection of inborn errors of amino acid metabolism. Future clinical applications might include determination of heavy metals, analysis of fatty acids, measurement of prostaglandins, and identification of bacteria.

*Principle of operation*. In mass spectrometry the sample is converted to the gaseous state and then ionized. The many positive ionic forms produced are accelerated toward a mass analyzer. In the mass analyzer, the positive ions are separated according to their mass-to-charge ratio (m/e ratio) resulting in a spectrum of masses (rather than a spectrum of light as seen in the spectrophotometer). The mass spectrum is "scanned," during which time the detector generates data representing each ionic species' mass and relative abundance in the sample being analyzed. These data can be interpreted with respect to compound identification, quantitation, and structural composition. This overall process is represented in the block diagram shown in Fig. 11-5. Each functional unit

represented in this diagram may use one of several available techniques to accomplish the desired effect. However, only the component most commonly used for clinical applications is discussed.

The sample in the gaseous form is introduced into the ionizing chamber. An electron beam is directed through the ionizing chamber and bombards the sample molecule. When an electron strikes the molecule, energy is transferred from the electron to the molecule. If the energy transferred is enough to eject an electron, the molecule becomes positively charged. If the energy absorbed by the molecule is enough to break one or more bonds, the molecule fragments into ions of constituent elements. For example, if CO is bombarded with high-energy electrons, the molecule will yield $CO^+$, $O^+$, and $C^+$ ions. Also, free electrons, negative ions, and neutral atoms may be formed, but these are separated from the positive ions by positively charged plates and a vacuum system. The positive ions are attracted to a negatively charged plate that directs the ions to an accelerating tube. The positive ions are accelerated through electrostatic fields and result in a narrow beam of high-velocity ions. This beam is a mixture of ions of various masses. The beam then travels through a field-free region and enters the mass analyzer. The mass analyzer is commonly a magnetic field. The ions enter the magnetic field and interact with the field, and the path of the ion is bent. The degree of ion deflection depends on its m/e ratio. The smaller the m/e ratio the greater is the degree of deflection. If analyzing carbon monoxide, greatest deflection occurs in order of the following list: $C^+$ (m/e = 12), $O^+$ (m/e = 16), and $CO^+$ (m/e = 28). Once the separation according to m/e ratio is achieved, the relative abundance of each ionic species must be determined. If the ions were permitted to impinge upon a photographic plate, the position on the plate would be indicative of the m/e ratio and the intensity of the area would be directly proportional to the relative abundance of the ion in the fragmentation of the molecule. Photographic plates have been used in this way; however, electronic de-

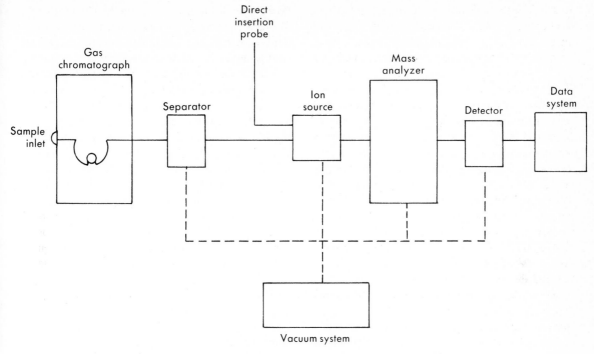

*Fig. 11-5.* Major components of typical GC/MS System. (Courtesy Hewlett-Packard Co.)

tectors are preferable. A narrow slit is positioned in front of an electronic detector, and the ionic species are swept across the slit. This is accomplished by one of two ways. The first is to maintain a constant magnetic field strength while decreasing the accelerating potential. Ions will be swept by the detector in order of increasing m/e ratio as the accelerating potential is decreased. The second and preferred approach is to maintain a constant accelerating potential while increasing the magnetic field strength (increase the current through the electromagnet). Ions will be swept by the detector in order of increasing m/e ratio as the magnetic field strength increases. The magnitude of the electronic signal from the detector is directly related to the relative concentrations of ions.

### Components
*Sample inlet.* The function of the sample inlet is to introduce the sample very slowly into the mass spectrometer system in the vaporized form. Different samples require different sample inlet systems. Gases can be transferred directly into the sample inlet. Liquids may be vaporized by the low pressure in the sample reservoir, or a heated inlet may be required to volatize the liquid sample. Temperatures must be regulated according to the sample; thermal destruction of the sample must be avoided. Solids must be directly introduced if they can be thermally vaporized. Frequently a derivative of a compound is volatile when the compound itself is not. Such a derivative can be used to enable the mass spectrometric analysis of a compound if the derivative retains all important structural features of the compound.

Required sample size for direct insertion is usually 1 $\mu$g or less, and for gas chromatographic-mass spectrometer interfaced systems, amounts down to 10 ng can be used. The gases diffuse slowly from the sample reservoir through a minute hole into the ion source. This slow leak of sample limits the number of molecular collisions with each other and with the ion source walls.

Liquid and particularly gas chromatographic separation before sample introduction into the mass spectrometer increases the analytical power of mass spectometry. Complex mixtures can be mass spectrometrically analyzed if they are first separated by gas chromatography. The interface between the gas chromatograph and the mass spectrometer must decrease the pressure of the sample at the mass spectrometer inlet and eliminate the carrier gas. A variety of devices can be used to introduce chromatographic effluents into a mass spectrometer.

*Ion source.* The function of the ion source is to efficiently ionize a sample into as many different ion species as possible to obtain maximum information from the mass spectrum of the sample. The electron impact source is most commonly used for ionization of organic compounds.

An electron gun (heated filament and accelerating electrode) is used as the source of energetic electrons (usually 50 to 70 eV). These electrons bombard the molecules leaked into the ion source, causing fragmentation of the molecule into multiple ionic forms. The positive ions are repelled from the ion source toward the accelerator. In the accelerator, through the attraction of the plates at differing potentials, the positive ions are focused and accelerated toward the mass analyzer.

*Mass analyzer.* Two types of mass analyzers used are the magnetic deflection type and the quadrupole filter.

In the magnetic deflection–type analyzer, the positively charged ions of fixed velocity travel at right angles to a magnetic field. The ion is deflected. The degree of deflection depends on the ion's m/e ratio, the lighter the m/e ratio the greater is the deflection. Thus, a spectrum of the different ions is formed according to the m/e ratio of each ionic form.

In the quadrupole mass filter the positively charged ions enter an area between four parallel rods. Two opposite rods carry a negative dc potential, and the other two carry a positive dc potential. A radiofrequency (rf) voltage is placed on one set of rods, and a rf 180 degrees out of phase with the first is placed on the second set of rods. At a particular ratio of dc to rf potential, only ions of one m/e ratio can pass through this field without striking one of the rods. Thus, by changing the ratio of dc to rf potential, a mass spectrum can be formed.

*Detector.* The electronic detector is an electrode upon which the positive ions impinge. When an ion strikes the electrode, an electrical pulse is amplified that is then presented to the readout mechanism. The magnitude of the electrical impulse is representative of the relative quantity of ion in the compound being analyzed.

*Data display and interpretation.* Data can be presented in several forms. Pen-and-ink strip chart recorders can be used if the scan rate is slow. For fast scans, oscilloscope display and photographic record can be used. Several galvanometers of different sensitivities can be used to present data on photosensitive charts. The most frequently used data handling system is a computer. Data are collected and interpreted in the computer, and the interpretation is presented to the operator.

# CHAPTER 12

# *Automation in hematology*

Twenty years ago the average medical technologist spent an appreciable part of every day counting red blood cells and white blood cells in ruled areas of a slide chamber to estimate the average number of red and white cells in a cubic millimeter of a patient's blood sample. In most laboratories a total of 30 counts a day for one technician was considered a heavy day's work.

In performing a red cell count, the technologist counted about 500 cells, out of a total of nearly 5,000,000 cells per cubic millimeter. The inescapable error due to random sampling, plus a multitude of dilution and preparation errors, glassware-calibration errors, and human errors of judgment and fatigue, could add up to a very large total error indeed. One of the most significant changes that have been made in laboratory equipment has been the introduction of devices for counting red and white blood cells quickly and accurately. These devices have arrived at a high state of mechanical efficiency and have become so trouble free that the technician employing them may be totally unaware of their operating principle.

Before the advent of today's counting instruments a few attempts were made at estimating a cell population by various indirect methods. The Leitz Photometer used the total absorbance of the suspended red cells in a simple dilution of blood as an indication of red cell population. This method assumed that all cells were equal in size, that the serum was essentially colorless, and that no clumping existed. In practice this method turned out to be useless except as a very rough screening method.

An instrument called the *Hemoscope,* which worked on a sort of nephelometric principle of light dispersion, was produced. This, too, failed to solve the problem.

Now, in addition to devices for counting red and white blood cells, advanced instrumentation makes it possible to determine red cell volume and hemoglobin and to estimate, from these parameters, the various indices that describe the red cell. A device to give information similar to the red cell sedimentation is available. Several companies have introduced highly automated systems to differentiate between types of normal white cells and enumerate them. It is probably only a matter of time before a complete blood count will be performed by one instrument and this information, along with the patient's identification, be entered directly into a computer for immediate reporting and storage. Some of the principles and ideas that make these things possible are examined.

## Particle counting

The instruments now in common clinical laboratory use depend on one of two principles. One type of instrument counts by means of a light signal, using a magnifying lens with or without the dark-field principle. The Coulter principle uses cells to interrupt a flow of current between two electrodes and counts the signals thus produced. Several variations of these two general ideas have been made, and a great deal of research into the physics and mechanics of cell counting, sizing, and identifying has been conducted. Much more will probably be done in this field in the next few years to further relieve the tedium of individual observation of cell and particle number, size, and type.

## Coulter cell-counting devices

*Early Coulter counters.* Technologists are greatly indebted to Joseph and Wallace Coulter for the introduction and refinement of sophisticated methods of cell counting. The illustration and description of this system, which Wallace Coulter prepared for presentation to the National Electronics Conference in 1958, is of some historical interest and is a very lucid explanation. The principle, with many refinements, is still basically the same as it was at that time. With his permission the following excerpt is reprinted in detail, and his original accompanying illustrations are used.

Figure 1 [our Fig. 12-1] shows a simple arrangement for holding the sample, establishing sample flow and "metering" the flow so that an electronic counter can be activated as a selected sample volume is drawn thru and scanned by the orifice. A dilute suspension of cells *(E)* is contained in a sample beaker. The tube *B* carries the aperture *A* thru which the sample is drawn. *C* and *D* are the electrodes. When stopcock *F* is opened, an external vacuum source (and waste discharge) *(P)* initiates flow thru the orifice and causes the mercury *J* in the manometer to assume the position shown with the mercury in the open leg of the manometer drawn slightly below the horizontal branch. When stopcock *F* is closed, the unbalanced manometer functions as a syphon to continue the sample flow thru the orifice. As the mercury in the open leg rises into the horizontal branch, it makes contact with a wire electrode *(L)* sealed in the manometer wall and energizes a high speed decade counter which begins counting all pulses which reach or exceed the threshold level. A few seconds later the mercury column makes contact with a second wire electrode *(M)* which stops the counter. The syphoning action continues until the mercury column comes to rest at a level near that of the mercury in the reservoir. Contact *K* provides a ground return path for the start and stop electrodes. The contacts *L* and *M* are very carefully located so that the volume contained in the tube between the contacts is ½ milliliter. As a consequence of the arrangement the counter is actuated as ½ milliliter is drawn into the system. In practice the horizontal section is a U tube in the horizontal plane so that contacts are near together. By this means the vacuum in the system at the start and stop contacts is kept substantially equal so that any elasticity in the system due to bubbles etc. will introduce less than $^{1}/_{10}$th percent error in the syphoned volume under the worst conditions.

The function of inlet *O* and stopcock *G* which is normally left in the closed position is to allow rapid filling of the system when setting it up instead of depending upon the relatively slow flow thru the orifice.

Figure 2 [our Fig. 12-2] is a block diagram of the electrical functions and Figure 3 [our Fig. 12-3] is a photograph of a model now in use in a number of laboratories. The pulses produced at the orifice are amplified and displayed on the oscilloscope screen and appear as vertical lines or spikes as shown in Figure 4 [our Fig. 12-4]. The height of an individual pulse spike from the baseline is a measure of relative size of the cell producing the pulse (except for coincident passage to be discussed) and since the rate at which they are produced is several thousand per second, the viewer obtains an immediate impression of the average cell size and cell size distribution. The threshold control dial located below the oscilloscope screen enables the operator to select the height or level above the baseline which if reached or exceeded by a pulse will result in the pulse being counted. The height or level corresponds to a particular cell size. When the syphon activates the counter, all cells of this particular size or larger present in half milliliter drawn thru the orifice will be counted. Cells below this minimum size will not be counted. In addition to a display of relative cell size the oscilloscope also indicates the effective level or setting of the threshold control by brightening that portion above the threshold level, of any pulse which reaches or exceeds it and which of course would be counted. In Figure 4 [our Fig. 12-4] the threshold level is shown intermediate between the height of the smallest of the desired pulses and well above the small irregularities on the baseline which represent the passage of very small bits of debris and any extraneous electrical disturbances which may be present. The screen indicates, at a glance, a wide discrimination against undesired debris and electrical background noise and correct functioning of the threshold circuit in relation to the particles to be counted. For the particular sample represented the threshold control setting could be varied considerably without affecting the count. For routine cell counting the threshold control is left at a sufficiently low setting to count the smallest cells likely to be encountered and need not be

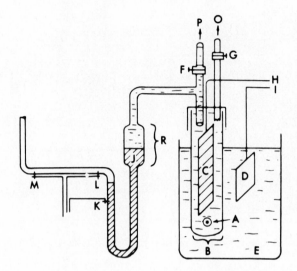

**Fig. 12-1.** Principle of the Coulter Counter. (From Coulter, W.: High speed automatic blood cell counter and cell size analyzer, Chicago, 1956, Coulter Electronics, Inc.)

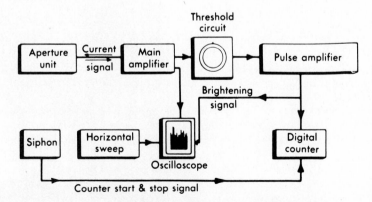

**Fig. 12-2.** Electronic circuitry of the Coulter Counter (as in Fig. 12-1). (Courtesy Coulter Electronics, Inc.)

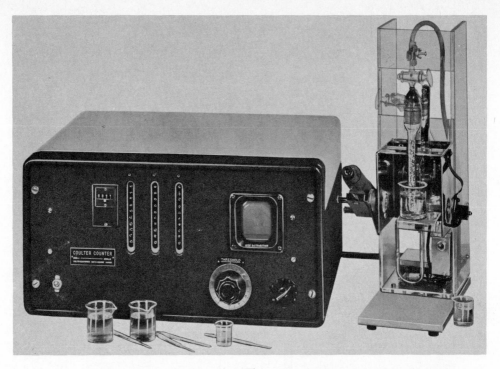

**Fig. 12-3.** Model A Coulter Counter (as in Fig. 12-1). (Courtesy Coulter Electronics, Inc.)

**Fig. 12-4.** Pulse pattern on oscilloscope screen (as in Fig. 12-1). (Courtesy Coulter Electronics, Inc.)

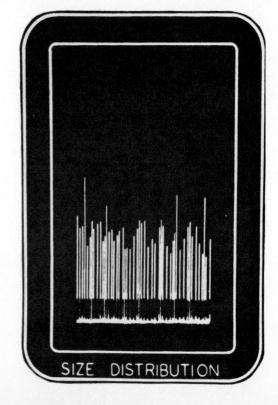

reset for different samples. The minimum function of the oscilloscope display is to provide a check of overall instrument performance in a manner which requires only an instants observation and is readily understood by the average medical laboratory technician.

The Coulter Counter pictured in Fig. 12-3 was known as the *Model A*. It was hand wired and used a total of 30 vacuum tubes. This was the original Coulter Counter that was introduced and used in the early 1960s.

The Model A was soon superseded by Models $F_N$, ZBI, and others that used solid-state circuitry, printed circuit boards, and digital electronic displays (Fig. 12-5). As can be seen, the manometer glassware and suction pump were included in the case. The digital and mechanical registers of the Model A were replaced, first by glow tubes in the Model F and then by numerical readout tubes in the Models $F_N$ and ZBI. The sensitivity controls were mounted on the front panel. The viewing

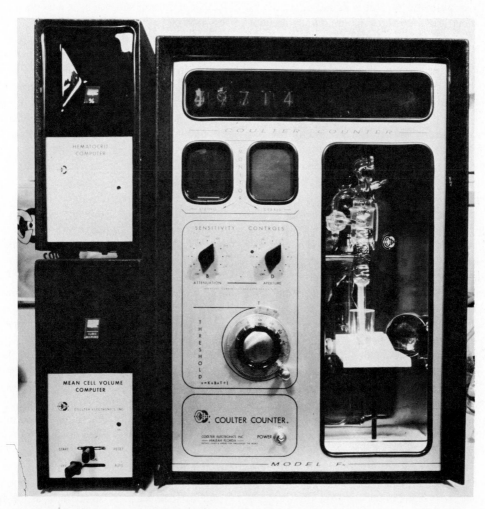

*Fig. 12-5.* Model $F_N$ Coulter Counter shown with hematocrit computer and mean cell volume computer. (Courtesy Coulter Electronics, Inc.)

lens for observing the orifice (mounted on the manometer stand of the Model A) was replaced by a viewing screen. The most important changes, however, were in the electronics. All tubes were replaced by transistors, and printed-circuit boards were used throughout.

Problems associated with these earlier instruments involved control of the vacuum system and a tendency to pick up ac broadcast signals from motors and fluorescent lights, causing high background counts. This latter problem could occasionally be resolved by proper gounding.

All electrically powered laboratory equipment should be grounded, and laws in most states require a three-pronged plug on all units, the third prong being the ground. It happens at times that the third slot of the wall receptacle is not actually grounded. This can happen in old buildings especially and in parts of buildings where wiring has been haphazardly added. The grounding can be checked with a voltmeter by measuring between the hot side of the circuit and the ground line. If no current registers, the ''ground'' is not actually grounded.

In spite of the small problems that may occur with the Coulter Models F and $F_N$, these have been highly reliable instruments, and problems are almost always attributable to diluent, glassware, or dilution error. Use of Coulter's Isoton Diluent, Isoterge Detergent for cleaning the instrument, and disposable plastic beakers almost guarantees immunity from these problems.

*Coulter Counter, Model S (Coulter Electronics, Inc.).* When the second edition of *Elementary Principles of Laboratory Instruments* was going to press, the Model S was just coming into production. At that time I predicted that it would have ''a major impact on the clinical laboratory.'' That prediction seems to have been borne out. The majority of all clinical laboratories of any appreciable size are now using this equipment or a newer modification, and it is considered a standard device in most hematology departments. Indeed, in most laboratories, it is a black day when the Model S is out of service—which, fortunately,

occurs seldom if proper maintenance and service are provided. Many busy laboratories now have at least two Model S counters to back each other up in case of failure, even though the counting rate, if fully utilized, provides for a very large number of blood counts to be performed in a day.

On first examination this seems to be a complicated system. Like most systems, when it is examined part by part, it is much simpler than one would first suppose. The electronics may be beyond comprehension for many, but the general idea behind each subsystem is easy to grasp (Fig. 12-6).

In discussion of the Coulter principle of particle counting it has been explained that a particle passing through a small orifice interrupts an electric current, giving a blip or signal that can be counted. Both red and white cells are counted in this way. Cells of each type are drawn, at a constant rate, through three aperatures at once. The three internal electrodes, one in each aperture tube, are associated with one common external electrode immersed in the fluid that is being drawn through the apertures. Thus, there are three *white cell counts* (WBC) and three *red cell counts* (RBC) performed during each cycle of the instrument. These are compared, and, if results are within reasonable limits, the three are averaged. If one count is out of limits, the other two are used, but if the three are widely separated, no result is reported. If a result is rejected, a red ''voting light'' over the oscilloscope screen, associated with that orifice tube, comes on so the operator knows to check for foreign material in that orifice. Unless there is a problem with blood clots or a similar hazard, these lights seldom come on during the count cycle. The manner of preparing the blood dilution for red and white cell counts will be explained presently.

While the blood is being diluted for the white cell count, a hemolyzing agent is added. The bath from which the white count is drawn is optically clear and presents an optical path of about 1 cm from front to back. A small light at the front of the bath acts as an exciter lamp and, at the time the white cell count is being taken, a photocell behind

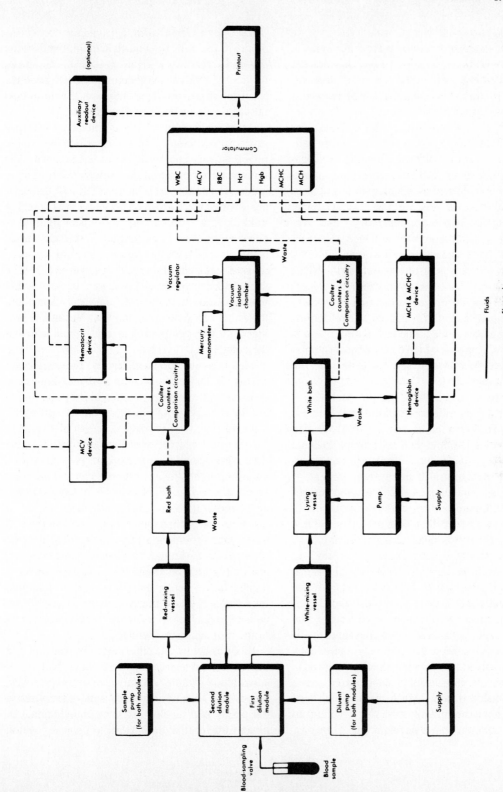

*Fig. 12-6.* Block diagram of the Coulter Model S blood-counting system. (Courtesy Coulter Electronics, Inc.)

the bath is measuring the optical density of the hemolyzed blood solution. From this information a *hemoglobin* (Hb) value can obviously be obtained.

As pointed out, while cells are being counted, each cell produces an electrical signal (which is actually the instantaneous decrease of the orifice current). The size of this signal is an accurate measure of the electrical resistance offered by the cell, and this is a function of the cell's volume. Measuring the total of all of these electrical signals and then dividing their total by the number of impulses (or cells) provides a very accurate average signal that corresponds to the average cell volume. Applied to the red cell–counting sequence, this technique reveals the mean red cell volume (MCV).

Methods for obtaining four parameters—RBC, WBC, Hb, and MCV—have now been discussed. Three other parameters are calculated from these four measured values. To find the mean corpuscular hemoglobin (MCH), the hemoglobin value is divided by the number of red cells per unit volume. This can be done electrically, using the electric signals just measured.

The hematocrit is defined as the packed cell volume, or the percentage of a blood sample that is red cells. This value is usually obtained by centrifuging a blood sample until cells are packed and measuring the volume of the red cell pack, as a percentage of the total. If the average volume of the red cells in the sample (MCV) and the number of cells (RBC) are known, multiplying these will indicate the total red cell volume in a given volume of blood. This is a highly accurate *hematocrit*. There is a problem, since measuring this way was not possible in the past and the cell packing that normally is done leaves interstices between the spherical cells even if there is absolutely ideal centrifugation. Since there is only an electrical value from the Model S that is analgous to a value that is not too well defined, the normally determined value is simply assigned to the electrical signal; in other words, the instrument is standardized with a known hematocrit value. Much research has been done to better define this situation, but it is more an academic problem than a practical one.

The *mean corpuscular hemoglobin concentration* (MCHC) tells how much hemoglobin there is, on the average, in a given volume of cell space. Obviously this can be determined from the electrical information corresponding to the mean corpuscular volume and the hemoglobin.

After this survey of the origin of all of these seven parameters, the system by which the sample travels to each measuring point is examined. The fluid-handling system of the Model S is extremely accurate. The degree of automation and the number of operations involved present a very complex fluid-moving problem. All movement of fluid is either by pressure or by vacuum. There are a great many valves that, on signal, open or close to move the diluted sample in the right direction. The command center for all these is a bank of small induction motors accessible from the back at about the center of the counting module. Vacuum is provided by the pump in a separate module under the counter.

Measurement of samples is by *segmented stream*. If the sample were in a tube having a very consistent and accurate internal diameter, a highly accurate sample could be measured by cutting off a precise, highly reproducible length of this tube. This is, in principle, what is accomplished by the measuring valve. The valve core is a metal cylinder, through which an accurate channel has been bored lengthwise. This cylinder is tightly fitted, at its ends, against plastic block faces. Holes in the block faces correspond to the holes in the cylinder, thus providing a pathway for fluid through one end block, through the channel in the cylinder, and through the other block. If the cylinder is rotated on its center axis, however, a stream of fluid through this pathway would be cut off, and an accurately measured sample would be retained in the channel of the cylinder.

Blood is drawn into this device by vacuum and the valve is turned, cutting off the accurately measured blood sample. As the valve turns, however, the sample channel is aligned with other holes in the plastic end blocks, and a measured stream of diluent washes the blood along to its next position and performs the necessary dilution at the same time. In this way the blood sample is first diluted and moved to a chamber on the right side of the counting module. From this chamber an aliquot is withdrawn and similarly measured and rediluted for the red count. This sample is placed in a bath on the left side of the machine. Both the original sample (white cell dilution) and the rediluted red count sample are now swirled into an additional chamber to facilitate mixing. Before moving to the counting bath, the white cell dilution goes to a hemolyzing bath where a few drops of a hemolyzing agent are added. Both the red cell and white cell dilutions now proceed to the respective counting baths where the orifice tubes will draw off samples at a controlled rate for the counts previously described. Between counting cycles the counting baths and orifice tubes are well rinsed with diluent. The block diagram in Fig. 12-6 may make it easier to understand the counting cycle.

It is hoped that this condensed and simplified explanation of the Model S hematology system

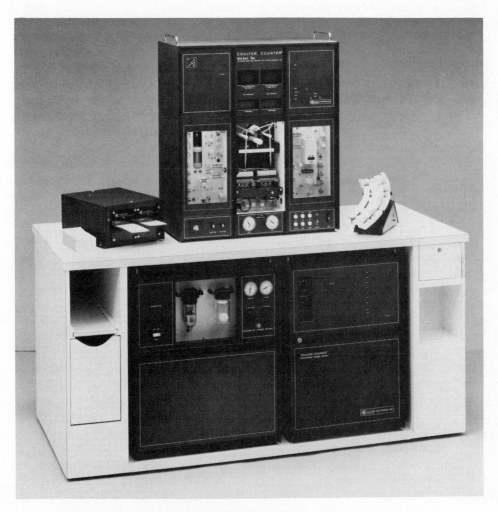

*Fig. 12-7.* Model Ssr. Coulter cell counter. (Courtesy Coulter Electronics, Inc.)

will make possible a fairly clear idea of the rationale involved. This system has proved to be very accurate and highly reproducible. The amount of laboratory work time saved is impressive, and the improvement in accuracy in hematology, in general, is a substantial contribution to better patient care.

The engineering of this instrument has proved to be superb, and many systems have now been in continuous use for 10 to 12 years, performing hundreds of counts per day with relatively little down time. There is a tendency to forget that this type of performance was virtually unheard of in any clinical laboratory equipment 20 years ago.

*Coulter Model Ssr. (Coulter Electronics, Inc.).* The original Model S has been improved and modified over the years, and new models with several additional advantages have been added to the line.

The Model Ssr. (Fig. 12-7) has improved fluidics and more stable electronics. Self-priming and self-flushing functions have made this instrument easier to maintain and have eliminated most of the service problems encountered on the Model S. The Model S has been discontinued as a separate model.

The Model S+ includes all of the advantages of the Model Ssr. with the addition of platelet counting and the capability of graphically recording platelet and red cell size distribution. Both instruments have improved electronics and fluidics, which further improves reliability. The precision of these instruments is outstanding when proper maintenance is provided.

*Hemac Laser Hematology Counter (Ortho Diagnostics Instruments)* (Fig. 12-8). The Hemac blood counter introduces revolutionary new technology into cell counting. Actual cell counting

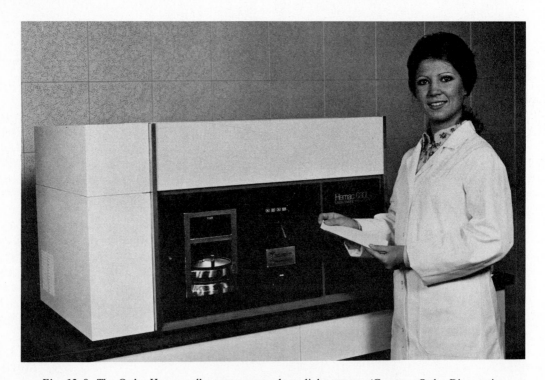

*Fig. 12-8.* The Ortho Hemac cell counter uses a laser light source. (Courtesy Ortho Diagnostics Instruments.)

depends on the optical principle just discussed, but the light beam used is a low-powered helium/neon laser beam. The advantage of the laser is its extremely sharp focus of discrete, monochromatic light. This sort of light, focused to about 20 $\mu$l, is ideal for cell counting because the beam approaches the total diameter of the aperture through which the cells will pass.

The aperture itself incorporates a unique idea. The sample stream, bearing the cells to be counted, is the center column in a high-speed stream of liquid passing through the light beam.

The method of achieving the very narrow stream of diluted sample through the counting area is one of the unique features of the instrument. The diluted sample comes together with a stream of isotonic fluid in a funnel-shaped flow cell (Fig. 12-9). The configuration of the cell and the precise regulation of flow pressures are such that the sample stream becomes an 18 $\mu$m column at the center of the larger stream of isotonic fluid. This laminar flow system maintains the cells in an effective fluid aperture at precisely the center of the laser beam (Fig. 12-9).

Blood is drawn into the sampling valve and split into two streams. One stream is diluted with a lysing solution and passed to the flow cell, where *white cells are counted* as they interrupt the laser beam.

The second part of the sample is diluted with isotonic solution and further split into two streams. One of these streams is further diluted and is passed through the laser beam in its turn. As *red cells* pass through the beam they are *counted* and their size determined by the degree to which they occlude the laser beam. This sizing information is totaled to report the *hematocrit*.

The remaining part of this second stream is further diluted with a hemoglobin diluent that converts the hemoglobin to *cyanmethemoglobin,* which flows to the special colorimeter where it is measured. This colorimeter is in itself unique. An LED, providing light at 539 nm, is used as the radiation source, and a photomultiplier is used as a detector.

The electronic system calculates MCV, MCH,

and MCHC. All seven parameters are reported using less than a hundred $\mu$l of blood. Dilution of the sample is less than one would expect—white cells, 1:19, and red cells, 1:3969—and a rather large number of cells are counted. On the average about 25,000 red cells and 7000 white cells are counted. The amount of diluent used is surprisingly low. All solutions for one count total only 13.8 ml.

The Hemac is an accurate instrument for performing blood counts. The counting speed of about one sample per minute seems quite acceptable, and the instrument appears reasonably easy to use and maintain.

*Parameter hematology analyzer (Ortho Diagnostic Systems).* Following up in the success of the Hemac, Ortho Diagnostic Systems introduced this newer version that allows a speed of over 100 samples per hour using a 100 $\mu$l sample size (Fig. 12-10). The on-board computer stores patient data and automates the quality control data handling. It can tabulate and display patient data or selectively recall and print out patient information including histograms. Abnormal results are flagged. A less expensive version called the *EL-7* that lacks the computer capabilities and the platelet counting is also available.

*H-6000 System (Technicon Instrument Corp.).* Over the past two decades Technicon has introduced a considerable number of blood-counting instruments including the SMA-4 and SMA-7, the modified 4-A and 7-A, the Hemalog and Hemalog-D, and the HS-90 System listed in earlier editions. These instruments generally counted on the principle of detecting cells in a flowing stream by a light-scattering technique. In the Hemalog an ingenious, in-line hematocrit centrifuge was introduced, an automated prothrombin time analyzer was added, and a flowing stream–differential counter was made a part of the sophisticated and complex system. The differential counter fixes and stains cells in four flowing streams that pass through laminar cells where cells are sensed and classified on the basis of their staining characteristics.

Technicon has now introduced the H-6000 Sys-

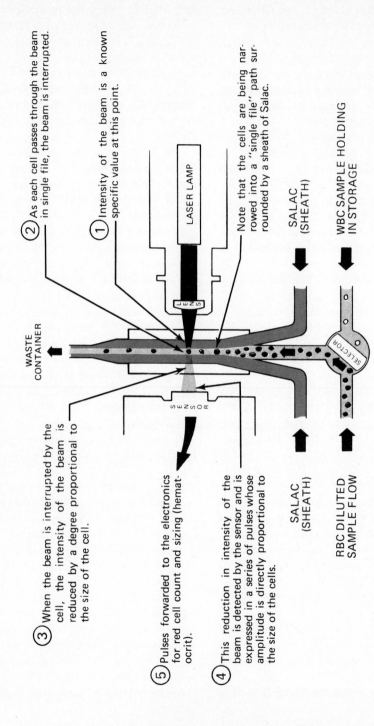

② As each cell passes through the beam in single file, the beam is interrupted.

① Intensity of the beam is a known specific value at this point.

Note that the cells are being narrowed into a "single file" path surrounded by a sheath of Salac.

SALAC (SHEATH)

WBC SAMPLE HOLDING IN STORAGE

LASER LAMP

LENS

WASTE CONTAINER

SENSOR

SELECTOR

③ When the beam is interrupted by the cell, the intensity of the beam is reduced by a degree proportional to the size of the cell.

⑤ Pulses forwarded to the electronics for red cell count and sizing (hematocrit).

④ This reduction in intensity of the beam is detected by the sensor and is expressed in a series of pulses whose amplitude is directly proportional to the size of the cells.

SALAC (SHEATH)

RBC DILUTED SAMPLE FLOW

*Fig. 12-9.* Flow cell of the Hemac cell counter. (Courtesy Ortho Diagnostics Instruments.)

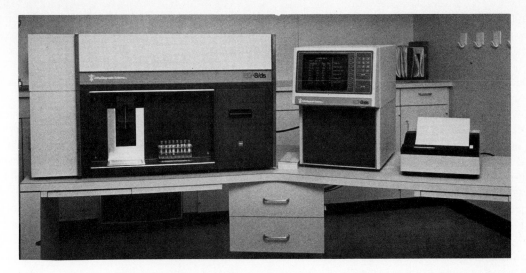

*Fig. 12-10.* A recent model of the ELT-8 Hematology System. (Courtesy Ortho Diagnostic Systems, Inc.)

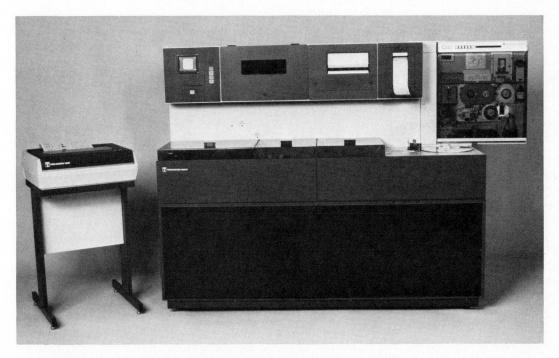

*Fig. 12-11.* The Technicon H-6000 System, which provides a complete blood count from one work station. (Courtesy Technicon Instrument Corp.)

tem (Fig. 12-11). A carousel-type automatic sampler is equipped with Technicon's excellent IDEE patient/report identification system. The prothrombin time device is not included, but the sophisticated computer system provides a complete report of the complete blood count, histograms of RBC and platelet size distribution, and graphic representation of a 10,000-cell differential on the basis of stain and size characteristics.

If this sort of system proves itself, it will have a considerable impact on the staffing of hematology laboratories, since a single work station would be required to produce complete blood counts at the rate of 60 samples per hour. Until now, Technicon's systems have not captured a large share of the hematology market. It will be interesting to see how this new entry is accepted.

*Quality control of cell counters.* In the use of cell counting equipment, considerable attention must be paid to quality control. In nearly all of the more sophisticated systems voltage is an important consideration. All of the manufacturer's recommended checks should be followed carefully each day. Such checks as power supply voltages, six-way attenuation, and ramp and precision checks may be involved. If air pressures or vacuum are involved in fluidics, these must be checked regularly. Background counts must be made regularly. At each work shift the proper calibration of the instrument must be ensured in some way. At least once each day assayed controls should be run. Reagent quality is important. Different lot numbers of reagent or reagents improperly stored may cause variations in counting. If a number of tests are run during a work shift, it may be advisable to repeat earlier samples from time to time to check for electronic drift, protein buildup around orifices, pressure changes, or other inadvertent changes that have gone unnoticed.

Because of the nature of the equipment, more attention must be paid to preventive maintenance and inspection. Valves, lines, chambers, and electrodes must be regularly checked for leaks, wear, and dirt. Cleanliness and regular service to the equipment can save hours of downtime and hundreds of dollars in repair bills. Where precise measurement is critical to results, pipetters and dilutors must be checked regularly for both accuracy and precision.

Backup equipment is generally needed for those times when counters fail or are being repaired, serviced or recalibrated. Such equipment should also be regularly checked and serviced and should be used occasionally to ensure that it is serviceable and in calibration. It is advisable to correlate backup equipment with regularly used instruments by running some samples in parallel and comparing results. Where results vary appreciably, data may need to be analyzed to determine the amount of bias regularly observed in the backup equipment and the degree of imprecision one may expect.

## Differential counting by pattern recognition

Automated counting of white cell differentials by computer-directed pattern recognition has become fairly common. Although the process involved is somewhat complicated, the general idea is fairly simple.

A device resembling a television camera first scans the image. This scanning process, like the electron gun in a cathode ray tube, records one point at a time. This information is primarily binary information: 0 or 1 for black or white. A sampling of these points is made so that perhaps 10,000 points in a $20 \times 20$ $\mu$m square might be considered, using three color filters for additional information. This mass of information is placed in storage and analyzed.

*Principle.* The classification of cells is based on information concerning size, shape, color and density that is acquired by electronic analysis of microscopic images. The blood smear is scanned until a cell is located, then the image is broken down into a large number of data points. Each point is analyzed for information, which is fed to a computer where the cell is classified on the basis of the characteristics mentioned above. The various instruments use different approaches for the acquisition and analysis of data.

Three companies produce instruments of this

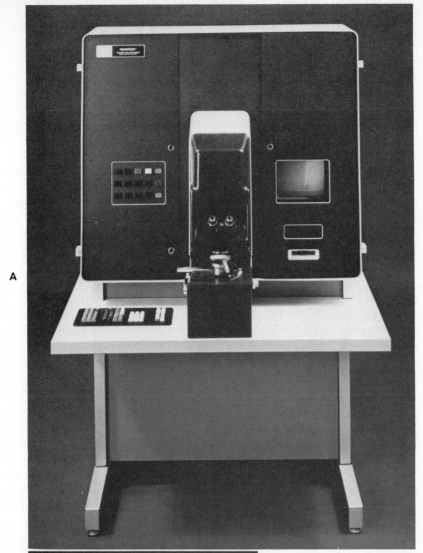

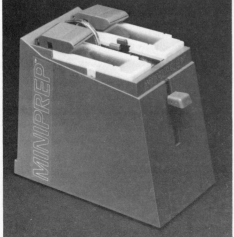

*Fig. 12-12. A*, Hematrak differential cell counter. *B*, Miniprep wedge slide maker for preparing blood films. (Courtesy Geometric Data Corp.)

type. Each company has some modifications, which have or can be added. The general characteristics of each company's instruments are described in the following paragraphs.

It is the general concensus of hematologists that any of these systems can perform reliably on normal blood smears, thus greatly reducing the tedium of manual differential cell counting. With any of these systems some abnormal cells require review. Better programs and more experience are permitting more dyscrasias to be recognized by electronic pattern recognition, but review will probably always be required.

*Hematrak (Geometric Data Corp.* (Fig. 12-12, *A* ). The first models of this instrument were introduced in 1973. Prior to this, the Larc Classifier by Corning had been the only instrument of this sort. The Larc is no longer manufactured. Blood smears for the Hematrak may be made by hand or by a proprietary, semiautomated, wedge-type instrument called the *Miniprep* (Fig. 12-12, *B* ). Spun smears can also be used. Because of the importance of counting a clean, monolayer film of cells, the Miniprep is recommended by the company. Slides are stained in a proprietary stainer and loaded into cassettes for counting. The cell is automatically scanned to locate 100 cells, which are analyzed. Platelets are counted and erythrocytes evaluated at the same time.

A standard Zeiss microscope frame and optics are adapted to the instrument. A scanning stage and motor-driven focus adjustment are provided. In the camera position a CRT is mounted. The flying spot of the CRT scans the slide until a cell is located. At that time the scan frame is reduced to the approximate size of the cell, and this window is scanned. Transmitted light is detected through the microscope's condenser by three photomultiplier tubes filtered to wavelengths of 425 nm, 530 nm, and 595 nm. The information from the 425 nm phototube is primarily used to electronically eliminate red cell interference. Information from the other two detectors is transmitted to the microprocessor for analysis. Image data is digitized to six density levels. All of the data concerning location, density and color are fed through the computer program, which classifies and tallies the cell. Platelets are counted, and RBC morphology is evaluated during the instrument's cycle.

A more sophisticated version of the Hematrak, called the *Model 590,* provides Price-Jones size distribution information and can display histograms on the screen.

*Diff-3 System (Coulter Biomedical Research Corp.)* (Fig. 12-13). This system was developed by Perkin-Elmer Corp. using extensive experience and expertise acquired in aerial photoanalysis. Coulter Biomedical Research acquired the instrument and has further developed it. It was first introduced in 1976.

Blood smears are prepared using a proprietary spinner that provides a highly reproducible monocellular layer. This is stained by a modified Ames Hema-tek slide stainer and loaded into cassettes. One hundred cells are located and analyzed.

A special proprietary microscope is used. Light is provided by a substage 60-watt tungsten lamp. Data are acquired through a 64-element photodiode array at 510 nm and at 580 nm, using a semaphore filter arrangement. Data acquisition is sequential and is digitized into 64 energy levels. The acquired data are transmitted to the computer where they are analyzed. Goulay logic (Fig. 12-14) is applied as part of this program to establish contiguity for better cell recognition. Platelet counting and red cell morphology are provided.

The computer of the Diff-3 can be programmed for other applications, whereas the other two instruments have dedicated systems.

*ADC-500 (Abbott Laboratories).* This instrument, introduced in 1977, is the newest of the three systems. Like the Diff-3, the slides are prepared using a proprietary spinner and a modified Ames stainer but are loose stacked into a carrier. Two hundred cells are examined by this system.

A specially designed microscope uses a 150-watt xenon arc substage lamp as a light source. Data are collected simultaneously by a 50-by-50 photodiode array at wavelengths of 412, 525, and 560 nm. Image data are digitized at 64 levels,

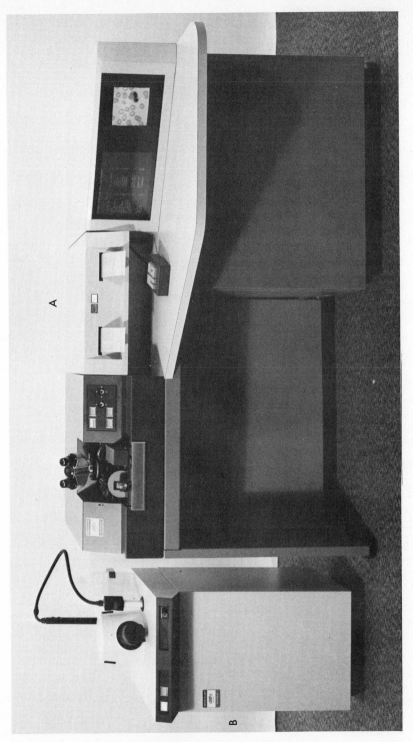

*Fig. 12-13. A,* Perkin-Elmer's new Diff-3 differential counting system. *B,* The free-standing Perkin-Elmer slide spinner uses a curtain of water around the spinning head to control the production of aerosols. (Courtesy Perkin-Elmer Corp.)

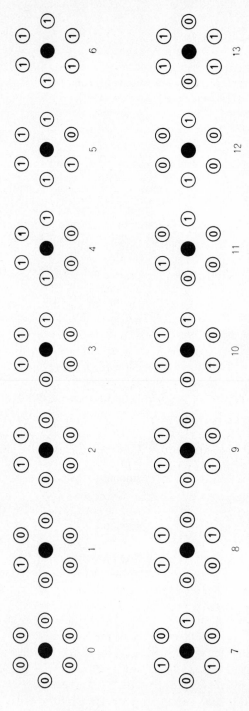

*Fig. 12-14.* Golay pattern transforms analyze each image point in terms of the binary state (1 or 0, meaning black or white, respectively) of the six other points that are nearest it in the hexagonal image-point lattice that constitutes the cartoon. There are 14 possible orientation-independent nearest-neighbor patterns, or surrounds. (They are numbered from 0 to 13 for computer processing.) (Courtesy Perkin-Elmer Corp.)

and the accumulated electronic information is fed to the computer for analysis and reporting.

*Quality control of differential counters.* Automated pattern-recognition differential counters are essentially maintenance free. As with any equipment, careful inspection for damage or maladjustment should not be neglected. Test slides are provided, and these should be run each day and whenever the instrument has been repaired or otherwise disturbed. Results of test slides should be compared with previous findings, and changes must be accounted for.

## Coagulation devices

The phenomenon of blood or plasma coagulation occupies a considerable amount of time and attention of the technologist. The principles involved are, of course, complex and not within the purview of this book. The measurement of the actual coagulation process is somewhat less complicated and, within some limits, is amenable to instrumentation. There are a number of problems, however. The nature of the clot formed and the sensitivity of occult activators and inhibitors that may affect coagulation render the process somewhat less concise than colorimetric analysis, for example. Certain fairly arbitrary tests of a general nature may usually be done safely by these devices. Specifically, prothrombin time measurement and partial thromboplastin time measurement are relatively reliable with automatic devices.

Any of several characteristics may be used to establish the fact that coagulation has occurred. The clot changes the viscosity, electrical conductivity, transparency, and fluidity of the sample. The clot has a cohesiveness and tensile strength and all or any of these characteristics can be measured. In practice, most of the devices produced in the United States work on one of three principles. The first of these depends on detection of the change in conductivity that occurs when a clot forms. The second detects a change in viscosity as the clot affects the motion of a mass or particles placed in the reaction tube. The third directly senses the change in optical density when clotting occurs.

*Fibrometer (Bio-Quest [Division of Becton, Dickinson, & Co.]).* For the past several years the Fibrometer has been the leader in the field of automated coagulation procedures. The test is performed in a plastic cup that is held in a thermostatically controlled block. A gun-type measuring pipette is used to rapidly introduce the patient's serum into the reagent mixture. An electric switch activated by the pipette's plunger causes a timer to start and also causes a mixing head to lower over the cup. Two small sensing agitators mix the test solution at a regular rate until coagulation occurs. Normally the coagulum appears precipitously, causing a sudden change in conductivity of the test solution. The change in the very small maintenance current between the probes causes the timer to stop.

In general the device works well. Very little maintenance is required. A small amount of grease on the pipette plunger of the gun helps keep it functioning smoothly. The metal barrel of the gun comes off the plastic handle with a slight pull, exposing the plunger. If the plunger knob is turned in the 0.2 ml position and depressed, the tip, with a small O-ring seal, will protrude enough to allow light lubrication.

At times, the Fibrometer head fails to drop into place as it should. A very light application of grease and thorough cleaning of the drop shaft under the mixing head help to keep it functioning smoothly. Bio-Quest has been extremely good about keeping these instruments in repair, and the instruments have been almost trouble free in service.

*Medical Laboratory Automation, Inc. models.* The Model 600 automates most of the coagulation functions (Fig. 12-15). Up to 50 plasma samples can be pipetted into a sample carousel, where they are held at 8° C until they approach the test station. As the sample arrives at the pretest area, the temperature is raised to 37° C. In the test position, reagents at 37° C are added automatically and the test cycle begins. The change in OD of the reactants is measured and monitored by a second detector. The result is printed onto a paper tape with the sample identification number. A computer jack

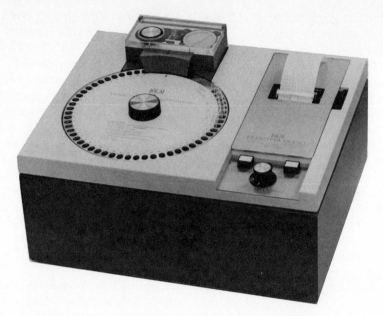

*Fig. 12-15.* Automatic Coagulation System, Electra 600. (Courtesy Medical Laboratory Automation, Inc.)

is also available for on-line testing. A number of these units are in use and have proved satisfactory. Results are highly reproducible unless the reagents are inconsistent. The saving of time is probably somewhat less than one would suppose unless large numbers of prothrombin time (PT) and partial thromboplastin time (PTT) tests are being performed. This might be said about many automated systems that are underutilized, however.

MLA has produced several other models on the same principle. A smaller unit called the *Electra 620* requires each sample to be manually introduced. Discharge of the sample through the light path triggers the timing mechanism. A double detection system prevents false end points. Test times are read out on a digital display. This model has had rather wide acceptance.

A newer, more advanced model called the *Electra 700* has recently been introduced. This instrument is designed to do PT, PTT, and fibrinogen assays, including saline dilutions and other coagulation tests. Different-colored cuvettes initiate PT

or PTT test sequences. Temperature probes in four locations monitor both refrigeration and incubation areas and provide a printed record of the readings. There is a self-check "confidence" test that monitors the clot detection system and records results. Patient reports are rendered on a printed tape that indicates duplicate runs and the average clotting time. Used cuvettes automatically fall into a disposable catch bin. Since reagents are refrigerated on the machine, there is no need to make up or take out reagents for each run. This model would seem to be an extremely convenient instrument that should have the same precision and reliability as the earlier models.

*Coagulation Profiler (Bio/Data Corp.).* This company emphasizes the fact that the rate of change of optical density during clot formation is as important as the time required for clot formation to occur. For this reason their instruments are provided with a strip-chart recorder on which the actual change in absorbance or optical density is shown. In the Model CP-8 is a cold block that can

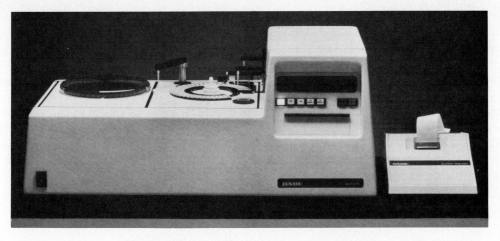

**Fig. 12-16.** Dade Auto-Fi Coagulation Instrument. (Courtesy Dade Division, American Hospital Supply Corp.)

store 54 samples at 4° C. Instrument status and test procedures are displayed during use on a panel. Two tests can be run simultaneously. Samples and reagents are pipetted into the test well, where the temperature is maintained at 37° C. As coagulation occurs, the absorbance change is sensed by cadmium sulfide photoresistive cells and is recorded on the chart paper as a function of time. By using the charted information during a coagulation with thrombin, the total fibrin can be calculated. Also, the dynamics of the clotting mechanism can be visualized. Standard and microsamples may be used. PTs and PPTs can be done simultaneously, saving considerable technician time.

*Platelet Aggregation Profiler (Bio/Data Corp.).* Various coagulation disorders can be attributed to the abnormal tendency of blood platelets to stick to each other or aggregate. This characteristic may be induced or amplified when various substances are present. Bio/Data Corp. has developed this instrument, which compares the absorbance of a platelet-rich and a platelet-poor sample. A differential amplifier receives the two signals and feeds them to the amplifier system of a chart recorder where the aggregation process is recorded. This instrument has proved to be of

considerable value in studying platelet functions under varying conditions and with certain additives.

*Auto-Fi Coagulation Instrument (Dade Reagents, Division of American Hospital Supply Corp.)* (Fig. 12-16). This is one of the few really new instruments that have been introduced in the past few years. The principle on which this instrument works has been suggested in the literature from time to time, but this is the first time, to our knowledge, that a commercial instrument has employed the idea. As the clot is formed, two parallel threads are pulled through the reaction chamber. When a clot is formed, it adheres to the threads and is pulled between a light source and a detector, which stops the timer. Although the nature of the reaction is quite simple, the instrument itself is somewhat more intricate.

The Auto-Fi is designed to perform PTs, PTTs, and fibrinogen tests and can be used for factor assays. The detection system operates in the same way for all these tests. Selector switches determine which reagent pump or pumps will operate and what the maximum test time will be. In the case of fibrinogen, thrombin clotting time is determined and compared to a graph of standard values plotted on log/log paper. Factor assays may be run, selecting the proper test button for one or two reagents, and the appropriate maximum test time or a manual mode can be used.

Samples are refrigerated in disposable sample cups before the test is started, on the sample carousel. From the sample cup, plasma is moved by the sample pump, using a disposable tip, to the test tray where it is mixed with the reagent(s). As the reagent is pushed into the cup, it is mixed with the plasma and the cotton thread and is carried between the light source and the detector. Interrup-

tion of light to the detector stops the timer and causes the printer to record the result. Reaction trays and reagents are incubated at 37° C, and the reagents are continuously mixed. Test trays will accept 10 consecutive tests, and the carousel holds 40 sample cups.

This is a large and expensive instrument that is designed for coagulation departments with a rather large testing load. It has not had widespread acceptance, possibly because of the cost and its relative complexity.

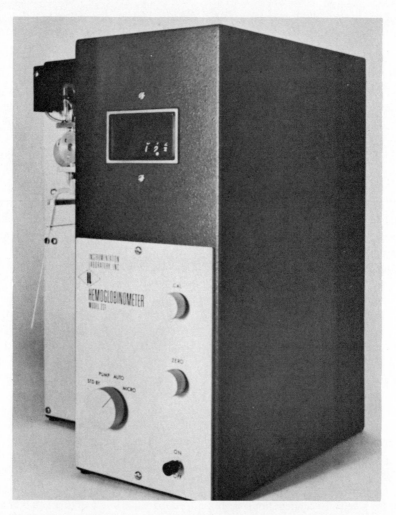

*Fig. 12-17.* Hemoglobinometer, Model 231. (Courtesy Instrumentation Laboratory, Inc.)

***Preventive maintenance and quality control.*** Considerable quality control is necessary with all coagulation equipment. Temperature is very important, and one or two degrees variation can produce significant error. The reaction well should be monitored each day. Timing must be quite accurate; therefore, timing watches and timing cycles of instruments must be rechecked frequently. The fluid measurement should not be assumed accurate in automated instruments. Some means should be devised for occasionally checking both accuracy and precision, since the volumes of patient plasma and reagents are obviously critical to test accuracy. Coagulation tests should be run in duplicate and should not be reported unless results agree within predefined limits. Probes or other materials that come in contact with the test system must be free of contamination.

## Hemoglobin-measuring instruments

*IL Hemoglobinometer, Model 231 (Instrumentation Laboratory, Inc.)* (Fig. 12-17). There are many special-purpose colorimeters on the market, and a number of these are designed specifically for reading hemoglobin. The Model 231 is particularly well designed and uses a slightly different rationale. The *isobestic* wavelength of 548.5 nm is used. This is the point at which oxyhemoglobin, carboxyhemoglobin, and reduced hemoglobin all read at the same concentration (Fig.

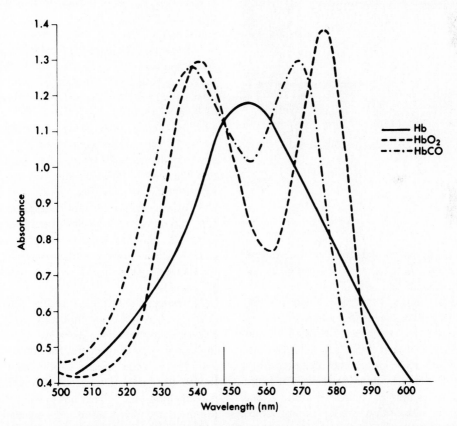

*Fig. 12-18.* Spectral scans of oxyhemoglobin, carboxyhemoglobin, and reduced hemoglobin. Note that any of the three would read the same absorbance at 548.5 nm if present in the same concentration. This is called the *isobestic point* for all three. (Courtesy Instrumentation Laboratory, Inc.)

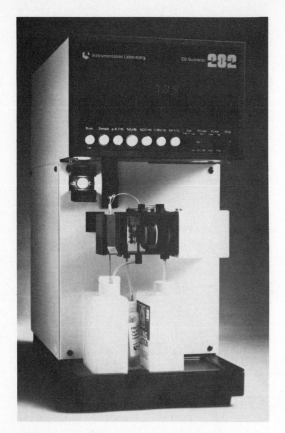

*Fig. 12-19.* Co-Oximeter, Model 282. (Courtesy Instrumentation Laboratory, Inc.)

12-18). An artificial standard is used to calibrate the instrument. A blood sample is automatically aspirated, diluted, and read at 548.4 nm; the resultant concentration is exhibited on a digital dial. The process requires about 15 seconds. A narrow-band pass interference filter is used. The interference filter, isobestic point, and automatic mechanical dilution provide accuracy that exceeds the accuracy of most hemoglobin methods. The instrument has the further advantage of flushing itself automatically a few minutes after the last sample is read. The IL Model 231 Hemoglobinometer is an outstanding example of special-purpose colorimeters designed for one specific function.

*IL Co-Oximeter 282 (Instrumentation Laboratory, Inc.)* (Fig. 12-19). A natural outgrowth of the Hemoglobinometer has been the Co-Oximeter. This instrument is able to record total hemoglobin at 548.5 nm. By ratioing the absorbances at 568 and 548.5 nm, the carboxyhemoglobin is measured. Oxyhemoglobin is measured in like manner, from the ratio of absorbances at 578 to 548 nm. This instrument is of particular value in cardiac catheterization, distinguishing between the output of the right and left sides of the heart and differentiating conditions in which there is mixing. A review of Fig. 12-20 will facilitate understanding the instrument's operation.

*OSM2 Hemoximeter (Radiometer A/S, Copenhagen)* (Fig. 12-20, *A*). This instrument is similar to the Co-Oximeter. A 20 $\mu$l sample of blood is automatically sampled from a capillary, syringe, or Vacutainer. The blood is then diluted and hemolyzed by ultrasound and the hemoglobin values read at 505 and 600 nm. The former is also an isosbestic point for hemoglobin and oxyhemoglobin; appreciable difference in the two forms exist at 600 nm, so the oxygen saturation is easily measured. The difference in absorbance at the two wavelengths is sensed by the same detector as the two filters are rotated rapidly between the light source and photocell (Fig. 12-20, *B*). After the absorbance is read, the total hemoglobin and percent saturation are calculated and electronically displayed, and the sample is flushed from the system. After automatic rinsing, the system is ready for another sample. The entire cycle requires about 50 seconds.

*Fibrinogen Analyzer (Sherwood Medical Industries, Inc.).* The determination of plasma fibrinogen has been done many ways, but most of the standard techniques are inaccurate, time-consuming, or inconvenient. This instrument seems to give reasonably good correlation with the Kjeldahl method and to be easy to use. Buffer and thrombin/calcium reagent are manually mixed with the patient's plasma and inserted into the instrument. At the end of 20 minutes the instrument reads the optical density of the clot, which is con-

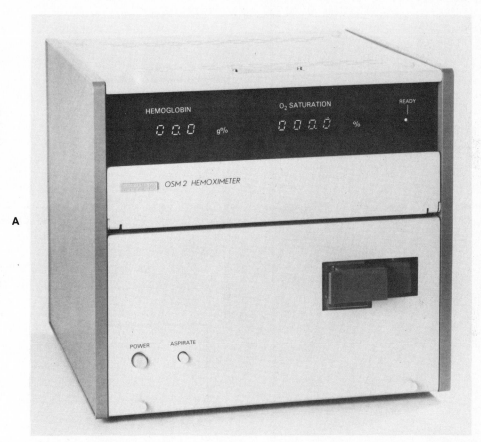

*Continued.*

*Fig. 12-20. A,* OSM2 Hemoximeter. *B,* Functional diagram showing the rationale of the OSM2 Hemoximeter. (Courtesy Radiometer.)

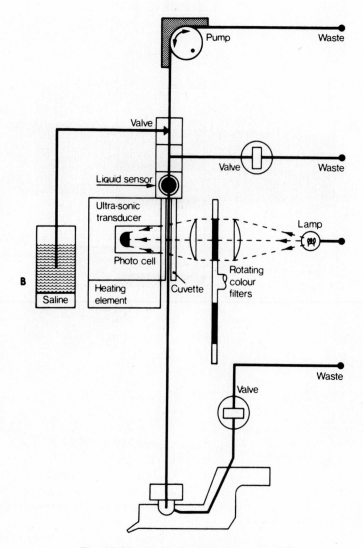

*Fig. 12-20, cont'd.* For legend see page 235.

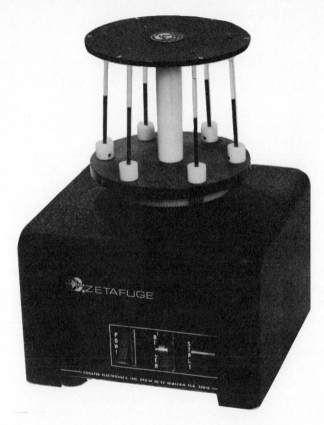

*Fig. 12-21.* Zetafuge. (Courtesy Coulter Electronics, Inc.)

verted into milligrams of fibrinogen per 100 ml of plasma.

The instrument itself is a relatively simple photometer set up to continuously monitor the density of the fibrin clot. A zero reading on the initial mixture is taken before clotting starts. This information provides a test blank to eliminate absorbance of icteric and chylous plasma, etc. Absorbance units are converted electronically to milligrams of fibrinogen.

## Automated sedimentation rate

Technologists and doctors often fret about the time that is required to complete a sedimentation rate. In an article on the zeta sedimentation ratio, published in the August 1972 issue of *Laboratory Medicine,* Drs. Brian Bull and J. Douglas Brailsford have presented an interesting idea. The sedimentation of cells can be speeded up by centrifugation, and, if all variables are properly controlled, a value can be determined that correlates well with traditional sedimentation values. Apparently the effects of temperature, vibration, etc. on the sedimentation rate are eliminated in this 3-minute method.

*Zetafuge (Coulter Electronics, Inc.)* (Fig. 12-21). Coulter's Zetafuge is intended to provide a means of properly performing this new test. The instrument is shown here. Results have been shown to correlate well with classical sedimentation rate results.

# CHAPTER 13

# Automation in chemistry

During the 1950s many medical laboratory workers were putting forth efforts to simplify procedures and save work time. Some of these efforts led to automatic pipetters, sequential samplers, shakers, and rotators, which were the first tentative steps toward automation of methods. A small company called Technicon Corporation introduced a tissue processor that moved surgical specimens through the steps of fixation, dehydration, and embedding in a timed sequence. This was done rather simply by mounting a metal disc on a clock movement so that it completed one rotation in 12 hours. Notches along the circumference of the disc actuated microswitches at specific times, turning small induction motors on and off. The motors, by a chain of gears and levers, caused the raising, lowering, turning, and agitating motions required.

These devices worked well and were quickly followed by others that performed mechanical functions in some sort of timed sequence in an automatic fashion without human involvement. There is really nothing particularly difficult or mysterious about these machines that do work by using gears, levers, cams and wedges in familiar ways. Almost all of the automation that is discussed in this chapter involves this sort of mechanical function in conjunction with various electrical devices such are discussed in earlier chapters. It is true that some of the modern marvels of automation seem mysterious, but when each step is examined, in its function, there is very little that does not seem reasonably simple. Many of the instruments are incredibly sophisticated because of the number of individual simple tasks that are performed. Saying that each of these tasks is in itself simple does not in any way detract from the impressive engineering involved in combining them into an integrated and practical working tool.

As automation has progressed, it has become possible to perform large numbers of analyses and accumulate quantities of data. In many cases, the sophistication of analytical devices has brought out many details requiring complicated decisions. Both the orderly storing of data secured through automation and the making of complex decisions can be done well by computers. Automated systems present details—changes of time and temperature, variations in chemical concentrations, etc.—to computer circuits for storage and retrieval at a later date or for use in further operation or computation. Modern automation makes use of mechanical ingenuity, electronic technology, and data handling.

During the past 10 years the state of the science of electronics has progressed very rapidly as solid-state components and integrated circuits mounted on printed circuit boards have almost completely replaced the hand-wired, vacuum tube instruments of earlier years. These remarkable advances have made possible much smaller, more accurate, and more trouble-free instruments. Miniaturization, which has been an important by-product of the electronic revolution, has made possible the combination of many functions into one cabinet or instrument. Electronic noise that plagued measurement of electronic signals has nearly disappeared as a routine problem, and the dissipation of large amounts of heat and the collection of electrostatic dust have mercifully greatly diminished as instrument problems.

Miniaturization and better manufacturing techniques have contributed to lower the relative price of instrumentation, so that most laboratories are now able to buy many specialized devices that would have seemed impossible 15 years ago. These size and price trends have probably contributed largely to the development of a great many specialized, dedicated small instruments for performing a single test or small group of tests—for example, glucose analyzers, BUN analyzers, and enzyme analyzers. Many of these are discussed in other chapters, even though they may indeed contribute substantially to the automation of chemistry.

The use of special-purpose electrodes as an analytical tool has gained considerable importance. The analysis of many substances has been dramatically shortened and simplified by the use of ion-selective and modified pH electrodes. Devices using this important, modern diagnostic approach are considered in Chapter 10. In all probability the trend toward electrode analysis will accelerate during the coming years.

Microprocessors or minicomputers have been incorporated into a large number of the new instruments. These sophisticated, small logic circuits have made possible such conveniences as automatic zeroing, automatic calibration, failure of instrument subsystems and components, and step-by-step, electronically displayed operating instructions. This would seem to be the largest change that has occurred during the past few years.

It seems quite possible that the next generation of devices—or the next—may make many analyses almost as easy to operate as the automatic coffee maker, and it may, in fact, be possible for the receptionist or the janitor to operate them. We believe it is extremely important that the laboratory scientist understand each of these devices, its rationale of operation, and its limitation. There is a regrettable tendency, on the part of manufacturers and vendors, to advertise these devices like radios

and coffee makers without supplying any details of operating principle or design. Technologists and other laboratory scientists need to inquire, examine, and study to thoroughly understand the tools with which they work.

In this chapter only the more automated chemistry systems are considered.

## Technicon's moving-stream principle

Historically the first real automation of clinical chemistry was done by the Technicon Corp. using a combination of clever, innovative ideas. The first idea involved in the Technicon approach is that samples can be picked up in a stream of fluid and moved along a tube by a peristaltic pump, through various changes, and finally be analyzed colorimetrically. For this concept to work, steps must be taken to segregate the samples in the moving stream and ensure that cross-contamination between samples does not occur. If a nonwettable plastic tube is used, there is a very small holdback effect if bubbles of air large enough to completely fill the lumen of the tube are introduced regularly. Mixed with diluents and reactants, the sample passes along the tube in small segments separated by air bubbles. This technique works well, and holdback with cross-contamination is effectively eliminated. There are a few places, such as in the colorimeter, where air bubbles cannot be tolerated. At these points the air is bled out of the tube through the vertical arm of a T-shaped fitting called a *debubbler*. Where the stream must run any distance without bubbles interspersed, a holdback is experienced. Keeping such distances very short minimizes this problem.

A second idea used by most of the Technicon systems is dialysis of the sample. Blood serum is, of course, rich in proteins. Proteins precipitate with heat or with strong chemicals such as acids. Precipitated protein would render a solution cloudy and would produce a substantial error in colorimetric readings. Since most of blood chemistry methods in use in the 1950s depended on heat or on acids, some way had to be found to eliminate protein. The Technicon solution was to pass the stream of sample across a membrane, parallel to a moving stream of fluid with a lower tonicity. As the two streams pass on either side of the membrane, certain substances dialyze across the membrane and pass from the sample stream into the new stream called the *dialysate*. It should be obvious that not all of a substance will pass across the membrane, but the amount that does pass is a function of its concentration in the sample stream.

Since the concentration of material in the dialysate is not a linear function of the material in the original sample, some means must be found to correct for this error. If a series of standards are run through the entire system and a curve is constructed by plotting their concentrations against their absorbance values, unknown samples can then be read on this curve. If an infinite number of points could be plotted, the method should provide excellent accuracy. Since this is not practical, values must be interpolated between established points on the curve. The resultant values are not absolute by any means but are clinically acceptable by almost any standard.

These early AutoAnalyzer systems produced by Technicon Corp. consisted of several components connected into a train. A typical system might include the following:

1. A sampler that could insert a plastic sampling tip into a different sample each minute and hold it there for a given time while the sample was aspirated at a constant rate.
2. A peristaltic pump that advanced a stream of sample, reagents, air, and diluent along separate plastic tubes by rolling steel rollers forward and pressing the tubes shut.
3. A dialyzer that allowed dialysis to occur between two moving streams in a temperature-controlled unit.
4. A unit where solutions passed through long coils to prolong their stay in a temperature-controlled bath.
5. A colorimeter where the absorbance of the test solution was measured in a flow cell.
6. A recorder that drew a curve, using the output of the colorimeter.

Later systems have employed these basic components, modifying them as need dictated.

As the interest in automation increased, Technicon adapted its systems to perform multiple analyses on a single sampling, and numerous modifications and improvements have been made. It has been possible to reduce the sample size significantly with a parallel reduction in reagent consumption. The large and awkward dialyzers have been replaced by quite small modules using a small, easily replaced membrane. The once cumbersome and problem-plagued peristaltic pumps have been replaced by better-designed, smaller units. Many other modifications have been introduced that have improved flow characteristics. Many of these changes have been incorporated into the current AA II Series. In the mid-1960s various multichannel systems were introduced.

The most dramatic early multiple system was the SMA 12/30 (Sequential Multiple Analyzer), which could perform 12 simultaneous routine colorimetric tests on one sample and could introduce samples at the rate of 30 per hour. In due time this unit was replaced by the SMA 12/60, which doubled the number of samples per hour and again reduced the sample and reagent requirement substantially. The principal innovation that made it possible to do sequential tests was the Technilogger, which allowed the recorder to accept the output from the photocells of three colorimeters in rapid sequence as the appropriate analysis came to completion in that instrument. This process is then repeated as the next three tests are completed. The obvious problem comes in phasing tests so that they come to completion and into the proper colorimeter flow cell at the correct moment. Since one sample is being tested for 12 constituents each minute, there is a period of only 5 seconds in which each result can be recorded. If the flow through the system, for one constituent, is slightly longer than for another, the test with the shorter line will come to completion, each test cycle, a little earlier; after a number of tests it may get considerably out of phase. Fig. 13-1 shows how the recorder charts sequential tests on a single sample.

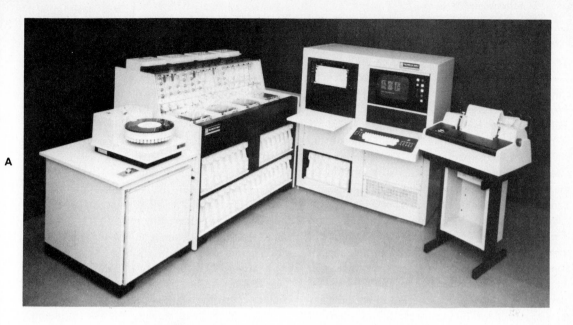

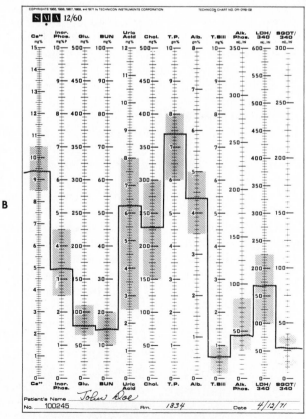

*Fig. 13-1. A,* SMA II. The unit on the left resembles the earlier SMA 12/60. *B,* Recorder chart from SMA 12/60. (*A* courtesy Technicon Instruments.)

Another Technicon system, introduced about the same time as the SMA 12/60, was the SMA 6/60. This system tests for glucose, urea nitrogen, chloride, carbon dioxide, sodium, and potassium. The first four of these tests use classic colorimetric methods that present no particular problem of instrumentation. Sodium and potassium, however, are done by flame photometry. The sample is diluted in a lithium (internal standard) solution by the proportioning pump and fed directly into the flame. Although flame photometry is a pretty well-developed science, there are many problems inherent in the continuous operation of a flame photometer in automated equipment. Maintaining a constant, even flow of fluid into the atomizer, maintaining flame characteristics, and eliminating carry-over between samples have all been problems. The SMA 6/60 does these things relatively well but not without a considerable amount of maintenance and occasional problems.

Reading the colorimetric values in the moving stream of Technicon's systems has not been any particular problem, once the *flow cell* was perfected. The debubbled stream passes through a narrow, horizontal glass tube, the ends of which are optically clear. Light, focused exactly on the front of this tube, passes through the solution for a prescribed distance (usually about 10 mm) and exits at the back where it strikes a photocell. The fluid enters via a connecting arm at the bottom at one end and exists in the same manner at the top and at the opposite end. Except for the flow cell, the colorimetry is not remarkable. The exciter lamp is monitored by a reference photocell, and the error signal between the photocells is amplified and activates a recorder pen.

Various other devices have been incorporated in Technicon chemical analyzers but the preceding, in essence, is the rationale of the system. Space does not allow for consideration of all the details of construction, methodologies, and modifications of each of the systems to be discussed; each automation system could be the subject of a large volume.

Certain advantages and disadvantages should be considered in this survey. The AutoAnalyzer was the first really workable automated chemistry system, and for many years it was virtually without competition. This fact alone has given this system considerable authority, and the company had years of experience in this field before most competitors entered it.

The idea of dialyzing the sample to get away from the problems of deproteinization is a solid advantage that other systems have had difficulty overcoming. Newer methods that can be performed successfully in the presence of protein are being developed; therefore, this is a less important point than it was at one time, but the advantage is still significant.

A principal disadvantage of the system is that plastic tubes become fatigued and distort, and they fail to carry the same volume, especially when pump characteristics change. The system requires a great deal of maintenance; a thoroughly competent analyst still requires a rather lengthy training on the system before he becomes proficient. There is no selectivity, and all tests must be done on each sample. Consequently there is no saving of reagents if tests are not needed. Also, the system is not easy to activate for a small number of tests or for a single sample.

***Technicon SMA II (Technicon Instrument Corp.).*** An updated version of the SMA 12/60 was introduced in January of 1977. Sampling was increased to 90 per hour with a corresponding reduction in sample and reagent required. A small computer/printer is a part of the total system. Through a keyboard, the operator can enter work lists and standard values and recall data, all of which are displayed on a CRT. The computer standardizes phases and computer correction factors and causes the printer to print out individual reports on a special form that can be used for the patient's chart. The operator can request that only selected tests or predefined profiles be printed out. The computer also is capable of some system troubleshooting.

***Technicon SMAC (Technicon Instrument Corp.)*** (Fig. 13-2). The next addition to Technicon's line of *Sequential Multiple Analyzers* was the SMAC. This major instrument incorporates

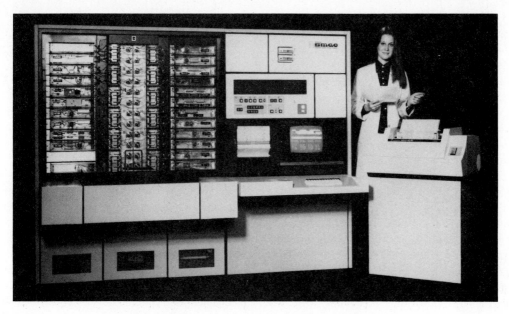

*Fig. 13-2.* SMAC system. (Courtesy Technicon Instruments.)

the principles of the earlier instruments into a much improved computer-monitored and -controlled system capable of accepting 150 samples per hour and performs up to 20 analyses on each sample. Each methodology has its own *manifold;* these are stacked one above the other in two panels in a block of 20 tests. The computer has self-diagnostic features that identify and localize operational problems. Start-up and shutdown procedures are computer controlled. With each batch of calibration standards a magnetic tape casette is provided, which feeds standard values to the computer to automatically calibrate each method. The SMAC's computer can be interfaced to other computer systems using ASCII language.

In the SMAC, flow lines have been reduced in most cases to 1 mm in diameter and all tubing kept as short as possible with very compact flow systems and cartridges. More bubbles are used, which improve performance considerably.

The sampler uses *eight-place racks* in a special centrifuge head. Additional racks can be continuously added to the sampler in an open-ended pattern. Serum aspirated by the sampler is immediately diluted and passed into a *riser,* which extends from the sampler, at the bottom of the system, to the last manifold at the top. *Peristaltic pump rollers,* at the level of each manifold, draw off the allotted portion of the diluted sample from the riser and move it to the *analytical cartridge,* where the diluted sample and reagent meet to pass through the same sort of analytical steps used in the SMA instruments. The *dialyzer* uses very small grooves and a thinner membrane for efficient transfer.

The colorimeter *flow cell* has a volume of only $2 \mu l$, and bubbles are not removed from the fluid stream passing through. The *computer* recognizes the absorbance information attributed to the bubbles and disregards it. *Fiberoptics* is used to transmit light from the source to the flow cell and on to a central colorimeter, which continuously monitors each flow cell in sequence.

The first SMAC Analyzers installed, understandably, had new-model problems, but the majority of these seem to be worked out, and the SMAC appears to be an efficient and economical computer-operated system of very large capacity.

New methods are being added to supplement the 20 tests originally offered. Sodium and potassium are analyzed with specific-ion electrodes similar to those used in the Stat-Ion.

Patient information is entered into a CRT terminal in the SMAC's operating panel along with the specimen number, and all test information is collated by the computer, printed on special forms, and placed in magnetic tape storage for analysis and/or transfer to a larger computer system.

*Technicon SMAC II System (Technicon Instrument Corp.).* The newest generation of Technicon analyzers was introduced in April of 1981. It is the SMAC II System. This chemistry analyzer, like the SMAC, performs up to 20 chemistries per sample at a rate of 150 samples per hour, requiring a total of 450 µl of sample for a full profile. The system is fully automated, incorporating distributed data processing with two host computers and up to 10 functional microprocessors. This additional computer power delivers greater quality control, data handling, and data-reporting capabilities. Quality control is done automatically on-line and is printed out on a schedule designated by the operator. Data storage and retrieval capabilities include 5000 files for patient demographics and 7000 files with a capacity of 40 results per file for any inputed laboratory results. Patient results can be reported in any of 32 formats. Information access is not a problem with the availability of up to five data terminals and three remote printers for the system.

Other changes in design from the SMAC include a fivefold decrease in the number of moving parts in the sampler; shortened reagent stream; addition of a probe wiper in the wash receptacle to minimize carry-over; improved accessibility to analytical cartridges; refrigerated sample reservoirs for controls, calibrators, and stats; and an improved sample identification system using bar code labeling. Operational improvements include automatic setting of the initial timing adjustment; short-sample optical detection; continuous optical monitoring for obstructions (for example, clots) at the beginning rather than the end of the test run; and computer interfacing, which permits user flexibility in formatting.

## Discrete chemical analysis

Automation was established in chemistry with the continuous-flow concept. Other approaches followed. Automated systems were developed that mechanized the old established manual steps in analyses. The samples were handled separately, or discretely, from each other, and therefore the system was called *discrete analysis*. In these systems an automated transport system moves the samples through each automated processing step. These processing steps are the same as were done manually: pipette sample; add reagents; mix; incubate; read, most commonly spectrophotometrically; calculate concentration; and record results. The difference now is that these steps are performed by mechanical or electronic devices under the control of a computer.

Another generation of discrete analyzers includes those using the principle of centrifugal analysis. This is a class unto itself and is discussed separately later in the chapter.

Numerous automated systems are commercially available, and others are in the developmental stages. Only a few automated systems will be described. These systems are representative of some different approaches in discrete analysis.

*Automatic Clinical Analyzer (ACA) III (E.I. DuPont de Nemours & Co.).* The Automatic Clinical Analyzer (ACA) III is the third generation of a well-established, field-proven technology (Fig. 13-3). This system takes an approach to chemistry automation that is different from any other system on the market. The reagents are prepackaged in a small plastic package, or kit, which acts as a reaction vessel, as well as a cuvette, for reading the colorimetric test at the end of the run. These units are remarkably complex packages, as may be seen in Fig. 13-4. A pack header and reagent envelope make up the test pack. The header is used to attach the pack to the transport chain, which moves the pack through the processing steps. The header may contain a column for sample prepara-

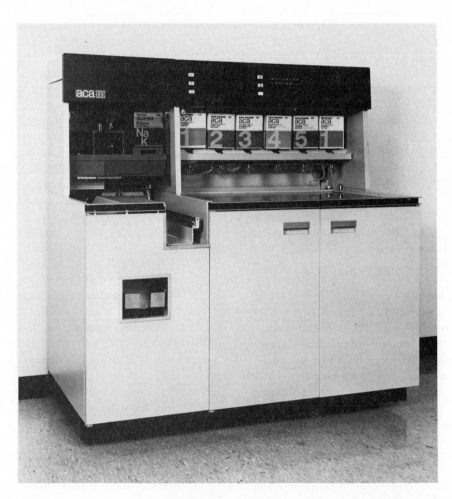

*Fig. 13-3.* The Automatic Clinical Analyzer (ACA) III. (Courtesy E.I. DuPont de Nemours & Co.)

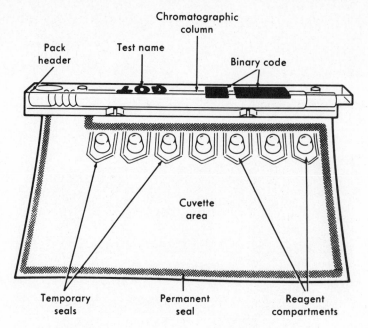

*Fig. 13-4.* The "pack" used on the Automatic Clinical Analyzer. (Courtesy E.I. DuPont de Nemours & Co.)

tion, such as for removal of interfering constituents from the sample prior to its introduction into the pack's reaction chamber. Also, the test name is identified both in binary code and abbreviated alphabetic form. Temporary seals are used around reagent compartments containing tablet or liquid reagents. A permanent seal forms the reaction chamber.

Serum samples are placed in rectangular cups, and a card on the side of the cup is filled out with the patient information as shown in Fig. 13-5. Anything written on the card is photographically reproduced on the final report form (Fig. 13-6), providing positive patient identification.

Processing of a test pack is completely microprocessor controlled. The block diagram in Fig. 13-7 shows the functional components involved in pack processing. As soon as the system is activated, a sample cup and test pack are moved into position in the filling station. A decoder reads the pack header binary code. This identifies the

test for the analyzer and instructs it as to the method specifics for this analysis, such as sample size, diluent selection and volumes, incubation period, and wavelengths of photometric measurement. Pack processing begins. A sample is picked up by a needle and injected into the test pack. Through the sample needle, appropriate diluent is delivered by selective action of computer-controlled solenoid switches. Filling of the pack will vary with the test pack in question. When one is filling a pack using a column immediately after sample injection, a portion of the diluent is also injected into the column fill–position (shown to the right on pack header); then the remainder of diluent is injected into the fill position directly into the pack (shown to the left on pack header) (see Fig. 13-4). Any number of 42 available tests can be performed in any order on a patient. The report slip size limits the number of tests that can be run after each sample kit to about 12.

Each pack in turn follows the same processing

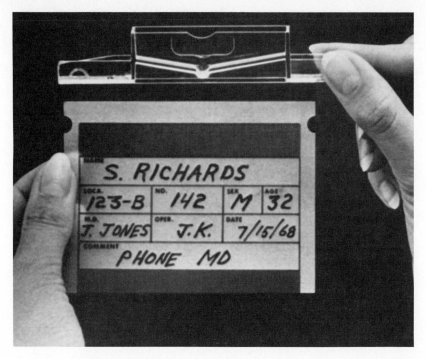

*Fig. 13-5.* Sample cup and identification card used on the ACA. (Courtesy E.I. DuPont de Nemours & Co.)

steps. From the filling station the pack header is pushed onto the transport chain. The pack is transported through the temperature-controlled processing chamber. In two preheater stations the test packs are warmed to 37° C. Next in breaker mixer 1, the pack is sandwiched between two metal plates, and four bullet-shaped protrusions crush the tablets in the first four reagent compartments. These reagents are mixed with the sample and diluent by a patting action of the two metal plates. The pack then is transported through five delay stations during which time the reaction develops. In breaker mixer 2, the last three reagent compartments are opened and the contents mixed with the reactant mixture in the pack. From here the pack is transported to the photometer. It is sandwiched between two metal jaws that molds a 1 cm cuvette into the optically transparent pack material as shown in Fig. 13-8. The smaller of the two

circular cells is an excess fluid cell, which is monitored to determine if solution volume in the cuvette is adequate. If not, an error code is noted on the printout. The photometer has a quartz-halogen lamp as a light source, a rotating wheel with 12 positions for interference filters, and a phototube detector. Absorbance readings are taken, concentration is calculated by the computer, and the results are printed on the report slip. Finally, the pack is moved from the photometer and dropped into a waste container. The initial test result is generated in about 7.5 minutes, with subsequent results generated every 37 seconds.

Sodium and potassium are done with ion-selective electrodes. A 170 $\mu$l sample is drawn from the sample cup and aspirated directly into the electrode measuring chamber. Results are visually displayed in 56 seconds and printed on the patient report slip in about 7 minutes.

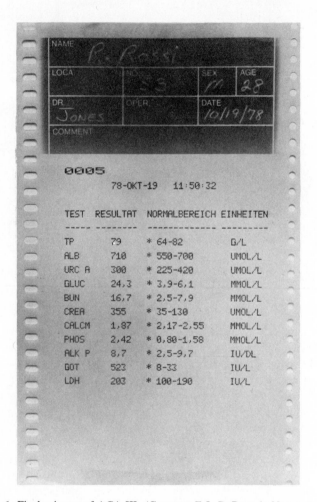

*Fig. 13-6.* Final printout of ACA III. (Courtesy E.I. DuPont de Nemours & Co.)

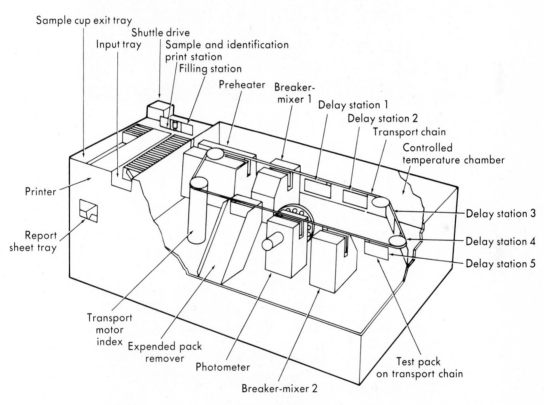

Sample cup exit tray

Shuttle drive

Input tray

Sample and identification print station

Filling station

Preheater

Breaker-mixer 1

Delay station 1

Delay station 2

Transport chain

Controlled temperature chamber

Printer

Report sheet tray

Delay station 3

Delay station 4

Delay station 5

Transport motor index

Expended pack remover

Photometer

Breaker-mixer 2

Test pack on transport chain

*Fig. 13-7.* Functional components involved in ACA pack processing. (Courtesy E.I. DuPont de Nemours & Co.)

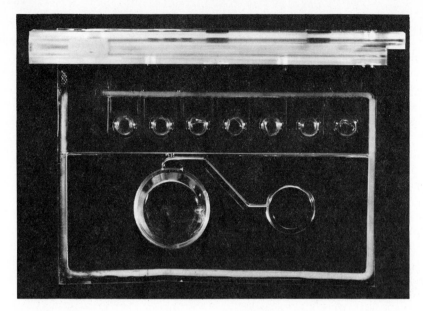

*Fig. 13-8.* Molded cuvette in ACA pack. (Courtesy E.I. DuPont de Nemours & Co.)

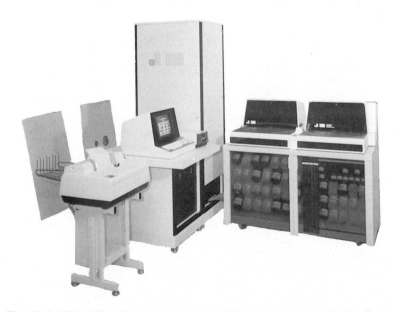

*Fig. 13-9.* KDA Micro Chemistry Analyzer. (Courtesy American Monitor Corp.)

This is, of course, a very simplified explanation of an intricate process performed by a highly engineered instrument. The precise planning and construction of all details, from the pack design to the photograph processing of labels, is fascinating to the student of automation. The first ACA was introduced in 1970. Reliability at this point seems to be high, and comparisons of test results with other methods indicate good accuracy and reproducibility. A self-check system detects many potential errors in instrument operation. The computer monitors processing sequence and acts as a command center for initiating steps in each test cycle. It processes the photosignal and converts it to a digital test result. Also, procedural and troubleshooting directions are provided by the computer for operator use.

This is a highly automated, microprocessor-controlled analysis in which the operator has very little to do with the actual processing of the test. One would suppose that a person could be trained to operate the ACA in a short time with relatively little difficulty. There is no extensive start-up procedure, operational checking, or standardization run prior to the start of actual sample testing. Each channel is calibrated every 3 months or with a change in the lot number of reagents, whichever comes first.

*KDA Micro Chemistry Analyzer (American Monitor Corp.)* (Fig. 13-9). This instrument consists of a chemistry console, a communications console, a card reader, and a printer. The chemistry console performs the mechanical operations, including sampling, reagent dispensing, mixing, incubation, and absorbance readings. Within the console is refrigerated storage for reagents. Two turntables are located on the chemistry console. A specimen turntable has 100 positions for specimen cups. The cups extend into a cold water bath to preserve sample integrity. As the cups are rotated past the sampler, patient samples are automatically pipetted from the sample cup into test tubes on the test turntable. With rotation of the test turntable, the test tubes pass under 26 dispensing and two mixing stations. A selection of 63, 31 of which are refrigerated, is selectively dispensed in appropriate volumes from pressurized reagent bottles through reagent lines. Flow through these lines is controlled by computer-controlled solenoid valves. Tests can be performed at ambient temperature or incubated at any of three programmed temperatures. The test tubes are surrounded by water at the selected temperature. After reaction completion, the test solution is transferred to a 1 cm square flow-through quartz cuvette where absorbances are measured. The monochromator consists of a tungsten-halide temperature-controlled ($10°$ to $14°$ C) light source and interference filters in the range from 340 to 760 nm. The detector is a vacuum photodiode. Data in concentration units are displayed on the CRT, and the data are stored on a ''floppy disc.'' When the run is completed, the printer prepares charting reports, with or without multiple copies. When a batch mode is used, report forms are omitted, and the cup position and its test value are printed. Test tubes are automatically discarded at the end of each analysis.

A keyboard and a CRT display screen provide a two-way communication system with the computer. A punched program card is used to select the proper reagents, volume of serum, mode of operation, reagent volume, sequencing of reagent dispensing and mixing, incubation time, and temperature. This system uses a number-based patient identification system. When blood is drawn, a numbered label from the machine-readable requisition card is detached and placed on the tube of blood. At the beginning of the test run, all request cards are fed through the card reader. The computer arranges the requisitioned tests in series and reports the sequence on the CRT screen. With this information, specimens are placed in their assigned positions. While the tests are being processed, patient demographics are inputed through the keyboard. Twenty-seven tests are available for the KDA, with sample volumes ranging from 5 to 174 $\mu$l. The rate of analyses is up to 900 chemistries per hour.

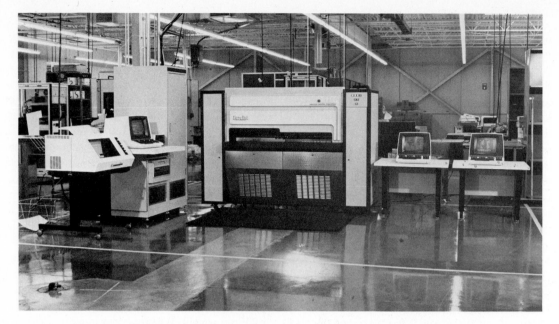

***Fig. 13-10.*** Parallel Analytical Chemistry System. (Courtesy American Monitor Corp.)

***Parallel Analytical Chemistry System (American Monitor Corp.).*** This is a 30-channel, high-speed, computerized instrument (Fig. 13-10). It performs analyses at a rate of 240 patients per hour, with 1 to 30 tests per patient or up to 7200 tests per hour. Only 750 $\mu$l of sample is required for a panel of 30 tests.

Analyses are performed basically as was described for the KDA Micro Chemistry Analyzer with the additions of a positive sample identification system, a different sample transport, greater computer capabilities, and a flame photometer for sodium and potassium assays.

Mark sense requisition cards are used for indicating tests, profiles, or panels to be done; recording patient demographics; and labeling the specimen tube with a unique 10-digit requisition number with bar code. Each requisition card has two bar-coded labels with adhesive backing for labeling specimens. Requisition cards are read by the card reader, and the original bar-coded labeled tubes are placed randomly in the 150-position

transport rack. Specimen labels on the transport are read by a bar-code reader and matched with the requisition. Only the tests indicated on the requisition will be performed.

The computer can store up to 25 previous standard runs per channel, including absorbance readings for standards and blanks, slope, intercept, and the standard error of estimate. A special interference channel is available for correcting sample interferences such as icterus, turbidity, hemolysis, and lipemia and for obtaining accurate initial absorbance readings for rate reactions.

***Kodak Ektachem 400 Analyzer (Eastman Kodak Co.)*** (Fig. 13-11). Kodak has developed a revolutionary approach to chemistry with the use of dry film–based slides for colorimetric assays by reflectance spectrophotometry and potentiometric measurements using film-formatted, single-use ion-selective electrodes. Chemistry slides now available total 12, including colorimetric blood serum analyses for glucose, BUN/urea, calcium, uric acid, amylase, total protein, albumin, and

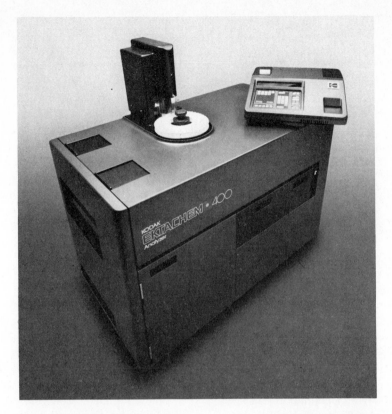

**Fig. 13-11.** Kodak Ektachem 400 Analyzer. (Courtesy Eastman Kodak Co.)

triglycerides and potentiometric slides for sodium, potassium, chloride, and carbon dioxide. Several colorimetric and kinetic enzyme assays are under development.

The Ektachem chemical slides are about the size of a postage stamp and are packaged in direct-loading cartridges containing 50 slides each (Fig. 13-12). Rate of analysis is 500 tests per hour in any of three operator-selected modes: Stat, discrete, or batch.

A colorimetric chemical analysis is initiated with a 10 $\mu$l drop of serum automatically delivered onto the surface of a multilayered thin-film slide. The top film layer is a white, microscopically porous spreading layer that distributes the serum evenly over the film. The spreading layer is selectively penetrated by sample components that move

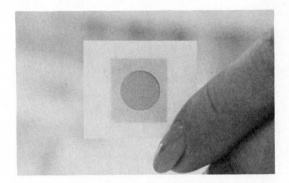

**Fig. 13-12.** The Kodak Ektachem clinical chemistry slide for colorimetry contains all the reagents needed to perform specified colorimetric tests in the clinical laboratory. (Courtesy Eastman Kodak Co.)

into a reagent layer. Typically, an enzymatic reaction results in formation of a dye proportional to the sample analyte of interest. The spreading layer functions as a white optical diffuser against which the dye intensity is measured by reflectance spectrophotometry and the concentration of analyte is determined.

Potentiometric measurement of electrolytes is performed with a unique single-use ion-selective electrode slide. Kodak has adapted the Ag/AgCl electrode to a film format for measurement of potassium, sodium, chloride, and carbonate. The slide consists of two identical thin-film ion-selective electrodes joined by a paper bridge. A 10 $\mu$l volume each of reference fluid and patient sample is applied to one of the separate film sections. This essentially creates a pair of electrochemical half-cells. The two fluids form a liquid junction by capillary flow through the paper bridge, this functioning as a salt bridge. Depending on the sample viscosity, the junction is formed after sample placement in about 20 to 30 seconds, and a stable analytical potential is reached in about 3 minutes. The electrode is connected within the analyzer to a voltmeter containing an algorithm to translate the measured potential difference to milliequivalents of electrolyte.

The analyzer consists of a chemistry unit and a control unit. Slide- and sample-handling mechanical and electrical systems are contained in the chemistry unit. The unit accommodates 16 slide cartridges. Functions of the chemistry unit include cartridge positioning, transfer of slide to metering station, sample delivery, and transport to appropriate incubation station for reaction development, to readout station, and finally to slide-disposal container.

The control unit includes a keyboard, display panel, thermal printer, and card reader. The keyboard is used to program, start, change, or stop the function of the analyzer. The display panel provides verification of input data and is an alternate output device. The thermal printer is the primary output device for test results. The card reader is used as an alternate input device.

Four different computers control the analyzer functions. A control-unit computer is the coordinating unit in that it receives commands, directs specific functions of other computers, and displays data on a 40-digit display panel. The second computer directs and synchronizes operations of the chemistry unit. Temperatures, humidities, and voltages in the chemistry unit are monitored and controlled by a third computer. These three computers interface with the fourth computer, which formats received data for the output device. Specified operating conditions are monitored by sensors, and deviations are reported to the operator by the control-unit computer.

Operation of the system is fully automatic once the patient samples are pipetted into sample cups and loaded into the 40-cup trays for insertion into the analyzer. The sample cup is divided into four sections, or quadrants, each of which holds 10 cups. Sample identification by cup position, tray number, and quadrant position is entered into the analyzer. Cartridges are loaded into the analyzer and automatically scanned by the analyzer for verification of test and position of cartridge.

Both colorimetric and potentiometric tests can be run in any combination in calibration, batch, or select mode. The batch mode programs the same test for a number of consecutive samples; the select mode programs a number of individual tests for each patient sample; and the stat tests can be performed as batch or select. The operator keys in test selection, mode, and identification information. The analyzer automatically compares each slide supply with the number of requested test for verification of sufficient number of slides to complete testing.

Automatic processing begins. The appropriate slide cartridge is moved to a dispensing station, and the slide is presented to a distribution station that has blocks on alternate positions for colorimetric or potentiometric slides. The slides are positioned at the metering station, a 10 $\mu$l drop of serum is deposited onto a colorimetric slide; on a potentiometric slide, equal volumes of serum and reference are used. The slides are transported to a

37° or 25° ± 0.2° C preheater for colorimetric and potentiometric slides, respectively, before being moved to incubation stations of the same respective temperatures.

After incubation, the colorimetric slides are transported to a reflectance spectrophotometer where a series of measurements are made and converted to concentration. At the read station, potentiometric slides are lifted to connect the contacts of an electrometer, which measures the potential difference between the ion-selective electrodes in the slide, and the electrolyte concentration is calculated.

After the slides have been read by either method, they are transported to and dropped into a disposal drawer in the analyzer. Test results are stored by the control-unit computer until all tests for each patient sample are completed, and the test results are then thermally printed for each patient.

## Centrifugal analysis

Dr. Norman Anderson introduced a new concept to chemistry automation with the development of the first centrifugal analyzer at Oak Ridge National Laboratory in 1968. The principle of centrifugal analysis is based on the rotation of a radial array of cuvettes so that each cuvette interrupts the path between a stationary light source and photodetector. While each cuvette is in the light beam (wavelength preselected), its contents are photometrically read and the absorbance stored in a computer. A rotor containing 20 cuvettes and rotating at 500 rpm allows absorbance readings of each cuvette every 100 msec. At this speed of data acquisition, readings are considered to be taken essentially simultaneously. Therefore, the optical system can be regarded as a multiple beam-in-time spectrophotometer with double-beam spectrophotometer-blanking capabilities. One of the 20 cuvettes in the rotor contains a blank, usually water. Each time the blank is read, 100% transmission is adjusted electronically. And each time the solid portion of the rotor interrupts the light beam, 0% transmission is electronically ad-

justed. This minimizes the chance of results being affected by drift in the measuring system. Another operational feature that contributes to the precision of the absorbance values is that the large number of absorbance readings obtained in a short time on each sample are averaged; this is referred to as *signal averaging*.

The centrifugal systems not only read fast but also initiate the test reactions almost simultaneously. By design of the rotor, sample and standards are separated from the reagents in separate compartments in each cuvette sector until rotation of the rotor forces the solutions into the cuvette at the outermost perimeter. Simultaneous mixing occurs within a few seconds, and absorbance readings can be obtained within seconds of reaction initiation. This capability coupled with rapid readings make centrifugal analyzers a good choice for kinetic analyses.

The first generation of centrifugal analyzers contained permanent rotors with a radial array of cuvette chambers made of parallel plates of optical quality–quartz secured together by outer metal plates. These heavy rotors required the use of large motors for the necessary rotational force. The permanent rotor required automatic washing and drying operations between test runs and additional cleaning procedures to prevent protein coating of the optical surfaces. Availability of materials for lightweight, disposable rotors resulted in a number of improvements now seen in second-generation centrifugal analyzers. The analyzers are smaller because of the use of smaller motors with lightweight rotors, elimination of automatic washing mechanisms within the instrument, and miniaturization of computers. Disposable rotors also provide the added advantages of eliminating possibility of contamination with sample carry-over from the previous run.

The acceptance of centrifugal analysis technology during the 1970s is evidenced by the number of comercially available centrifugal analyzers, a few of which are described briefly.

*Centrifichem (Union Carbide Corp.)* (Fig. 13-13). Tests are preprogrammed and may be se-

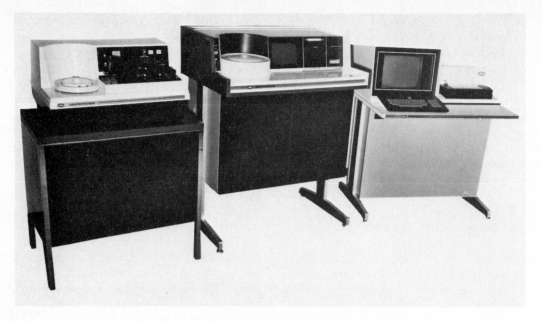

*Fig. 13-13.* Centrifichem. (Courtesy Union Carbide Corp.)

lected by test code. The reusable rotor will accept 30 samples. Seven interference filters select wavelengths in the range of 292 to 720 nm. Results are displayed on a CRT, which can exhibit a bar-graph display of real-time absorbance, and are printed on a paper tape by a quiet, thermal printer. The analyzer washes and dries the rotor at the end of the cycle so that it can be immediately reloaded for a new test run.

A pipetter is available with which a rotor can be loaded with samples and reagents in about 4 minutes. Sample size can vary from 1 to 50 $\mu$l, and reagent use is 250 to 350 $\mu$l per test. Changing the system can be accomplished in about 15 seconds with almost no reagent waste. A sample error not to exceed 1% is claimed.

A computer system is designed to process data from two analyzers simultaneously. Patient data and test requests can be entered for the day's work. The computer will organize the test sequence and assign cuvette positions. When testing is completed, all tests for each patient will be printed out on individual report forms. Abnormal results

will be flagged, and quality control statistics will be generated. Interim reports on individual patients can be called up at any time. Absorbance readings may be printed out for review of photometric information. The quality control data may be stored and accumulated on a long-term basis if desired. This system is now marketed as the Baker/Centrifichem System (Baker Instruments).

*Rotochem IIa (American Instrument Co.)* (Fig. 13-14). The Rotochem IIa must be thought of as a system more than as a simple instrument, since it is made up of a number of modular units. The Roto-fill II is the sample/reagent dispenser that can pipette samples, diluent, and two reagents into all 15 compartments of the rotor in 85 seconds. The centrifugal analyzer has a tungsten-halogen source, six interference filters, and a vacuum diode detector. A log-to-linear converter processes the photosignal before feeding it to the computer module, which not only processes, calculates, and reports analytical data but also controls the system. A PDP-8A minicomputer is the heart of this module. All essential information, including reports of

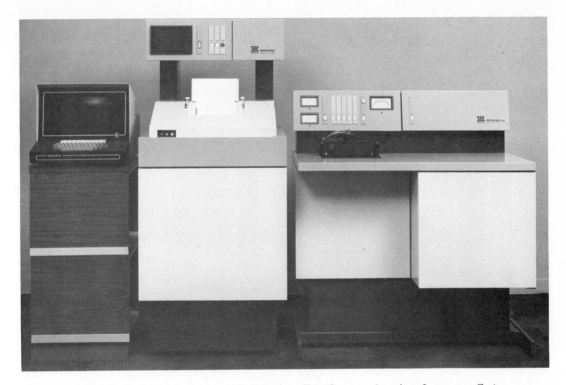

*Fig. 13-14.* American Instrument's Rotochem IIa. (Courtesy American Instrument Co.)

analyses, is reported on a 150-line-per-minute printer, which can give up to six clear carbon copies. Communication with the analyzer and computer is by way of a CRT and keyboard. Peripheral storage is available on a "floppy disc" to handle as many as 250 patients with 50 tests each. Fortran IV is the computer language used.

*Gemeni (Electro-Nucleonics, Inc.).* Fig. 13-15, *A*). This instrument can be programmed to perform any of 32 tests. When a coded test card is inserted in a card reader, the microprocessor selects the appropriate wavelength, incubation time, sample blanking, data points for kinetic enzymes, and calculations for the method requested.

A disposable 20-place cuvette disc may be loaded using automatic pipettes at a loading station. The disc is then positioned in the analyzer and the standard value dialed in on a thumb wheel. When the RUN button is pushed, sample and re-

agent are thrown together into the cuvette portion of the disc where readings are made. The chamber is a circulating air, thermoelectrically controlled temperature environment of 37° C. End-point reactions are read and concentrations calculated by the microprocessor, which causes the reports to be printed on report forms opposite assigned sample numbers. In the case of kinetic reactions, 20 readings are taken, the linear portion of the curve is identified by the microprocessor, and the units of activity are calculated.

The photometer consists of a tungsten-halide exciter lamp, seven interference filters (340 to 650 nm), and a solid-state detector. The card reader detects the punched holes, using photo-Darlington detectors to sense the light from LEDs. There is a separate integrated circuit (chip) in the microprocessor for each method used. These are located on the four easily replaced computer boards. The

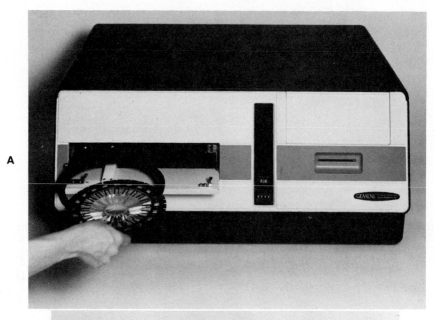

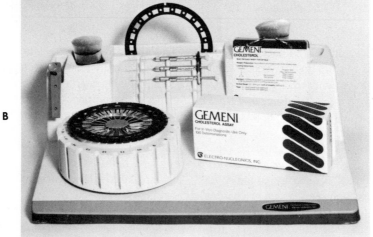

*Fig. 13-15. A*, Gemeni Centrifugal Analyzer, showing the disposable cuvette disc being inserted. *B*, Gemeni loading station. (Courtesy Electro-Nucleonics, Inc.)

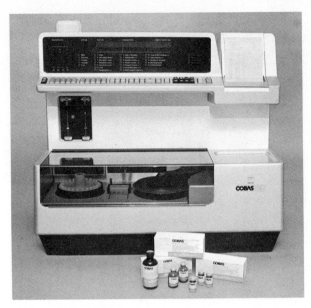

*Fig. 13-16.* COBAS BIO. (Courtesy Roche Analytical Instruments, Inc.)

power supply is modular and can be replaced easily, using four screws and a plug. The printer-reader and the built-in diagnostic circuitry are also modular and easily replaced. Troubleshooting is programmed and easy to follow. Service of the unit is very simple. The fan filter needs to be washed and dried occasionally, the filter wheel should be cleaned as needed, and contacts on printed circuit (PC) boards might need to be burnished after considerable time in use.

The units in use seem to be generally satisfactory and trouble free. The Gemeni functions well for batch testing or stats and could be used for performing small groups of profiles by running each group of samples through each test mode desired.

*Flexigem (Electro-Nucleonics, Inc.).* This system was introduced in 1981. It is microprocessor-controlled, with 32 preprogrammed chemistries and the capability of storing 30 additional procedures of recall access. It uses a 20-place disposable rotor disc. Wavelength selection in the range from

340 to 650 nm is accomplished with eight interference filters. Analysis can be run at any of three temperatures, 25°, 30°, or 37° C. Available are 10 calculation algorithms, 4 curve fit routines, 30 multistandard curve storage capacity, and 6 standards capacity for automatic calculation of assays. With these design and operating features the system is targeted for handling multiparameter standard curve of EMIT, ELISA, and turbidimetric immunoassays.

*COBAS BIO (Roche Analytical Instruments, Inc.)* (Fig. 13-16). This microprocessor (64K)-controlled unit can perform 30 preprogrammed tests with 19 different selectable parameters. It uses a 30-place disposable rotor with horizontal cuvettes, which permits use of variable programmable light path lengths.

A built-in pipetting station (Fig. 13-17) is used to automatically pipette samples and reagents in volumes specified during programming of test channels. The reagent module, with a removable plastic cover, can accommodate up to two reagents

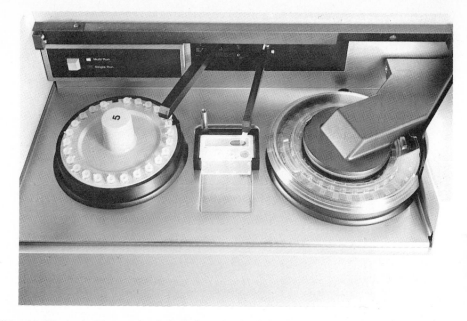

*Fig. 13-17.* A pipetting station is built into the COBAS BIO. (Courtesy Roche Analytical Instruments, Inc.)

and three standards. The sample discs hold 25 samples. Each sample is contained in a sealed tube that is pierced by the sample probe.

The optical system (Fig. 13-18) uses a xenon flash lamp as a light source. The output of the lamp is monitored and corrected for intensity fluctuations by a reference diode. A grating monochromator provides wavelengths in increments of 1 nm ranging from 290 to 750 nm. Four different cutoff filters are automatically positioned for stray light reduction. Data are available in any of seven different printout modes.

***Multistat III MCA and Multistat III F/LS (Instrumentation Laboratory, Inc.).*** The Multistat III is available in two models for different measurement technologies—the MCA for absorbance and the F/LS for fluorescence, light scattering, and absorbance. The basic Multistat III system consists of two modules, the analyzer, and a pipetting station for loading the rotor. In this loader, if required, a second reagent can be pipetted. The Multistat III uses a 20-place disposable rotor. Two

temperatures are factory preset in the range between 25° and 45° C, usually at 30° and 37° C. The system is controlled by a built-in minicomputer that also functions as the data processor. Analyses programs are stored on magnetic tape cassettes.

The Multistat III Micro Centrifugal Analyzer (MCA) is used for absorbance measurements only. The light source is quartz halogen, and wavelength selections are made with eight interference filters in the range from 340 to 690 nm. The F/LS model is used for fluorescence and light scattering as well as absorbance measurements. The MCA cannot be upgraded to the F/LS system. The difference in the MCA and F/LS is in the optical system. The rotor of the F/LS is designed with three optical surfaces in the cuvettes, top, bottom, and the surface radially out from the rotor. The excitation light from a high-intensity xenon arc is diffracted by a diffraction grating (300 to 700 nm), and a selected band of light is focused through a slit and onto the third optical surface to impinge

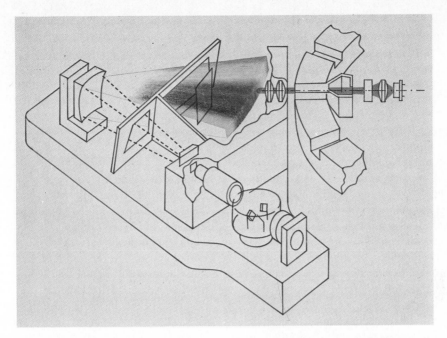

*Fig. 13-18.* The optical system of the COBAS BIO. (Courtesy Roche Analytical Instruments, Inc.)

upon the sample. The monochromator also includes five different stray light interference filters. Light from the quartz-halogen–absorbance source must be physically blocked with a large-diameter cover over the rotor during use of the excitation source. A photomultiplier is used for photodetection. For light scatter measurements, nonlinear curves necessitate running a number of standards from which the computer calibrates a curve-fit.

## Future trends in chemical automation

The automation of clinical chemistry procedures has occurred almost entirely within the past 20 years. The process seems to accelerate each year as more breakthroughs occur in electronics and other fields. Many of the techniques of space exploration have been translated into faster, smaller, more accurate instruments in other fields, and it is no accident that the fallout of the space program

has been realized during the years of fastest development in laboratory automation. As mentioned earlier, some hesitancy is being noted on the part of administrators and laboratory directors to invest heavily in today's automation, in anticipation of next year's developments. Many thoughtful laboratory people are wondering what is the prudent course in the present situation.

Several points seem obvious. With almost 80% of laboratory expense relating to personnel costs, automation that saves any appreciable work time is a good investment. At the same time, one wonders at the logic of writing off the largest percentage of a $50,000 to $100,000 investment in 3 to 5 years because of obsolescence. This practice has been ingrained into our thinking. At the same time, the public is asking for increasing amounts of free or low-cost medical service. Public funding, however, seems almost inadequate to finance the service promised or desired. There is continuous criticism of the cost of medical services. Pressure on hospitals to cut costs is increasing at the same time that the demand for improved services is being voiced.

As the capability to perform large numbers of automated tests is increased, the demand for other tests is stimulated, and there is often a lag period before these new tests are ordered in quantities sufficient to stimulate the production of automated equipment. Many people have tended to project the increase in total numbers of tests, types of analyses, etc.—to prophesy infinity in these areas. While progress will no doubt continue to be made, there is reason to doubt that straight-line projections of laboratory activity are valid. Most explosions of knowledge ultimately tend to simplify problems rather than render them more complex.

Within the past 10 years the impact of microprocessors, electrode analysis, and the greatly expanded use of integrated circuits has been felt. It seems entirely reasonable to assume that small dedicated instruments can be economically produced for nearly every test performed in quantity and that the rationale of such instruments can be integrated into profiling systems of high reliability. The next few years should be extremely interesting.

The roles of computers and data handling in the laboratory have not yet been discussed, but it is difficult to think about the future of laboratory automation without taking their influence into account.

As more data are accumulated, more time is consumed also in identifying patients, collecting blood, and processing and reporting information. It would seem, then, that the most fruitful field for development would be in these areas. The next chapter points out that automated devices for fast processing of requests, more certain and rapid patient and sample identification, and faster data handling are being built into complex systems that integrate with chemistry, and other, processors. This would seem to be the immediate direction of development. Many of these devices are modular in concept but flexible enough to tie in to different configurations.

It would seem that the best system will be the one that can handle the largest volume of tests the most rapidly and that is the most flexible, the most economical, and the most capable of automating the entire laboratory performance. Competition will probably largely eliminate systems that are not satisfactorily accurate or reliable. As time goes on, it seems imperative that preoccupation with numbers, volume, data flow, and techniques be overcome and that there be a thoughtful evaluation of the cost effectiveness of all this, as it relates to patient well-being and care. Maybe then we will start to differentiate many of the meaningful observations from the trivia.

# CHAPTER 14

# Computers in the laboratory

## Overview

A decade ago computers were magic boxes that seemed to do everything without effort, and everyone looked forward to the time when all of their problems would be solved when they got one. Suddenly computers are everywhere. Computers make plane reservations, handle utility and insurance bills, diagnose car engines, and even add up grocery bills. Home computers for the family budget, income tax, and Johnny's homework are now commonplace. We have found that they are not magic and they do not solve everything, but they certainly make many of life's chores easier.

Rather early in the development of computers, several people believed that the computer would be the perfect solution to the problems of handling the numerous reports generated by clinical laboratories. Several companies, large and small, undertook to develop systems for the laboratory. Fifteen years later not a single one of those original companies is producing computers for this use.

There are probably a number of reasons why this has happened. The flow of information in the hospital laboratory is a somewhat more complex pattern than most early developers supposed. At that time much of the standardization of methods and automation of analysis was not yet in place. Hospital billing systems and patient records were much less uniform, and hospital laboratory people were not ready to work with computers. The computer industry itself was not ready for the type of problems it found.

With the passage of time many changes have occurred in the laboratory, in hospital accounting and organization, and in the computer industry that encourages the development of laboratory computers. Many larger laboratories now have some phase of their operation computerized. However, there are numerous ways automated data handling, microprocessors, minicomputers, and similar devices, all called computers, can serve the laboratory. In this chapter we shall look at how these devices function and what they can do for us.

*Early hospital computers.* When the first hospital systems were designed, it was apparent to the planners that many records and reports were transmitted throughout the hospital and that handling of these had become so burdensome that it impaired the ability of technologists, nurses, and doctors to economically provide good care. On first examination, it seemed reasonable to suppose that all of these data could be easily handled by one large computer, which, after all, could easily digest millions of bits of information.

One of the first problems encountered was that there were hundreds of places in the hospital where orders, reports, and records were generated or received. At that time terminals for entering information or getting information from the computer were quite expensive and often bulky. Aside from the cost and space required, it became obvious that the computer time required to serve all these terminals was quite considerable. Computers are quite fast, but at that time the demands of many terminals on one central system slowed the process so much that no one had time to wait for the central computer to react. The only answer was to build larger computers, which became too expensive.

Another complicating factor was that work patterns were not organized. There was a general lack of standardization, and each nursing floor, doctor, and technician had their own preferences, systems, and imagined needs.

The frontal attempt to computerize all of a hospital's activities fell back in disarray. Some areas of the hospital worked reasonably well with computers. Accounting, for example, received charges from all over the hospital, entered them into one or two terminals, and printed out consolidated bills. These could be collected and cancelled from the billing process, and the whole cycle could be kept under control.

Producing a relatively simple small "computer" to perform a specific function was obviously easier to do. As better electronics, smaller and more efficient chips, and faster and more economical terminals were developed, these small devices became common in the hospital. Larger systems could not receive appropriate information from these specialized units and thus coordinate the hospital's activities.

*Modern hospital computers.* Modern day computers began as very large, self-contained, electronic data-handling systems. Early applications were primarily for tabulation and computation. The computer has evolved physically from the very large maintenance-intensive complex system using thousands of vacuum tubes to virtually trouble-free, highly sophisticated units miniaturized through advances in solid-state electronics and integrated circuits. Semiconductor technology in computers was responsible for substantial reductions in physical size, power consumption, and cost while at the same time increasing reliability and the scope and sophistication of applications.

Computer capabilities such as high-speed data manipulation, storage, and retrieval are used to manage the data explosion in the clinical laboratory. Laboratory computerization varies in extent and function. Roles of computers can be "contributory" or "dominant." A contributory role is one in which the computer processes or handles only data supplied to the system. The computer exerts no governing function. A computer system can handle the output from one or all analytical instruments in the laboratory. The data can be manipulated as required and stored or outputed in any preestablished format. A microprocessor or microcomputer may be built into the instrument to serve functionally as an extension of the signal handling device. The analog signal generated by the detector is converted to a digital signal which is the required input form for the microcomputer. After rapid completion of complex data manipulation and/or processing, the microcomputer output signal is converted from digital to analog form for driving a readout device.

A dominant role is exerted by computers that control operations of the instrument. Microprocessor-controlled instruments may perform many mechanical and analytical procedures under total control of their internal computer or, more accurately, the microprocessor. The dominant or controlling role of the computer has become very important in automation.

The extent and function of computerization in the laboratory is limited only by the requirements of the instrument or laboratory. Types of available computers are becoming increasingly more numerous. However, a basic review of computers will provide a general understanding of all digital computers. This review includes terms related to computers, the major components and their functions, and electronic representation of information.

## Computer terms

*Binary numerical system.* A binary numerical system is a system based on units of two compared with the familiar decimal system, which is based on units of 10. The binary system includes digits of 0 and 1.

*Bit.* The smallest unit in computer language, a bit is a binary digit, either 0 or 1. A computer bit can be compared with a letter in the alphabet.

*Word.* A word is a collection of bits. Languages based on alphabetic characters use ordered sequences of letters to form words that convey meaning. Similarly in the numeric-based computer language, the numeric digits of 0 and 1 (bits) in an ordered sequence form a word that is meaningful to the computer. The number of bits (commonly 4, 8, 12, 16, 24, or 64) in a computer word is restricted by the size of the computer. Minicomputers commonly use 16-bit words, and microcomputers use 8-bit words. The capacity of the computer memory is the number of words it can store. A computer with a 4K memory can store approximately 4000 words, and one with 16K can store approximately 16,000 words.

The computer word contains two pieces of information, an address in the computer memory and a datum and/or instruction. The address directs input data and instructions to a specific location in the computer memory. Compilation of addresses forms a large catalog system of contents in memory locations to make possible rapid retrieval of stored information.

*Byte.* The commonly used term "byte" is a computer word consisting of 8 bits.

*Nibble.* Nibble is a word used to describe a 4-bit word.

*Program.* A program is a sequence of specific instructions to be executed by the computer.

*Computer language.* The communication network of a computer does not have the complex networks of synaptic junctions for regulating passage of electrical impulses to appropriate brain centers as do humans. Instead, a computer has a very large complex of ON/OFF switches that must be set appropriately to regulate computer response to each binary code instruction. Effective communication with a computer is achieved only through use of machine language or machine code, which is binary coded words. Binary coded words constitute a language foreign to most humans. Therefore, programming languages were developed which were more closely related to al-phabetic-based language. The first was assembly language. Assembly language is a collection of letter codes relating to binary codes. This was still difficult to learn and cumbersome to use. High-level languages such as *Fortran* and *Basic* use familiar terms and abbreviations for inputing data and instructions into the computer. These languages, however, are foreign to the computer and must be translated into machine code by a computer program referred to as a "compiler."

*Microprocessor.* A microprocessor is an integrated circuit containing a miniaturized central processing unit called a *Microprocessor R.*

*Microcomputer.* A microcomputer consists of a microprocessor, memory, input device, and output device. Typically the words used are 8 bits, and the memory capacity is available in increments of 256 words. Eight memory increments total a 2048-word memory. Microprocessors and microcomputers are increasingly being used for control of automated analytical instruments. A microprocessor is dedicated to a single function defined by the permanent program designed into its construction. A microcomputer is not dedicated by design but can be programmed by the user.

*Minicomputer.* The result of miniaturization of computers, the minicomputer is a small computer capable of performing functions once limited to the large computer systems. A minicomputer commonly uses 16-bit words and has a memory capacity of at least 4K.

### Digital computer components

Major components of digital computers include an input unit, a central processing unit (CPU) that contains a control unit and an arithmetic/log unit (ALU), a memory, and an output unit (Fig. 14-1). The function of each component will be described briefly.

*Input unit.* The input unit transmits a digital signal to the computer. A variety of input devices are used, including output signals from analytical instruments, punch cards, electric typewriters, and

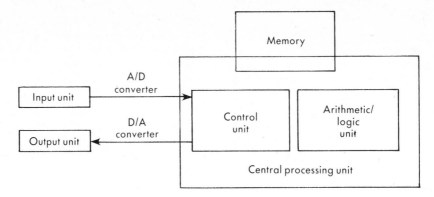

*Fig. 14-1.* Digital computer components.

magnetic tape or disc. Most of these input devices generate an analog signal that must be converted to a digital signal. This is accomplished by an analog-to-digital converter before the signal is presented to the computer.

***Central processing unit (CPU).*** As the name implies, the central processing unit is the center of activity. It contains the control unit and the arithmetic/logic unit (ALU). The control unit receives the input instructions and data, sequentially directs and controls computer operations as defined in the program stored in memory, transmits appropriate data and instructions to the arithmetic/logic unit for mathematical and logic operations, and transmits requested information to output and, when so directed, to memory.

***Memory.*** Computer memory stores instructions and data that can be retrieved for use by the central processing unit. Information can be stored in magnetic media such as magnetic tape or disc or in electronic memories using magnetic cores or integrated circuits. The slow access to magnetic storage is a disadvantage to their routine use. But since such storage is nonvolatile, retained in memory with loss of external power, programs and data can be stored for safe future reference. Memories using integrated circuits have very short access time but are volatile. With loss of power, stored information is lost.

***Output unit.*** An output device is used to display data in understandable form. Commonly used readout devices include meters, recorders, electric typewriters, and cathode ray tubes. These devices require analog signals to operate rather than the digital signal transmitted from the computer. Therefore, a digital-to-analog conversion is required prior to signal acceptance by the readout device.

### Logic circuit elements

Arithmetic and logic operations are performed in digital computers in circuits consisting of a network of gates. The logic gates distinguish between the binary digits 0 and 1 as low and high voltages such as 0 and 5 volts, respectively. The following presentation includes schematic representations, outputs resulting from inputs tabulated in a form referred to as a "truth table," and a brief description of the function performed by each of three logic gates: the NOT, AND, OR logic gates.

*NOT gate.* The NOT gate functions to invert a binary digit, changing 1 to 0 or 0 to 1 (Fig. 14-2 and Table 5).

*AND gate.* The AND gate accepts 2 bits at the input; both must be 1 (high voltage) to generate an output of 1 (Fig. 14-3 and Table 6).

*OR gate.* The output of the OR gate is 1 when

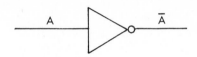

**Fig. 14-2.** Schematic representation for NOT gate.

**Table 5.** Truth table for NOT gate

| Input A | Output $\bar{A}$ |
|---------|------------------|
| 1 | 0 |
| 0 | 1 |

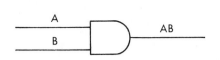

**Fig. 14-3.** Schematic representation for AND gate.

**Table 6.** Truth table for AND gate

| Inputs | | Output |
|--------|---|--------|
| A | B | AB |
| 1 | 1 | 1 |
| 0 | 1 | 0 |
| 1 | 0 | 0 |
| 0 | 0 | 0 |

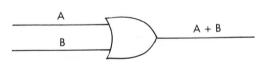

**Fig. 14-4.** Schematic representation for OR gate.

**Table 7.** Truth table for OR gate

| Inputs | | Output |
|--------|---|--------|
| A | B | A + B |
| 1 | 1 | 1 |
| 1 | 0 | 1 |
| 0 | 1 | 1 |
| 0 | 0 | 0 |

one of the input bits is 1 (high voltage) (Fig. 14-4 and Table 7).

Configurations of these three logic gates can be interconnected to obtain any desired logic functions.

## Levels of application

The use of computers in the hospital laboratory might be considered on three levels. The first has to do with the movement of information between the laboratory and the rest of the hospital; the second includes data management in the laboratory itself; and the third is at the instrument or bench level. As shall be seen, these are interrelated.

When working with computers, one must organize one's thinking carefully. Let us look at each of these levels of use in detail.

The sending of requests to the laboratory and the return of reports to patients charts was probably the first interest of the pioneers in laboratory computing. Efficiency experts have long deplored the wasted motion in hospitals of people carrying paper back and forth. In order for the process to work smoothly for the computer, the location of the patient needs to be known. Patients come and go in a short time and are frequently moved about; therefore, a current, accurate census must be kept. When reports are returned to patient's record, they must be arranged in some sort of order for easy access. Also, an interpretation of laboratory reports requires knowing what normal values the test procedure gives. Aside from the mechanics of reporting, the computer can very easily generate charges for the business office. The savings from inadvertently lost charges being retrieved nearly pays for many computer systems.

In the laboratory itself, the computer can do many more tasks. Receiving the orders from various nursing stations, the computer can record the time of receipt and organize requests into priorities and areas of the hospital for more efficient specimen collection. Labels can be prepared in advance to speed specimen collection. At the same time, work lists can be generated to alert laboratory sections or work stations about impending tests. The computer can provide a reporting format and can, if properly programmed, keep track of the status of the request and record test results through interfaces with test instruments. Reports coming from different areas can be organized into an easily read reporting format that includes comparison with previous days' reports. These organized report summaries can then be transmitted directly to the nursing floor for early incorporation in the patient's chart. If certain tests are delayed or overlooked, a "late list" or incompleted work list can be called up to alert the laboratory to the delayed reports. Perhaps one of the most important capabilities is the easily accessed file of tests ordered, tests in process, and tests completed. Rapid answering of queries about requests and reports can save a large laboratory thousands of hours of telephone time each year. From all the information passed through it the computer is able to generate very detailed, complete, and accurate analyses of the work load, reporting times and costs that are essential to good laboratory administration.

With the more recent development of integrated circuits and microprocessors, the computer now has a significant impact at the level of the laboratory work station. In many instruments the computer can now control the entire operating sequence, including such tasks as selecting the sequence at the touch of a button and choosing incubation temperatures, times, reagent quantities, and wavelengths. Standardization and calibration can be done automatically, and the system can perform self-checks and correct for errors or inform the operator of the nature of a problem. Quality control data can be accumulated and analyzed, and reports that are unacceptable can be automatically rejected. Results that are medically significant can be flagged. Completed patient data can be organized and collected. For example, all of the various tests on one patient can be printed out on a single report form along with normal values. If programmed to do so, the computer may also interrelate test information to cross-check instrument performance or patient diagnosis or condition.

In each of these three operating levels, much of the same information is used. The names and addresses of patients; times of ordering, collecting, and reporting; and test results for the entire hospital stay are common to all of these levels. It is here that the computer demonstrates its greatest efficiency. In one fast, easily accessed file a great deal of the information needed throughout the hospital can be found with the touching of a few keys. But in order for this modern miracle to take place, the entire process of requesting, collecting, testing, and reporting must be painstakingly analyzed and organized. The computer does *only* and *exactly* what it is told to do. It is much harder than we generally realize to reduce such a complicated process to an accurate description. Getting everyone to exactly define how and why things are done is half the task of setting up a computer system, and much of the benefit of the computer flows from this process of definition.

## Variations in laboratory systems

The physical components, or hardware, of a computer system have been described. For each location where a request or data is to be entered into the system, there must be an input terminal such as a typewriter or key-pad. Wherever information is desired, there must be an output terminal such

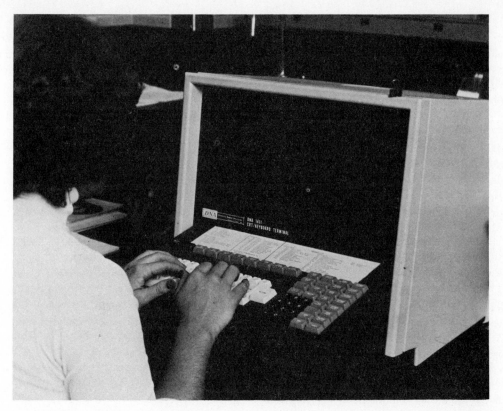

***Fig. 14-5.*** The cathode ray tube (CRT) device is one of the input/output (I/O) terminals through which one enters and extracts computer information. (Courtesy Diversified Numeric Applications, Division of AVNET.)

as a CRT (Fig. 14-5) or a printer. Whenever a test instrument is to give data directly into the computer, an interface must be designed and built. For each step in the process, steps in the computer program must be developed and written into the system. The cost of each terminal is considerable, and the number of nursing stations, departments, offices, and laboratory work areas adds up to a very large expense. Programming is possibly even more expensive; some decisions have to be made as to the economic feasibility of including various areas, processes, and data into the system. The system that is finally assembled may vary a great deal from hospital to hospital. At times systems are built up, starting with a single process

and adding pieces until a fairly complete computer installation emerges. It is not unusual for a hospital to have a central computer that maintains the hospital's census by having the admitting department enter all hospital admissions, discharges, and transfers. From this data base, each floor can order tests on its own keyboard that relays the request to a laboratory printer. This may be the extent of the hospital's system, but automatically charging the patient's account for the test ordered is so simple that it is usually done. Later some of the elements of a laboratory reporting and/or file storage may be added.

Some laboratory computers are designed so that they will do many of the processes described.

That is to say their programs have been written to define certain tasks for the computer and this is all they are to do. Systems of this sort are called *turnkey* systems. Other computers' functions can continually be changed by adding or modifying programs. Most hospitals do not have the resources to provide trained programmers, however, so many of the systems now being installed are essentially turnkey. Arithmetic/logic units for calculation and very limited programming may be provided as an option.

An acronym widely quoted in computer discussion is GIGO—"*garbage in, garbage out*"— which is a way to say that if the computer is given poor information, it will report the same. To control the data input most systems now have a *verification* process. All data entering the computer from a keyboard or an interface appears on the screen or printer and must be verified by a responsible person before it can go into storage or be reported.

Access to information in the computer must also be controlled at times. Since all patient information is confidential, there must be some way to prevent a hospital visitor, for example, from calling up patient reports. This *access control* is generally provided by giving authorized people or groups of people codes with which they can call up information appropriate to them.

The capability of computers has increased dramatically in the past few years. Also, the relative cost of performing most tasks by computer has decreased because of improvements in the state of the art and because of the increased market. As systems become more affordable and more common, there has been an increased acceptance of standardization, which in turn makes the process more economical. As noted before, computers are everywhere, and their impact on the laboratory in the next few years will be tremendous.

### Problems computers can help solve

To organize our thinking about the computer in the laboratory, let us tabulate some of the problem areas where data handling could help.

1. Large numbers of request slips come to the laboratory each day. These must be accepted and processed to the right places. Often some confusion exists about the identity or location of the patient.

2. A data base is necessary from which one can find out with certainty who is where and what work was ordered.

3. When blood is to be drawn, requests must be organized so that each person has a reasonable assignment of patients located reasonably close together.

4. Individual laboratories or work stations need to know what work to expect and to have it organized, so that time is not lost in organizing requisitions.

5. Properly identifying the patient and maintaining this identification throughout the drawing, labeling, transporting, separating, analyzing, and reporting steps are of critical importance.

6. Calculations take time and introduce the possibility of error.

7. Transporting reports from the work station or separate laboratory to some central laboratory reporting office is time consuming. Often the report is needed urgently and it may be at the work station, in transit, or in the office.

8. All reports on a patient must be collated so that one organized report is presented to the physician. This process also requires many steps in getting individual reports into patient's charts, which may be distant from the laboratory.

9. Filing of reports in some form for retrieval in a reasonable period of time requires many hours of time and still does not produce an error-proof, complete library of information.

10. Records or samples may be lost. The loss may not be apparent until it is too late to repair the damage.

11. Charging information must be relayed to the patient's billing record.

12. Statistical analysis of work performed is needed both for quality control and for management of the laboratory.

Although this listing is not exclusive, laboratory

workers can generally identify with most of these problems. Before we look at the systems that have been designed to attack these problems, let us think about the overall approaches which have been and are being made.

At the present time, the interest in data processing equipment in the laboratory centers on choosing the computer that can care for the processing of the laboratory's paperwork. A second large interest is in the techniques, systems, and equipment needed to pass information between autonomous data processing systems. For example, the laboratory system needs admitting information for building a data base, and it receives reports from the various analytical devices. At the same time, it generates quantities of billing information that must somehow be relayed to the billing computer.

## Minisystems for simple problems

As we have discussed various instruments, we have seen how much microprocessing is used internally to calculate, make choices, report instrument status and collate data. In discussing computerization it is hard to differentiate between devices that calculate, sort, compute, sense, and process. Let us consider a number of small devices that do some of these functions.

Calculators are, of course, everywhere, to the point that many people do not feel dressed without a minicalculator in their coat pocket or handbag. The very tiny circuitry of these devices can be used in all kinds of equipment to perform the same or similar functions.

There has been a great deal of interest in devices that can be taken to the patient's bedside to electronically read the patient's ID bracelet and generate a specimen label with identical information. Other similar devices would then read the specimen label to transmit the ID information into analyzers that would prepare reports using the same data, thus carrying positive identification electronically from patient to report. No one system has yet been perfected that resolves the basic problems and is still workable and economically feasible. It is nearly certain, however, that some

system of this kind will be perfected and put into use soon. Errors in sample or patient identification are the source of more serious patient damage by the laboratory than anything else. Malpractice suits are filed and won on the basis of this large problem, and the costs in settlements, court and legal fees, and lost time are astronomical. At least one system is under development that would electronically maintain identification fidelity from the patient through the laboratory reporting computer.

## Conventional laboratory systems

Full computer systems attempt to solve most of the problems mentioned earlier. Although they may vary considerably, most laboratory computer systems have about the same characteristics. Let us look at some of the routines common to nearly all these. All laboratory computers must start with certain basic information. These would include such details as the following:

1. A *catalog of all tests* in the laboratory. Since the names of these may be long, *mnemonic* designation (short form, for example, "glu" for glucose) or a code number may be assigned.

2. *Room and bed numbers*. These are used as addresses for patients so they can be found in the files.

3. *Normal values* for all tests. These may be printed on the report forms and may also be used to flag unusual test results.

4. *Formats* of the various sorts of reports that one will expect to see.

5. *Operating procedure* detailing how the system is to function.

In order for the system to work smoothly, all patients must be listed so that their requisitions and test results may be assigned to their files. Some procedure is initiated to enter all patients' names and basic identification information (age or birthdate, doctor, hospital, ID number, room assignment, and possibly more), and each day new admissions, discharges, and transfers are processed. At all times the system should have very close to the actual *census* of the hospital in its current files. If there is much discrepancy, the requi-

```
-------------------------------------------------------------------------
    SORENSON, PATRICIA L.            29 YEARS
    541-38-7406       GYN/403/C      FEMALE           125-DR. SMITH, CHARLES V.
    ADMITTED 06/11/74  DISCHARGED              RELEASED
```

*Fig. 14-6.* Patient's file information.

sitioning and reporting of tests and the admission of new patients becomes very complicated. Tests may be ordered after the patient's file is opened by calling his ID number or name to the screen (Fig. 14-6) and then entering the test name or code number.

When blood is to be collected, a *collection list* (Fig. 14-7) may be called, which may be simply a printing of specimen labels for all blood tubes. This list may be sequential by bed number or other criteria and may be broken up into nursing stations, groups of 10, or other listings.

Work to be done may be printed out by work station, laboratory, or test method on work lists (Fig. 14-8). Thus, all blood sugars might be listed together or all SMA 6/60 profiles or all routine chemistry tests ordered, depending on preference and the capabilities of the system.

When work is completed, test results are entered into the patient's record by again calling his file by requesting the ID number or name on the terminal. The computer collates all tests on a single patient and assembles them into an easily read format that can be called up on a CRT screen or printed by the printer.

At designated intervals during the day, *summaries* (Fig. 14-9) on all patients are printed and distributed to nursing stations. These may be cumulative summaries that present all tests that have been run on each patient since admission. To save printing time and paper, the cumulative report is usually not run more often than once per day and is supplemented by *partial summaries* that go back to the last summary printed and update it with work performed since its printing. On discharge, a *discharge summary* is printed, including all work done during the patient's hospital stay. Some sys-

```
 _____
|                                    |
|   COLLECTION LABEL WARD 3E         |
|   02/01/75       07:00 AM          |
|                                    |
|   TYPE: 1 COLLECTED BY TEAM        |
|_____|

 0195 | 0195  SMITH, GREGORY HE-0195
 HE-1 | HE-1  373024           3B-301
 - - + - - -  7 BLUE           02/01/75
 0195 | 0195  FIBRINGN
 HE-1 | HE-1

 0195 | 0195  SMITH, GREGORY HE-0195
 HE-1 | HE-1  373024           3E-301
 - - + - - -  7 LAVNDR         02/01/75
 0195 | 0195  PLATELET
 HE-1 | HE-1

 0087 | 0087  JOHNSON, CHRIS CH-0087
 CH-1 | CH-1  533096           3E-304
 - - - - - -  20 RED           02/01/75
 0087 | 0087  BIO SCRN
 CH-1 | CH-1

 0181 | 0181  JOHNSON, CHRIS HE-0181
 HE-1 | HE-1  533096           3E-304
 - - - - - -  7 BLUE           02/01/75
 0181 | 0181  FIBRINGN
 HE-1 | HE-1

 0105 | 0105  ANDERSON, JOHN CH-0105
 CH-1 | CH-1  533692           3E-310
 - - + - - -  20 RED           02/01/75
 0105 | 0105  BIO SCRN
 CH-1 | CH-1

 0183 | 0183  ANDERSON, JOHN HE-0183
 HE-1 | HE-1  533692           3E-310
 - - - - - -  LAVNDR           02/01/75
 0183 | 0133  CBC DIFF
 HE-1 | HE-1

 0125 | 0125  TAYLOR, PHILIP CH-0125
 CH-1 | CH-1  521644           3E-310
 - - - - - -  10 RED           02/01/75
 0125 | 0125  LYBUNGLU
 CH-1 | CH-1
```

*Fig. 14-7.* Set of specimen labels.

```
14:28          COAG/PT                    #120        DO NOT MARK HERE
4/12                                      P. 008      0 1 2 3 4 5 6 7 8 9 12 11
                                                      0 11 2 3 4 5 6 7 8 9 12 11
                 COMPLETED         TECH               0 1 2 3 4 5 6 7 8 9   100
*REPRINT*       ----------         ------             0 1 2 3 4 5 6 7 8 9   200
```

| ACC. # | NAME-ID-LOCATION-AL | RESULT | CODED RESULT/CONDITION |
|---|---|---|---|
| BX5109 ** WILLIAMS JOE<br>4/12  004676441  BTC-EYE<br>PT-CON  ( 1.0- 99.9) | 0<br>--.--<br>(SECONDS ) | |
| BX5109 ** WILLIAMS JOE<br>4/12  004676441  BTC-EYE<br>PT-PAT  ( 10.0- 13.0) | 0<br>--.--<br>(SECONDS ) | |
| BX5144 **<br>4/12  000070751  BTC-EYE<br>PT-CON  ( 1.0- 99.9) | 0<br>--.--<br>(SECONDS ) | |
| BX5144 **<br>4/12  000070751  BTC-EYE<br>PT-PAT  ( 10.0- 13.0) | 0<br>--.--<br>(SECONDS ) | |
| BX5150 ** FOSTER ERIN R<br>4/12  004560108  BTH-4NM<br>PT-CON  ( 1.0- 99.9) | 0<br>--.--<br>(SECONDS ) | |
| BX5150 ** FOSTER ERIN R<br>4/12  004560108  BTH-4NM<br>PT-PAT  ( 10.0- 13.0) | 0<br>--.--<br>(SECONDS ) | |
| BX5194 ** ESQUIVEL MARGARITO J<br>4/12  004118618  BTC-OTO<br>PT-CON  ( 1.0- 99.9) | 0<br>--.--<br>(SECONDS ) | |
| BX5194 ** ESQUIVEL MARGARITO J<br>4/12  004118618  BTC-OTO<br>PT-PAT  ( 10.0- 13.0) | 0<br>--.--<br>(SECONDS ) | |
| BX5224 ** TERRY LILLIAN<br>4/12  004628837  BTP-ER<br>PT-CON  ( 1.0- 99.9) | 0<br>--.--<br>(SECONDS ) | |
| BX5224 ** TERRY LILLIAN<br>4/12  004628837  BTP-ER<br>PT-PAT  ( 10.0- 13.0) | 0<br>--.--<br>(SECONDS ) | |

```
**=STAT INSERTS
A = CANCEL TEST      B = CHANGE TYPE      C = ADDITIONAL INF
H = HEMOLYZED        I = >                J = Q.N.S.
K = NO TEST          L = NOT INSY
```

Fig. 14-8. Computer-printed work list. This form, used with the Honeywell system, provides for test results to be marked in the machine-readable field at right. The document reader can then enter an entire page of results into the system in seconds. (Courtesy Honeywell, Inc.)

```
DR. RICHARD ERHART          MEMORIAL HOSPITAL          01/30/75 1821
DIRECTOR OF PATHOLOGY       INTERIM REPORT                    PAGE  1
LOC CCU-B2A                             MED. REC. NO.--   122353
AGE 50Y  SEX F  PHYS-MAKARI        A    KENNARD, JOAN L
-----------------------------------------------------------------------
   DRAWN                                   UNITS OF
DATE/TIME   SPECIMEN   TEST NAME    RESULT   RESULT    NORMAL RANGE
01/30 1412  SERUM    ACETONE
                     UNDILUTD     NEGATIVE
                     NEGATIVE     1:4
01/30 1412  SERUM    ALDOLASE         5.    MU/ML       1.  -     6.
01/30 1412  SERUM    AMYLASE        123.    UNITS      50.  -   200.
01/30 1412  SERUM    AUSTRALIA AN NEGATIVE
01/30 1412  SERUM    BILIR-MICRO    1.3     MG/100ML   0.2  -    1.5
01/30 1412  SERUM    BIOCHEM SCREEN-12
                     T.PROT         6.8     GM%        6.0  -    8.0
                     CALCIUM       10.1     MG%        8.3  -   10.5
                     PHOSPHORUS     3.4     MG%        2.5  -    4.8
                     CHOLESTEROL  250.      MG%      110.   -  300.
                     GLUCOSE       96.      MG%       75.   -  115.
                     BUN           12.      MG%        5.   -   25.
                     URIC ACID      5.7     MG%        2.5  -    7.0
                     CREATININE     1.0     MG%        0.7  -    1.5
                     T.BILIR        0.3     MG%        0.2  -    1.5
                     ALK.PHOS      43.      INT-UNIT  25.   -  110.
                     LDH          115.      INT-UNIT 100.   -  250.
                     SGOT          56.*     INT-UNIT   0.   -   40.
01/30 1412  SERUM    CAROTENE     198.      MCG/DL    60.   -  368.
01/30 1412  SERUM    CHLORIDES    126.*     MEQ/L     95.   -  107.
01/30 1412  SERUM    CO2           27.      MEQ/L     24.   -   32.
01/30 1412  SERUM    C P K         55.*     INT-UNIT   0.   -   35.
01/30 1412  SERUM    CREATINE       0.2     MG/100ML   0.0  -    0.6
01/30 1412  SERUM    IRON BINDING PENDING
01/30 1412  SERUM    TOTAL IRON S PENDING
01/30 1412  SERUM    LACTIC ACID    4.9     MG/100ML   3.0  -   12.0
01/30 1412  SERUM    L A P         11.      MU/ML      8.   -   22.
01/30 1412  SERUM    LIPASE         0.4     UNITS      0.0  -    1.0
01/30 1412  SERUM    ACID PHOSPHA   1.8     INT-UNIT   0.0  -    2.0
01/30 1412  SERUM    POTASSIUM      3.9     MEQ/L      3.5  -    5.0
01/30 1412  SERUM    SODIUM       126.*     MEQ/L    135.   -  145.
01/30 0830  WH BLOOD CBC
                     WBC            7.0     THOUSAND   4.5  -   11.0
                     RBC            5.00    MILLION    4.20 -    5.40
                     HEMOGLOBIN    14.1     GM        12.0  -   16.0
                     HEMATOCRIT    39.2     %         37.0  -   47.0
                     MCV           88.      CU MCRON  81.   -   99.
                     MCH           30.1     MCMCG     27.0  -   31.0
                     MCHC          35.4     %         32.0  -   36.0
                     BAND          12.*                0.   -    6.
                     SEG           30.*               36.   -   66.
                     LYMPH         50.*               24.   -   44.
                     MONO           2.*                3.   -    7.
                     EOSIN          1.                 1.   -    4.
                     PLATELET     ADEQUATE
```

*Fig. 14-9.* Patient's summary report.

tems purge information from memory after a pre-determined number of days have elapsed and use the discharge summary as a *hard-copy* record of the patient's file. Most companies provide some system of *archival storage* on magnetic tape or magnetic disc.

The statistical information entered into the system may be subjected to any of several types of review. One such screening would involve simply assessing and marking tests as *outside normal limits* (designated as *low* or *high*). Another judgment might be whether the value is "absurd." This sort of judgment can be thought of in several ways and limits set accordingly. The value might be judged as not compatible with life, indicating a serious laboratory error. Or the limit might be thought of as a "panic" level at which the physician must be notified immediately and the test repeated. Statistical analysis may be applied to the sample and reference values and any of a number of *quality control* documents prepared.

For management purposes it is desirable to have a *statistical report* of some kind, listing how many tests of each type have been performed in some defined report period. Analysis of the workload may also be calculated and reported. *Billing information* must be produced that will enable a bill to be prepared for the tests performed. This information might be in the form of a printed list of patients with their tests and amounts billed (hard copy). It might be relayed through connecting lines to a computer in the business office (hard wired). Or it might be transferred to magnetic tape, paper tape, or floppy disc to be read into another computer by an appropriate reading device.

Some computer systems also make available software or operating sectors by which *calculations* can be made or simple problems solved.

Most systems provide a number of conveniences for the monitoring of activity. *Incomplete lists* show what work has not yet been completed; these tests can usually be classified by departments, tests, or work stations. *Abnormal values* may be printed out on a separate list. *Work logs* may list

all work done, by test, department, or on another basis. *Census* of all patients with their hospital locations may be printed by nursing station as a *bed list,* or alphabetically. In short, once the information is in the system, it may be massaged and restructured to provide specific information. All these processes require implementation of programs in software. Smaller systems may easily be overwhelmed by program modifications that slow down or confuse smooth processing of essential data.

## Partial solutions

The past few years has seen many new companies enter the laboratory computer market and even more leave the field in disarray. At the present time, the situation seems to be stabilizing, with a few companies offering similar concepts.

Many laboratories are acquiring parts of a complete system with the idea of gradually adding hardware and programs. For example, the hospital may choose to place terminals at each nursing station so that requests can be printed on request forms in the laboratory. Work would then be reported on these forms and hand-carried to the nursing station for entry into the patient's chart. Another hospital might decide to have only terminals and a printer in the laboratory. Reports would be entered by hand on the computer keyboard, and the computer would only organize the data into a summary report, which might be hand-carried to the patient's chart.

Totally computerizing the laboratory and integrating it into a hospital-wide system requires a great deal of careful planning, time, and money. A number of such systems are now in operation. Until now, few of these systems have actually decreased the number of people required, but errors are greatly reduced and all sorts of information is more readily available. The overall effect has been to improve patient care and simplify the decision-making process for management, but it is questionable whether money has been saved. Probably the improvement in patient care and fiscal management will eventually bring about savings as computer systems become simpler, more standard, and more generally used.

## Environment

The importance of environment is often overlooked in planning computer operation. Most computers are extremely sensitive to fluctuations in line voltage and any type of interference in the sine wave pattern. A *clean line* from the bus bar should be dedicated to the CPU, and care should be taken that the line is not cut into in order to supply other electrical needs. Many laboratories have most electrical circuits overloaded, and changes are often made to borrow between circuits as equipment is added. To the electrician trying to find additional amperage to meet new needs, a line with only one outlet is a gold mine, and he will splice into it if it is not marked or safeguarded.

Most laboratories are crowded, and the crowding and normal activities of a busy laboratory produce a dirty environment. There may be heavy collection of dust, acid fumes, and high humidity, all of which can be very damaging to a computer. The CPU and disc drives are especially sensitive to problems of dirt, moisture, and corrosion. If at all possible these units should be housed in a separate room where dust can be kept to a minimum. Carpets contribute considerable lint, and heavy concentrations of paper handling and traffic tend to increase problems. Filters of some kind in the air-handling vents may prove helpful. Room temperature may also present a problem. As has been noted earlier, most solid-state components are inherently quite sensitive to changes in temperature. Ambient temperatures in excess of 27° C are quite likely to cause problems with many data-handling systems. For best operating results a temperature between 20° and 23° C is usually recommended.

When functioning properly, computers do not make mistakes. People make many errors in entering data and programming, but the device itself does not distort information when it is functioning properly. When it is not functioning as it should, it can alter results, wipe out thousands of records, and cause untold chaos. For this reason many computers have *fail-safe* systems that protect the memory and operating programs in event of electrical failure. Also, backup discs are generally made and records and data stored at frequent intervals so as to be immediately available in the event of damage or loss.

Computers cannot function well if the personnel involved in their care and management are not careful and thorough. The computer has no way to correct errors or omissions in entering data. The census must be assiduously maintained and all protocols followed in regard to operation and maintenance or the system is useless. Given adequate care, however, the computer can process data and solve clerical and logistic problems that can be solved in no other way.

## Are laboratory computers practical?

Because of the many benefits they can offer and the large cost involved, the decision whether to purchase a computer may be a difficult one. It has been reported that as high as 10% of laboratory reports may contain some element of error. Also, laboratory revenue may be seriously affected by a reported rate of 10% or 15% lost charges due to billing errors. Laboratory reports prepared by computer are certainly better organized and more readable. These arguments seem valid and convincing.

It cannot be assumed, however, that all errors will disappear when a computer is installed. Reports are only as good as the data entered into the terminal. Also, it should not be assumed that the computer will save much time. The experience of most laboratories has been that at least as much time is required for processing information. Also, backup records must be kept because the computer may lose information if it breaks down or if electric power is cut off. Fortunately, this sort of problem is less common now than it was a few years ago.

Since no time may be saved, the economic justification must usually be made on the basis of the saving of lost billing and in the improvement of service through faster, more legible reports.

Many new computer systems are being introduced. Since the state of the art is greatly improved, they are more economical, more trouble free, and have greater capability. It seems likely that most larger laboratories will be computerized in the next few years, and as relative costs decrease, nearly all hospitals will find it profitable and convenient to computerize their laboratories.

# CHAPTER 15

# *Instrumentation of nuclear medicine*

## *Radionuclides and radiant energy*

Isotopes are forms of an element having the same atomic number and similar chemical properties but differing in atomic weight and often in radioactive behavior. *Stable* isotopes vary in atomic weight but possess no imbalance of electric charge and hence exhibit no radioactivity or instability. An atom that possessed an additional or deficient neutron, for example, would change in weight but would still possess very similar properties.

The term *nuclide* is grammatically more precise than isotope, since isotope means any of two or more forms of an element. If there is only one form of the element, the term would be inappropriate. Nuclide refers to a specific type of atom characterized by its nuclear properties and its energy state. It is said to be a *radioactive* nuclide, or simply a *radionuclide,* if it is capable of giving off radiant energy in the form of particles or rays. As has been seen in an earlier chapter, *x-rays* are produced when inner-shell electrons are displaced. If protons are displaced from the nucleus, *gamma radiation* is produced. In the process of nuclear disintegration other forms of radiation may be produced. Of these, *alpha* and *beta* radiation are the most common.

Naturally occurring radionuclides have been known for many years. It was not until the explosion of the atomic bomb in 1945 that quantities of these radioactive materials became available for study. Construction of the cyclotron and the chain-reacting pile made possible the preparation of various radionuclides of nearly all the elements. Recent advances in chemistry have made it possible to substitute radioactive elements into a large variety of molecular structures. These "tagged" molecules can be used to follow the course of various physiological phenomena by the simple device of detecting the characteristic radiation in the tissues, exudates, etc. after ingestion. Thus, it is possible to follow many physicochemical processes occurring in an organism without interrupting or disturbing its physiological functions. Tagged molecules can be injected into the bloodstream; swallowed, or breathed into the lungs and followed as they circulate or are metabolized. In the very small amounts that are used for such measurements, these radionuclides are essentially harmless, and it is not necessary to subject the patient to any appreciable discomfort to measure or trace them.

Depending on the molecular physics involved, several different particles and forms of energy may be emitted by a radionuclide. The energy of these is generally rated in terms of two capabilities. The first of these is the *ability to penetrate*. Relatively heavy alpha particles may be capable of penetrating only a few centimeters of air, whereas more energetic gamma rays can penetrate many materials for some distance and can even pass through an inch of solid lead.

The second capability considered is the *ability to ionize* other atoms that are encountered. This capability of the particle is related to its energy, which is measured in *electron volts*. An electron volt is the measurement of power equivalent to the energy of one electron accelerated through a potential difference of one volt. This value is $1.6 \times 10^{-16}$ erg. It is a very tiny measurement, and the measurement *million electron volts* (meV) is more commonly used. The smaller term *thousand electron volts* (keV) is also commonly used.

*Alpha particles* are doubly ionized helium atoms with very high energy levels but very low penetrating power. Preparations emitting alpha particles are not commonly used as tracers for obvious reasons.

*Beta particles* are high-energy electrons or positrons. They have slightly more penetrating power than alpha particles but are stopped by a few meters of air or very light shielding. Their ionizing potential is relatively low but varies, depending on the decay reaction that produced them.

*Gamma rays* and x-rays are both energies of the electromagnetic spectrum. X-rays are much less commonly produced by radionuclides and are of little value in measurement.

Gamma radiation is the form of energy that is most commonly used in tracer studies in biological tissues. Radiation of this type is characterized by wavelengths of less than 1 Å. Compared with ultraviolet or visible light, these waves have very high energy, but compared with the ionizing potential of alpha particles (around 10 meV), they are fairly weak. However, they have high penetrating power, as mentioned earlier. The combination of these characteristics makes gamma radiation convenient for biological work. A gamma-emitting radionuclide injected into, or ingested by a living organism will not cause a great deal of ionization with resultant tissue damage. At the same time, the gamma ray energy will penetrate the tissues and utensils sufficiently well for their position and concentration to be easily detected.

The exact energy (wavelength) emitted by a particular radionuclide depends on the quantum mechanics of the atom in question, and only discrete energy levels are possible. It is thus possible to identify a radionuclide by its energy level or spectral emission. This identification process might be compared with spectral scanning in the visual region. By noting the amplitude of the energy at the characteristic wavelength (energy level), it is possible to quantitate by comparing the energy reading with suitable standards. This process is quite similar to that of spectrophotometry in the visible range.

Unfortunately, the energy peak for the radionuclide of an element is less clear-cut than the emission or absorption maxima of visible light. The gamma ray, with a very specific energy, may communicate all its energy to an electron that is ultimately the source for our photoelectric measurement. In this process, called the *photoelectric effect,* the energy of the photoelectron is equal to the energy of the gamma ray. In a considerable number of cases, however, the gamma ray may *collide* with an electron. The energy available for measurement in such a case is the net energy that will be dispersed. This process, called the *Compton effect,* yields a scattering of energies somewhat lower than that of the original gamma ray. Compton scatter and various other sources of radiation cause the definition of the specific energy of the gamma ray to be more difficult. In spite of this problem, the radioactive element can be quite definately indentified and quantitated with adequate instrumentation.

Radioactive nuclides are atoms in their excited states and, as such, are unstable. Over a period of time the atom returns to ground state, at which time emission theoretically ceases. Since this radioactive decay is a geometrical progression (first-order rate), the end point is infinity, and there is no such thing as a time at which the atom has returned to ground state. To describe the decay rate for various radioactive nuclides, the term *radioactive half-life,* or *physical half-life,* is used. This is the time required for the given radionuclide to lose one half of its radiant energy. Table 8 lists the half-life span of a number of common radionuclides. Note that one element may have more

**Table 8.** Half-life of various radionuclides commonly used as tracers

| Name of element | Symbol | Half-life |
|---|---|---|
| Iodine | $I^{121}$ | 8 days |
| Iodine | $I^{125}$ | 60 days |
| Gold | $Au^{198}$ | 2.7 days |
| Mercury | $Hg^{197}$ | 2.7 days |
| Mercury | $Hg^{203}$ | 48 days |
| Chromium | $Cr^{51}$ | 28 days |
| Cobalt | $Co^{57}$ | 270 days |
| Selenium | $Se^{75}$ | 127 days |
| Strontium | $Sr^{85}$ | 65 days |
| Technetium | $Tc^{99m}$ | 6 hours |
| Indium | $In^{113m}$ | 1.7 hours |
| Xenon | $Xe^{133}$ | 5 days |
| Iron | $Fe^{59}$ | 45 days |

than one form and each form may have its own radioactive characteristics.

The *biological half-life* of a compound is a measure of the disappearance of the compound itself from the organism and has no relation to its radioactive properties.

## Units of activity and standards

The activity of a radionuclide preparation is measured as the number of nuclear disintegrations occurring per second. The *curie* is the unit of activity commonly used. One curie is $3.7 \times 10^{10}$ disintegrations per second. This is a great deal of activity, and smaller units such as a *millicurie* and a *microcurie* are much more commonly used.

Exposure to radiation is measured in *roentgens*. One roentgen is the amount of radiation that, when passed through 0.001293 g of air under standard conditions, will produce one electrostatic unit of electricity per centimeter, of $1.61 \times 10^{12}$ ion pairs per gram of air.

In the calibration of devices for the detection of radioactivity, standards are necessary. Since all active nuclides are constantly in the process of decay, it is necessary to establish the activity of the standard in question at the time of use. Commer-

cially available nuclides of all types, including standards, carry a label giving activity at a specific date and hour. If the half-life is known, the decay rate can be applied and the current activity determined. Manufacturers often supply convenient decay charts that give the approximate activity at a particular time interval after assay.

Most of the commercially available preparations are given an assay value and decay rate that are quite adequate for clinical use. Absolutely standardized solutions are more carefully assayed and are hence more desirable for calibration purposes. They are, naturally, considerably more expensive. A *reference solution* is a solution that has been carefully measured in comparison with an "absolutely standardized solution."

Certain *solid standards* are available. These may be thin wafers of a long-lived nuclide that allow the setting of the spectrometer at a given point with good accuracy. They may also be *mock standards* whose radiation simulates the radiation of a commonly used element. For example, barium 133 and cesium 137 in a 12:1 ratio have an emission closely resembling that of iodine 131 if a filter is used to screen out extraneous levels.

## Measuring devices

There are several ways of measuring radioactivity, but relatively few of these have been used in practical working insturments in the biological sciences. Many specialized devices have been developed, using a few basic principles.

The simplest means of detecting radiation is undoubtedly by the use of photographic plates or film. The familiar *radiation-monitoring badges* worn by all personnel in x-ray and radionuclide work are the most common application. Copper and cadmium filters are placed over the film. If gamma radiation is present, the film will be darkened over its entirety. If the film is darkened only where the cadmium filter protects the film, the radiation is x-ray. If both cadmium and copper protect the film, beta radiation could be present.

The localization of a nuclide in tissue can be demonstrated by a film process called *autoradiog-*

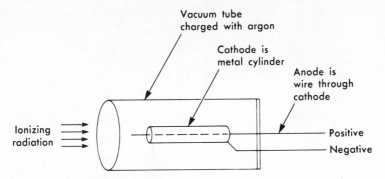

*Fig. 15-1.* Sketch of Geiger-Mueller tube.

*raphy.* If the tissue is placed on a film for a few minutes, the radiation from the nuclide will cause the film to blacken in the area adjacent to it.

The *ionization chamber* is another radiation-sensing device. The most common form of an ionization chamber is a gas-filled vacuum tube to which an ionizable gas such as argon has been added. The charge between the cathode and anode is kept just below the voltage necessary to ionize the gas. When radioactive energy penetrates the chamber, it provides just enough energy to produce ionization, and an electrical pulse is produced. These are called *Geiger-Mueller tubes* (Fig. 15-1). Small pocket chambers *(dosimeters)* that store the charge until the device is inserted into a meter socket are available. As the chamber discharges, the meter is deflected to indicate the absorbed charge. Many types of survey meters (Fig. 15-2) for detecting stray radiation and spilled radioactive material are made, using the idea of the ionization chamber. These chambers measure various types of radiation, depending on what gas is used in the chamber.

*Dose calibrators,* very accurate bench-top instruments designed to measure the amount of radioactive material to be given to a patient, often use ionization chambers as detectors. The energy level necessary to produce ionization can be set to correspond with that of any radionuclide, and the proper dose of any material can be determined by the ionization that occurs (Fig. 15-3).

Recently *metal oxide semiconductors* (MOS) have been found to provide an accurate and reliable means of measuring radiation. Meters using MOS detectors are economical and sensitive and are finding wide application.

The *Geiger counter,* so well known to the public, is constructed in a manner similar to that of an ionization chamber. The cathode is in the form of a metallic cylinder around the anode. A high potential (1000 to 2500 V) is applied. Ion pairs result from this very high potential, and other ionization is produced as high-velocity charges strike gas molecules. An avalanche effect is produced. As the cumulative charge is released at the anode, a pulse forms; the process may be repeated at a rate dependent on the intensity of the radiation. There is a brief dead time between discharges, and practical counting rates are not in excess of 15,000 per minute. This type of counter is best for beta radiation.

Beta radiation is used in some cases for in vitro testing. Since beta radiation has very low penetrating power, the means of its measurement must be somewhat different than for gamma rays. The beta particle is actually a high-energy electron ejected from the nucleus of an atom when a neutron is broken down. It possesses considerable ionizing potential but relatively little penetrating power. *Liquid scintillation counters* are the devices normally used to measure beta radiation. The sample is mixed with chemicals that scintillate, or emit

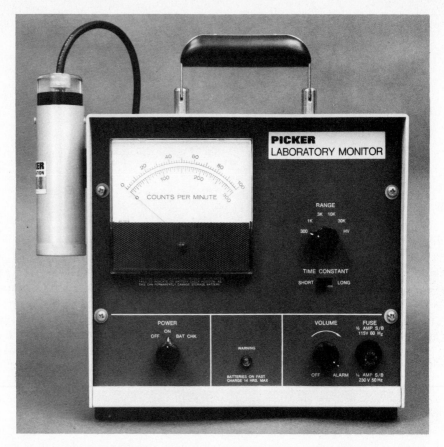

*Fig. 15-2.* Picker Laboratory Monitor. (Courtesy Picker Corp.)

light, when struck by beta rays. The mixture is then placed in a detector chamber between photomultiplier tubes that are capable of sensing the very weak light signals emitted. The chemicals used to generate the emission are complex organic compounds in aromatic hydrocarbon solvents. Since activities may be very low in samples of this type, counting may take a long time; sample changers are used to reduce the inconvenience in moving new samples into the counting chamber after lengthy counting cycles.

For detection of gamma radiation, *scintillation crystals* are the method of choice. The most widely used crystal of this kind is the *sodium iodide* crystal, activated with 1% thallium. *Anthracene, stil-*

*bene,* and several other organic crystals are also used. These crystals are optically clear and are usually 2 or 3 inches across in well counters. As the gamma rays strike the crystal, a very tiny scintillation is produced. The time is usually a fraction of a microsecond, and the total energy released may escape detection by the eye.

The scintillation crystal is enveloped in a foil that protects it from extraneous light and helps reflect the scintillation. The end of the crystal is sealed to the face of a high-quantity photomultiplier tube that detects and amplifies the impulses.

The crystal and photomultiplier are usually enclosed in a lead-shielded *probe* along with a preamplifier circuit that further amplifies the output of

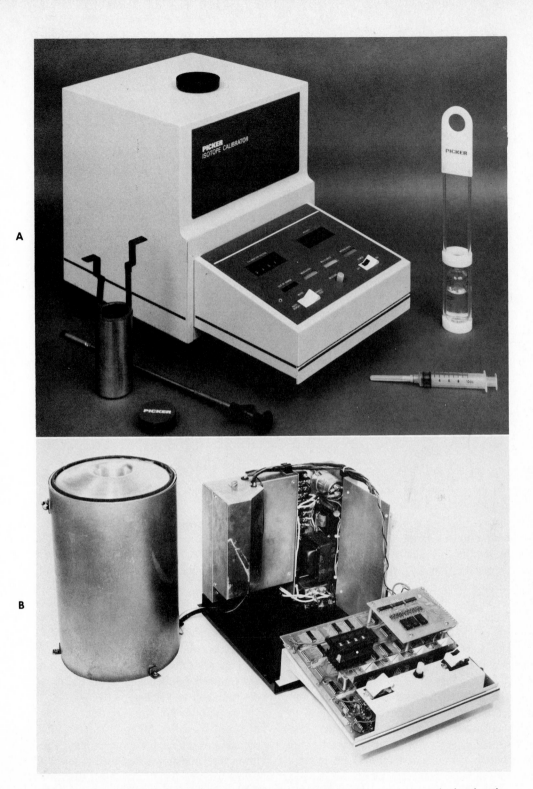

***Fig. 15-3. A,*** Picker Isotope Calibrator. ***B,*** Isotope Calibrator with cover removed, showing the heavily shielded well and microprocessor circuitry beneath the control panel. (Courtesy Picker Corp.)

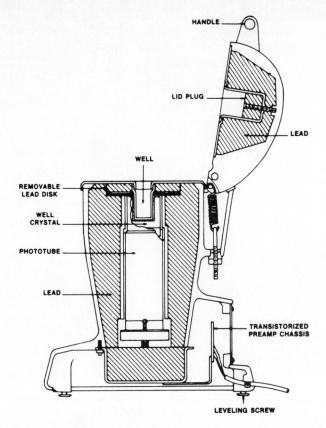

HANDLE

LID PLUG

LEAD

WELL

REMOVABLE
LEAD DISK

WELL
CRYSTAL

PHOTOTUBE

LEAD

TRANSISTORIZED
PREAMP CHASSIS

LEVELING SCREW

*Fig. 15-4.* Cross-sectional view of Scintillation Well Counter. (Courtesy Picker Corp.)

the photomultiplier. At the front of the probe, a thick sleeve of lead is usually placed in such a way that the crystal is protected from all radiation except that approaching it from an area determined by the opening in the sleeve. This protective lead shield is called a *collimator,* since its function is to collimate radiation onto the crystal. If the collimator is shaped like a funnel, all the radiation in the angle of the funnel will strike the crystal. If a series of very narrow holes is bored through a thick lead plate at the front of the crystal, only radiation that comes from directly in front of the crystal will reach it. *Counting wells* (Fig. 15-4) are, essentially, probes in which a crystal is hollowed out to permit a test tube to be inserted. This more intimate contact between the radiating substance and the crystal allows better counting sensitivity. A lead collar over the top of the crystal allows only an opening for insertion of the test tube. A high-voltage dc source of excellent quality is necessary to operate the photomultiplier tube. One of the leads to the probe or the well will be of high voltage—probably around 1000 V.

Signals from the photomultiplier in the probe or well are relayed to the main amplifier, where they are further amplified and may be processed to a discriminator and scaler.

The *pulse-height analyzer* (Fig. 15-5), or spectrometer, is the part of the system that allows identification of the nuclide from its energy level. The lower discriminator is designed to reject all pulses below a given level. The upper discriminator re-

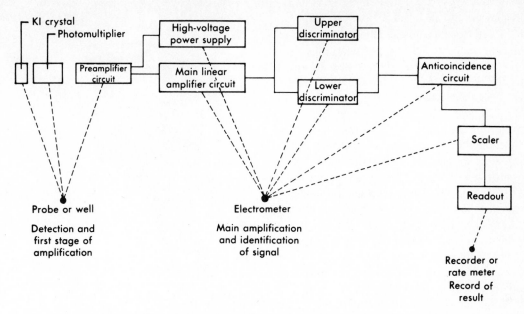

*Fig. 15-5.* Schematic representation of the elements of a pulse-height analyzer.

jects impulses higher than the lower discrimination level plus those in the *window* or *channel* width. By the use of the two discriminators, only the voltage analogous to the meV of the nuclide in question is passed through the discriminator or spectrometer. The number of emissions at this energy range provides quantitation of the isotope, and stray radiation and radiation from other elements are eliminated. This device, although operating on a different principle, functions as a monochromator similar to that used in the visual range.

The *scaler* is a device that combines several individual signals, by means of capacitors, to make them count as a single impulse. Two common types of scalers are in use. One is the *binary scaler,* in which the impulses are counted in each phase by twos, giving multipliers of 2, 4, 8, 16, 32, 64, etc. The other is the decimal or *decade scaler,* which passes each tenth pulse. The latter is obviously much simpler to use, but the former is more adaptable.

The readout of various well and probe devices

will depend on their application. Recorder tracings, printed tapes, magnetic tapes, and LED digital displays are used. Microprocessors have come into heavy use, and the raw data from radionuclide monitoring may be used in calculations. The readout may be presented finally as an LED digital display, printed report, CRT display, or magnetic signal to a computer. Modern equipment occasionally still uses ammeters, but they are almost gone from the scene.

An *anticoincidence circuit,* with the function of compensating for the coincidence of two scintillations at the exact same time interval, is included. The probability that two scintillations will coincide can be determined mathematically, and an appropriate signal correction is made. The various elements of a typical pulse-height analyzer are schematically shown in Fig. 15-5. This may help clarify the components and relationship just discussed.

Many detectors are equipped with timers, which are simply electrical devices that open and close the counting circuits, permitting the counting of emissions per minute or other time interval.

Radioactive isotopes are used in diagnostic medical applications, principally as *tracers;* that is to say, some radioactive element is "tagged" onto a molecule or other entity which is given to the patient. Since the element continues to radiate, it can be located in the body by means of collimated probes or be found in the blood, urine, and stool and identified by its characteristic radiation. Gamma emitters are best suited to medical work, since they have low ionizing potential and hence cause less tissue damage. They also have considerable penetrating power and can be measured through greater thicknesses of body tissue. Fortunately it is possible to measure very small amounts of gamma radiation with excellent accuracy, and spectrometers can accurately identify the radiation as characteristic of a given element.

With the increased use of microprocessors and various solid-state devices, it has become practical to have separate instruments to perform many specialized functions or tests. A review of some specific systems and measuring instruments will serve to demonstrate this diversity.

In the nuclear medicine laboratory it is necessary to have *monitoring equipment* capable of detecting spills and contamination. The Model 655-186 Portable Beta, Gamma Geiger Survey Meter (Picker Corp.) is an example. This instrument contains two Geiger-Mueller tubes as detectors. One of these is contained within the metal case of the instrument itself and is for detecting high levels of gamma activity. The other is in a probe on the end of a cable that allows the probe to be moved about to remote and inaccessible locations. This second tube is capable of measuring low levels of gamma and beta radiation. Beta can be discriminated from gamma by closing a metal shield on the probe. Counts per minute and milliroentgens (mR) are indicated on a meter mounted in the case.

The Model 655-011 Cutie Pie Survey Meter (Picker Corp.) (Fig. 15-6) is a hand-held instrument that is pointed, like a gun, at the suspected contaminated area. A very thin window on the ion-chamber detector allows passage of alpha and beta

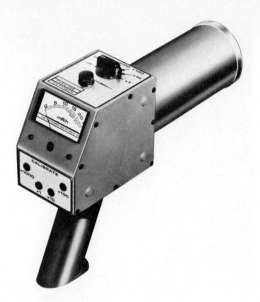

*Fig. 15-6.* The Cutie Pie Survey Meter is convenient for locating spills and other contamination. (Courtesy Picker Corp.)

radiation. When an aluminum cover is placed over the window, only gamma radiation will penetrate and be counted. A small meter at the back of the "gun" provides a readout and is calibrated in milliroentgens (mR) and electron volts (meV and keV).

As mentioned earlier, dose calibrators are needed to quickly and accurately measure the activity of the radionuclide being administered to a patient. The Digital Isotope Calibrator manufactured by Picker Corp. is an example of these devices. This is a compact, lead-lined box into which syringes, vials, bottles, or capsules can be inserted. A flexible remote handling tool is provided. Output from the Geiger-Mueller tube is calculated by solid-state circuitry and reported on an LED display as meV or keV. Measurement usually takes under a second.

Several companies have manufactured *instruments for calculating blood volume.* A measured amount of radioactive solution is assayed in a well counter and injected into the patient. Within a few minutes the radioactive material is pumped about

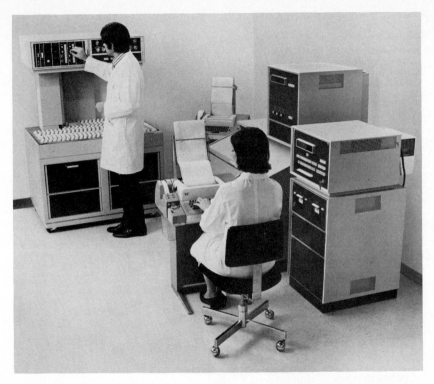

**Fig. 15-7.** Automated 300-sample gamma counting system with teletype and computer. (Courtesy Searle Analytic, Inc.)

the body by the heart, and mixing with the blood is complete. A sample of the blood is drawn and the radioactivity measured. A calculating circuit in the instrument determines the dilution factor and hence the volume of blood circulating in the patient's circulatory system.

### Radiochemistry

*Radiochemistry* methods use radioactive tagged substances that are employed in a large number of in vitro tests. The volume of these tests performed in hospital laboratories has expanded so rapidly that single-tube well counters are no longer adequate. Large volume counting systems have been devised to automate the measurement of many tubes. The MR 252 Gamma Counter (Roche Medical Electronics, Inc.) is typical of these devices. The spectrometer of the instrument is set up to provide optimum windows (upper and lower dis-

criminators) for eight different nuclides. A window is automatically set when the appropriate button is pushed, and the detector will only measure energy characteristic of the designated isotope. A sample changing system is provided that can move up to 252 sample tubes into and out of the detector without operator attention, and the time that the tube stays in the detector can be varied from 0.1 minute to 100 minutes. A seven-digit LED display shows sample identification, time, and counts per minute. A teletype can be attached to print out reports during several hours that the system may be left unattended. A built-in microprocessor provides many additional operating features such as calculation of percent of standard readings. The Model 1285 Automatic Gamma Counting System (Searle Analytic, Inc.) (Fig. 15-7) is an example of a somewhat more sophisticated system. Samples are handled in 36 tube racks that can be loaded, mixed, centrifuged, and counted without manual handling. These racks can be fed through an open-ended relay system that carries the rack to the detector area. A mobile detector moves to the tube rather than tubes being individually displaced. Three samples are counted at one time. Various tests can be mixed in the loading sequence and identified by a user ID card, by which the system identifies the patient, sample, method, and screening level. After reading activities, the instrument is able to make appropriate calculations. When standards are presented to the system and identified, standard curves are automatically printed out and subsequent samples related to the curve produced. When used with the PDS/3 Data Evaluation and Quality Control System (Searle Analytic, Inc.), nearly any type of in vitro radiochemistry testing can be automated and the calculation, reporting, and quality control computerized.

*RIA testing.* Perhaps the fastest growing type of test in the clinical laboratory during the past few years has been the *radioimmunoassay,* or *RIA,* test. The test is applicable to a large number of biologically interesting proteins. In this test the tagged protein substance (the antigen) of interest is complexed with its antibody, so there is no excess of either antigen or antibody. When a patient sample containing the substance of interest is introduced, tagged material is displaced from the antigen-antibody complex. This principle is known as *competitive protein binding.* After this reaction has

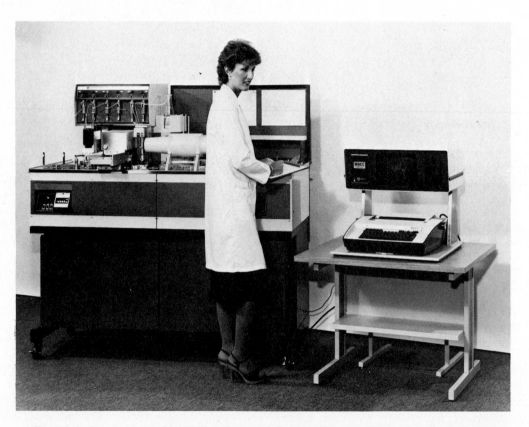

*Fig. 15-8.* Concept-4 with MACC Data-Reduction System. (Courtesy Micromedic Systems, Inc.)

taken place, it is possible to separate the bound and free samples and measure the radioactivity of each. If standards are run in the same way, the concentration of the protein in question can be calculated. The method is extremely sensitive, but the necessary materials are difficult to prepare. For this reason several companies manufacture kits for a variety of substances, such as digoxin, cortisol, digitoxin, gastrin, and insulin. There are almost unlimited possibilities for tests of this type, and the volume of tests ordered has reached the point where automated test systems are economically feasible.

The radioactive bound and unbound antigen from the test may be counted in a gamma-counting instrument such as has been described earlier.

The ratio of the two counts is then related to an activity curve, and concentration is calculated. The process of establishing the curve, using several duplicate standards is time consuming. The ratios must then be calculated and applied to the curve and concentration found. Quality control data must also be analyzed. All of this calculation is difficult and tedious, and computers have become important in speeding up the operation.

It was discovered that the antibody could be coated onto glass and dried. Kits are made that contain a separate antibody-treated tube for each test. The Concept-4 (Micromedic Systems) (Fig. 15-8) provides an automated RIA procedure using such coated tubes. Fig. 15-9 shows the test sequence of this instrument. Since the antibody is

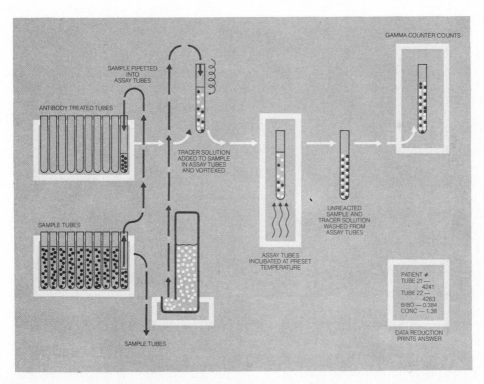

GAMMA COUNTER COUNTS

SAMPLE PIPETTED INTO ASSAY TUBES

ANTIBODY TREATED TUBES

TRACER SOLUTION ADDED TO SAMPLE IN ASSAY TUBES AND VORTEXED

UNREACTED SAMPLE AND TRACER SOLUTION WASHED FROM ASSAY TUBES

SAMPLE TUBES

ASSAY TUBES INCUBATED AT PRESET TEMPERATURE

PATIENT #
TUBE 21 —
4241
TUBE 22 —
4263
B/BO — 0.384
CONC — 1.38

DATA REDUCTION PRINTS ANSWER

SAMPLE TUBES

**Fig. 15-9.** The schematic illustration shows how tests are performed by the Concept-4 Radioassay Analyzer. (Courtesy Micromedic Systems, Inc.)

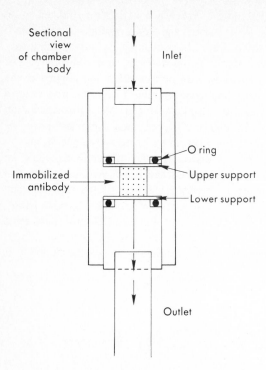

Sectional
view
of chamber
body

Inlet

O ring

Upper support

Immobilized
antibody

Lower support

Outlet

*Fig. 15-10.* Unique antibody chamber of the ARIA II RIA System. (Courtesy Becton Dickenson Immunodiagnostics.)

bound to the glass, centrifugation is not required. Two tubes are counted at a time. Data are reduced, and readings and calculations are reported out on the printer. The mechanics are similar to discrete sample chemistry systems that have been discussed.

The ARIA II (Becton Dickinson Immunodiagnostics) uses a different approach to automating RIA testing. Becton Dickinson has developed an antibody chamber (Fig. 15-10) in which the antibody can be permanently bound onto a porous material. Antigen can be bound and then eluted off without damage to the antibody, and the process can be repeated up to 3000 times before the chamber must be replaced. This unique chamber is at the heart of the ARIA II system. A full tray of 120 calibrators, controls, and specimens can be placed

on the instrument at one time. A separate floppy disc is provided for each test to direct the on-board computer that controls cycling of the pipettors and detectors and provides the data reduction logic. The antibody chamber allows extremely fast, efficient binding. During the cycle, the patient sample and tagged antigen are mixed and passed through the chamber. Unbound antigen flows through into the counting cell and is counted. The chamber and counting cell are flushed clear. Then an eluting buffer washes the bound antigen free from the chamber and it is counted. Calculation of the bound/unbound (B/Bo) ratio is calculated and the process is repeated. The entire cycle requires only about 2 minutes. Since the antibody is reused, this element of the test is highly reproducible.

## Measurements in vivo

By using a probe to detect the appearance or disappearance of a radionuclide, a physiological function may be measured. At one time many *renograms* were done in this manner, which is a good example to explain this type of measurement. If iodohippurate sodium (Hippuran), which has been tagged with radioactive iodine, is injected into a vein, it is quickly mixed with the blood. Since it is normally excreted quickly through the kidneys, its movement through the body provides a good measure of kidney function. If a probe is placed over each kidney and radioactivity is measured and recorded on a rectilinear recorder as a function of time, it is possible to clearly graph the arrival of the Hippuran in the kidneys and its excretion into the bladder. A similar technique may be used in many ways to show other functions.

It is often desirable to have an image or picture of an organ or part of the body showing the distribution of a radioactive tag. The process is called *imaging*. By using instruments that will be described, it is also possible to prepare images, or pictures, of the organ in fast succession so that the movement of the radionuclide can actually be seen in successive pictures. These pictures are made with devices called *gamma cameras*. Before

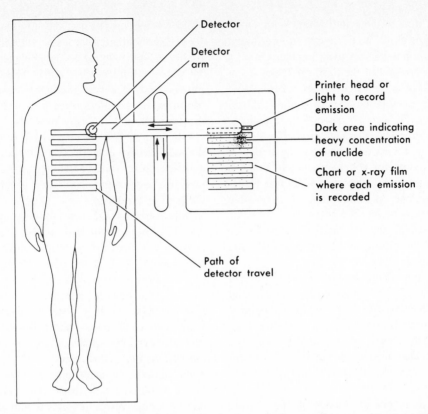

*Fig. 15-11.* Patient is scanned by probe carried on the end of a traveling arm. A tapper or light makes a record of the radioactivity detected.

we examine them, however, let us consider a somewhat simpler device called a *scanner*.

**Scanners.** *Rectilinear scanners* are being used frequently in medicine and biology to map areas of the body where an isotope may be concentrated (or excluded (Fig. 15-11). Various companies manufacture a scanner with two probes. These detectors scan both sides of the patient simultaneously to speed up the total scanning process and to define areas more sharply.

The rectilinear scanner provides a means of producing an image or map of the area under observation, but it has limitations. The time required to perform a scan makes it impossible to observe fast changes in isotope concentration. Also, the study of different areas or levels in an organ is very time-consuming and tiring to the patient. Some method has been needed for visualizing isotope distribution very rapidly. Also, a means of visualizing distribution in three dimensions was needed. The gamma camera and various refinements and additions have gone a long way toward answering these needs.

The construction of a single detector has already been reviewed. In this detector a crystal was cemented to the face of a photomultiplier tube. The gamma camera had one very large crystal with several photomultiplier tubes cemented in a symmetrical pattern to its upper side. Each scintillation will be sensed by more than one photomultiplier. The strength of the photosignals sensed by the various photomultipliers will depend on the proximity of the tube to the scintillation. With simultaneous signals of different strength from different locations, it is possible for the computer circuitry to locate the position of the flash on X and Y coordinates and position a light dot on a CRT. With hundreds of scintillations being plotted in this fashion, the CRT becomes a map of the radioactivity of the area under examination. If a *persistence scope* (a CRT with a phosphor coating that continues to glow for some measurable time) is used, this map can be examined while it is showing a large number of scintillations. It is possible to place a photographic film in front of the CRT and produce a picture for later, detailed examination. Polaroid pictures can be made rapidly and easily in this way.

Since this type of information can be gathered easily and quickly, it is possible to do sequential pictures (with a time-lapse camera, for example) at very short intervals and thus get a time-lapse pattern showing the progress of an event. By the same token, it is also feasible to focus at different levels of an organ and thus obtain some depth perception.

The patient is placed on a table beside the scanner. A probe, containing the gamma detector, is made to travel across the body area that is to be scanned. The scanner probe moves back and forth in parallel lines until every area has been sensed. This mapping pattern is called a *raster pattern*. The moving probe is suspended on a moving arm. At the other end of the arm is a *tapper,* which makes an ink mark on paper of each emission sensed. The resulting pattern shows the distribution of nuclide in the area scanned. In place of the tapper a small light may flash, exposing a photographic film. The developed film will, of course, provide a similar ''picture'' of nuclide distribution. Loci of heavy radioactivity or areas showing no activity may show the location of tumors.

*Cameras.* The Dyna Camera (Picker Corp.) shown in Fig. 15-12 is typical of the several gamma-imgaing systems in general use. The large drum-like head, shown at the left, is positioned over a patient. Gamma radiation from the patient strikes a large crystal near the surface of the drum face. The radiation causes scintillation—tiny flashes of light—in the crystal. Behind the crystal, 19 photomultiplier tubes detect these tiny light flashes, and each tube produces analogous electric impulses that are relayed to a computer where the position and intensity of each flash is processed into a CRT. A map of the distribution of the radioactivity is produced on the screen. When a photographic film is exposed to the CRT, a permanent image of the distribution of the isotope in the body is produced.

Improvements are constantly being made in gamma camera design that provide faster, sharper pictures with less effort. High-energy short-lived radionuclides like technetium ($Tc^{99}$) have also expedited these developments.

In order to study large areas, or the whole body, a whole-body imaging system is available. This system moves the patient under the camera head as the detectors sense radioactivity and record it on the CRT screen and on film.

*Tomography* is the technique involved in getting views of radioisotope distribution and concentration at various planar sections within an organ. It can be used with x-rays as well as isotopes. Various devices and techniques have been employed recently to accomplish this. Most of these involve some device for rotating a collimator with parallel holes drilled at the same angle. By triangulation the concentration of isotope at a given depth can be located. This idea may require a moment's thought. If a rod were pushed through one of the holes of the collimator and the collimator then made to spin, the rod would appear to be a cone. The point of such a cone will be farther from the collimator if the hole used is close to the edge of the collimator. As the holes approach the center of the collimator, the point of the cone (or focus of radioactivity) is seen closer to the collimator. By using the information received from all photomultiplier tubes of the gamma camera equipped with such a rotating collimator, the computer circuitry can establish the level of concentration of isotope.

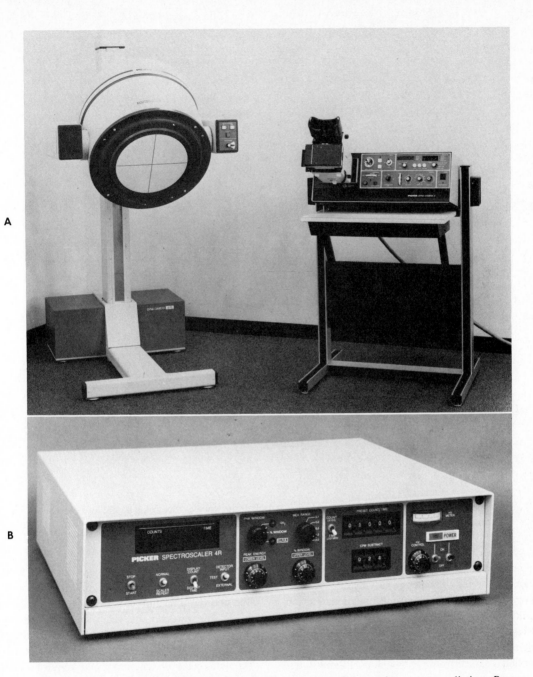

*Fig. 15-12. A,* Picker Dyna Camera, a scintillation camera for mapping gamma radiation. *B,* Close-up of the scaler showing control panel. (Courtesy Picker Corp.)

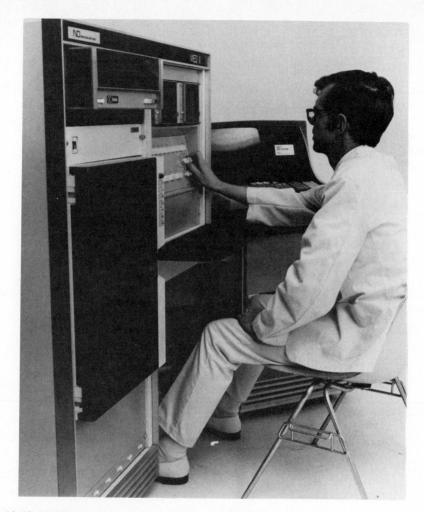

*Fig. 15-13.* Med II system for data storage and retrieval, designed to function with the Radicamera. (Courtesy Nuclear Data, Inc.)

Tomographic cameras produce high-resolution images in a series of planes at varying depths in an organ or tissue. This allows visualization of the size and shape of a formation such as a tumor. The mechanics by which this instrument works are complex. A collimator is used that focuses at a specified distance from the detector. Up-and-down movement of the detector and collimator will change the pattern of emissions detected. The normal X-Y scanning provides information for plotting emissions of these axes. Information from dual probes is analyzed on a highly accurate time basis, and the information is resynthesized to provide 12 tomographic images. The distance between the planes so defined can be selected, and a large area can be scanned.

Applications such as tomography require a high state of sophistication in both electronics and data handling. Special minicomputers have been developed and programmed to handle all manner of calculations and data handling that are inherent in nuclear medicine. Some applications are *data storage* and *playback systems* (Fig. 15-13) that can be used with gamma cameras. The circuitry of the camera locates a scintillation as an X-Y plot, and this information is then fed to the CRT to locate a point of light at an analogous position on the screen. The stream of electrical information passing from the detectors to the CRT can be stored on magnetic tape in exactly the same sequence and speed in which the CRT receives it. On command, the magnetic tape can then play back this stored information to a CRT at any later date for further study. Thus, it is possible to watch the kinetic accumulation of information on the screen and to reproduce it at will. Also, it is possible to isolate a specific *area of interest* on the matrix when the stored information is being played back and to blow it up to provide greater detail. It is also possible to stop the kinetic display of information at a specific point in time for detailed study.

New cathode-coating materials make possible the use of colors in the CRT screen. The image of an organ might show "hot spots" (areas of high isotope concentration) as red patches. Areas free of radiation would appear blue, and lower concentrations would be differentiated similarly. This might seem to be something of a gimmick, but its use has made the differentiation of diseased tissue considerably easier.

The field of diagnostic nuclear medicine is growing at an extremely rapid pace. New nuclides, more sophisticated instrumentation, specialized computers, and advances in radiochemistry and immunology are making the field extremely dynamic. A sizable book could be written about new equipment in this area. In this text we have looked hurriedly only at the principles involved in the most commonly used devices. It is hoped that this panoramic view of the field will stimulate your interest in this fast-growing specialty.

# CHAPTER 16

# Miscellaneous instruments

A walk through any medical laboratory reveals a large number of devices that have still not been discussed here. A complete cataloging and description of these would require a considerably larger book, and new gadgets each year vie for a place in the medical market. This chapter provides a quick look at a few of the more significant of these. Devices for heating and cooling, centrifuges, recorders, dilutors and new devices to automate the bacteriology laboratory are all important. These and a few other selected devices will be discussed.

### Heating and cooling devices

Water baths, incubators, ovens, refrigerators, and chilling baths are vital to the laboratory. Heat is generally produced by passing an electric current through a high-resistance wire or heating block. Heat production requires considerable electricity. A 2- or 3-gallon bath may draw 10 or 15 amps when it is heating up rapidly. Exposed wire coils are rarely used for resistance now, since they become oxidized or corrode and break easily after heavy usage. Where a block or panel of metal is used, the element rarely deteriorates.

Heat, once produced, must be transmitted to the area to be heated and evenly distributed there. In blood pH and blood gas analyzers, as well as in equilibrated sample compartments, the heat is often distributed by pumping water through tubes, around the samples. Circulating pumps are required to move the water. An impeller may be used to push the water forward or a positive pressure pump may be used. Valves are necessary to allow the fluid to continuously flow forward as it is pushed along by pistons, peristaltic rollers, or vibrators. Because of the mechanical problems inherent in pumps, valve mixers, and impellers, there is a tendency to use heating blocks of various kinds. With newer designs and careful engineering, these devices can, in most cases, maintain biological specimens at very accurate temperatures, and circulating baths are now seen much less frequently.

In conventional water baths the water may circulate simply by convection current. An agitator, mixer, or pump may be used to provide better mixing and more even temperature distribution, however.

In ovens, incubators, and air baths, the heat may be radiated through large metal surfaces, the air may move by convection, or a fan may be provided to maintain circulation. The accuracy of temperature control required will dictate the method used.

Several means are available for controlling the heating process. The oldest and simplest of these is the *bimetallic strip thermostat* (Fig. 16-1). Two metal strips with different expansion coefficients are fastened together at either end. When they are heated, one metal expands more than the other and causes the sandwiched strips to bend. This distortion is used to close or open a contact to a heater. In older ovens, heaters, and in some cheaper models the current was passed through the bimetallic element to the heater. This resulted in considerable arcing at the contact points, with dire results: either the contact points fused, causing the

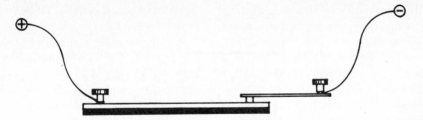

Bimetallic element at room temperature (contact to heater closed)

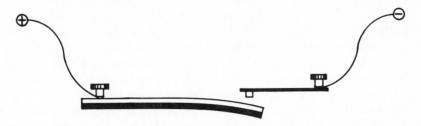

Same element at 37° C (contact to heater opens as element is distorted)

*Fig. 16-1.* Bimetallic thermostat.

heater to stay on until a fuse blew or the unit burned up, or the surfaces of the contacts got so rough, blackened, and corroded that they would not conduct and the circuit would not close. In an attempt to correct this deficiency, manufacturers used silver or platinum contact points, but this did not completely solve the problem.

Where these devices are used in newer controls, current is passed through a microswitch that is closed or opened by pressure of the distorted bimetallic element.

*Wafer elements* or *expansion elements* are composed of two circles of metal, fastened together to form a wafer. The outside of the wafer is constricted by a heavier ring. As the material expands, the metal discs buckle outward so that the thickness of the wafer increases. This expansion is used to depress a microswitch that opens or closes a circuit.

*Fluid-expansion elements* are used in many water baths. A liquid-filled probe is immersed in the water. The probe is connected to an expansion element in the control panel by a very fine capillary. As the fluid is heated, it expands, causing the expansion element to inflate, which, in turn, depresses the plunger of a microswitch. Corrosion or mechanical damage may cause leakage of the fluid from these elements. In most baths either the liquid-containing unit or the entire thermostat assembly can be replaced.

With all these devices, the microswitch may become defective and have to be replaced. This is usually a fairly simple task; many microswitches are standard items that are available in electrical supply outlets.

The devices for temperature sensing just mentioned are purely mechanical in nature. The *thermocouple* is slightly different. When two metals are brought into close contact, there is a rearrangement of electrons on their surfaces that produces a difference in electric potential between them. If a circuit between them is completed, a flow of electrons can be demonstrated with a sensitive meter. This effect is very marked in the case of certain metals; the rate of electron flow through such a circuit will vary considerably with temperature. This characteristic is used as a sensitive indicator of temperature change in the thermocouple. A very weak current can be amplified and used to activate a switch or a relay to control a heating cycle.

As explained earlier, the *thermistor* is a semiconductor component that allows current to pass at a rate dependent on the temperature. The current passed can be used to actuate an ammeter to indicate the temperature or to control the heating process itself. Thermistors can control temperature very precisely and have the advantage of having no moving parts. It is quite unusual for a thermistor to fail unless there is some other serious problem that burns it out. New equipment uses this type of control device almost exclusively; the mechanical thermostats are disappearing from use in laboratory instruments.

Cooling is done, in almost all cases, by refrigerator compressor, which uses the cooling effect of expanding gases. Cold spot platforms, for pouring paraffin blocks around histology specimens, have expansion coils embedded in an aluminum block. As the gas expands and cools the coils, the block is chilled. A thermostat in the block controls the compressor to produce more cooling or to discontinue it.

*Maintenance and quality control.* Careful control of temperature is absolutely essential for accurate laboratory work. A difference of one degree can alter enzyme or coagulation tests appreciably. Inactivation of sera must be done at an accurate temperature or immunologic procedures may be in error. Typical growth may not occur when bacteria are incubated at improper temperatures. Patient samples, blood products, media, and reference materials may deteriorate if not properly refrigerated. It should never be assumed that heating or cooling devices are maintaining the proper temperature. Most such devices should be checked at least once each day. The temperature should be recorded, since it is easy to neglect this surveillance if no record is kept. Blood and blood products for transfusion require refrigeration with temperature-recording devices and high- and low-

temperature alarm systems, as well as daily reading of a second thermometer.

Reading of many thermometers and the necessary recording of temperatures require considerable time each day. Several companies have developed central monitoring and alarm systems. These are generally designed to continuously record the temperatures of many devices or to record temperatures of each device at specific times each day. Acceptable temperatures for each device can be set. When these limits are exceeded, an audible and/or visible alarm is activated. Most of these systems consist of a central recorder and/or printer that is connected to a thermistor in each heating and cooling device by a thin wire. A multiplexer allows each thermistor to be checked in rotation at designated intervals. Such systems can be very reliable and save a great deal of time. However, their calibration and function should be monitored periodically.

As with all laboratory equipment, power cords, switches, and controls should be checked occasionally and the general cleanliness and condition of the equipment assessed.

## Centrifuges

Various types of centrifuges, for separating solid components from liquid suspensions by centrifugal action, are used in the laboratory. They are relatively simple. A few words on their construction and maintenance might prove helpful, however.

The centrifuge consists of an electric motor to which are attached a head and accessories for carrying samples. Usually the head turns on a spindle, which is an extension of the motor shaft. To this basic instrument various devices may be added. A *safety shield* around the rotating head is a necessity, since a broken head or similar disaster could throw fragments at a velocity of 500 mph, according to International Centrifuge manuals. An *on-off switch*, to interrupt the current to the motor, is an obvious requirement. A *timer* is commonly incorporated. Either a simple spring-driven clock mechanism that opens a switch at the end of a preset time cycle or an electric timer that performs the same function may be used. There is usually a switch that gives the operator a choice between continuous operation and operation using the timer.

A *brake* is often supplied. Some models make use of a *mechanical brake,* consisting of a leather shoe pressing on the rotor at some point. It is activated by holding down a lever or knob. Other centrifuges have an *electric* brake, which reverses the polarity of the current to the motor. When such a brake is held down past the time needed to stop the motor, the motor reverses direction and spins backward.

*Tachometers* are provided on many instruments to indicate speed, in revolutions per minute. A cable or flexible shaft attached to the motor spindle turns inside a flexible housing. It is attached to the meter movement at the other end. As the cable turns, it causes the needle to move upscale. If the cable is twisted or if it becomes dry or corroded, it may cause a ticking noise and the needle may jump erratically. Eventually the cable may break. Some centrifuges use electric tachometers in which a magnet rotates around a coil, producing a current that may be measured.

The speed of the centrifuge is controlled by a potentiometer or a *variac,* which raises and lowers the voltage supplied to the motor. The potentiometers may become defective and fail to provide a smooth transition between speeds, or they may open entirely and fail to function. The variac has a graphite brush or *wiper* that moves across its windings. This brush may become worn and may occasionally cause damage to the windings unless sufficient care is taken. Many small centrifuges have a multiposition switch that selects voltage steps by connecting taps on a transformer.

Most centrifuge motors are series-wound dc motors that turn faster as the voltage is increased. Diodes and capacitors are used to rectify the alternating current normally available. Some centrifuges use ac motors in which the speed is adjusted stepwise by reducing the number of poles in the magnetic field.

Electrical contact to the *commutator* in nearly all centrifuge motors is provided by *graphite brushes.* These gradually wear down as they press against the commutator turning at high speed. If the graphite is allowed to completely wear away, the retainer spring of the brush will make contact with the smooth soft brass surface of the commutator and cut grooves or scratches in its surface. A rough commutator surface will cause excessively fast wear of new brushes, and the graphite that is worn away may deposit about the contacts and cause arcing and burning; this decreases the efficiency of the motor and may damage it or, in extreme cases, may even start a fire in the motor.

If the commutator becomes scratched or worn so that there is excessive brush wear, it may be "turned down" on a lathe. A few thousandths of an inch of the soft brass is shaved off until the surface is smooth again. The metal is usually only sufficiently thick to allow this process to be repeated two or three times before the armature is destroyed. It is very important that brushes be checked frequently and replaced before damage occurs. Be sure that the proper size brush is used. A brush that is too small may become lodged between the brush housing and the commutator and cause considerable damage.

When an *armature coil* burns or shortcircuits or wires become broken, it can be rewound by an electric motor shop. Also, new commutator plates can usually be installed. Depending on the type of motor, difficulty in finding the proper replacement, and general condition of the rest of the motor, it may be cheaper to replace the motor. In general, small, standard motors can better be replaced. Occasionally the *field coils* of a motor may become damaged. They can also be replaced by an electric motor shop fairly easily in most cases.

The *shaft* of the motor, to which the head is attached, turns within *sleeve bearings* at the top and bottom of the motor. These bearings are designed to very close tolerance and must be kept well lubricated to prevent wear. Loose bearings may cause vibration and loss of motor efficiency. A dry bearing increases the load on the motor considerably, slowing the speed of the centrifuge and producing heat. Some centrifuges have sealed bearings with lifetime lubrication. The instruction book for the instrument should be read carefully to determine which bearings need grease or oil and where the lubrication points are located. The lubrication schedule should be followed religiously. *Ball bearings* are used in some motors. This type of bearing is somewhat more expensive and reduces friction considerably.

Badly worn bearings can be replaced, but this is generally a job for a careful electric motor shop or knowledgeable repairman. High-speed motors, in particular, are troublesome in this regard. Tolerances are very close, and centering and alignment are critical. Hematocrit centrifuges are especially troublesome, and the instrument with replaced bearings is often quite noisy.

Centrifugal force depends essentially on three variables: *mass, speed,* and *radius.* Since aqueous solutions or other solutions with a specific gravity close to 1.000 are usually involved, only the speed and radius must be considered.

The *relative centrifugal force,* or RCF, is calculated according to the formula

$$RCF = 0.00001118 \times r \times N^2$$

where r = the radius in centimeters and N = the number of revolutions per minute. The radius is measured from the center of the shaft to the inside bottom of the tube.

The speed is dependent on the voltage in most centrifuges, but efficiency (speed) is lost as resistance is increased. Resistance may include such items as air resistance and turbulence, dry or worn bearings, brush friction, and electrical inefficiency inherent in the design of the motor. The same centrifuge will achieve different speeds with different accessories and in varying states of repair. The calibrations often furnished on the speed control are only relative voltage increments and can never be taken as accurate indicators of speed. A tachometer or strobe light should be used to accurately determine speed. (A *strobe light* is a light that very rapidly turns on and off. When it is held over the spinning centrifuge head, it is adjusted to the frequency at which the head appears to stand still. At this frequency the light is on at exactly the instant when the centrifuge head is in the same position, during each revolution. The speed of the centrifuge in revolutions per minute is then obviously the same as the frequency of the strobe light. Allowance must be made for harmonics, of course.)

When the revolutions per minute have been determined, the RCF can easily be determined, by use of a nomograph (Fig. 16-2). This is faster and easier than using the formula and is sufficiently accurate for clinical use.

*Maintenance and quality control.* It cannot be overemphasized that proper maintenance is vital to the efficiency and long life of the centrifuge. The following rules are very important and are listed here for emphasis:

1. Check brushes often and replace according to the manufacturer's instructions well before they are completely worn away.
2. Be sure the proper brush is used. A brush that is too small may wedge between the brush holder and commutator and cause serious damage.
3. Keep the motor clean and free of carbon dust and debris.
4. Clean the inside of the bowl frequently and thoroughly. Always remove all traces of broken glass. Replace cushions in shields where glass has broken. Waxing the inside of the bowl helps keep down dust and dirt and reduces drag.
5. Lubricate bearings according to the manufacturer's directions. Never let a bearing become dry.
6. Use proper accessories and cushions for the instruments. Never run a centrifuge when it is out of balance or is vibrating.
7. Check the balance of accessories often. Numbering helps keep them in the proper position.
8. Unstoppered patient samples should never be centrifuged.

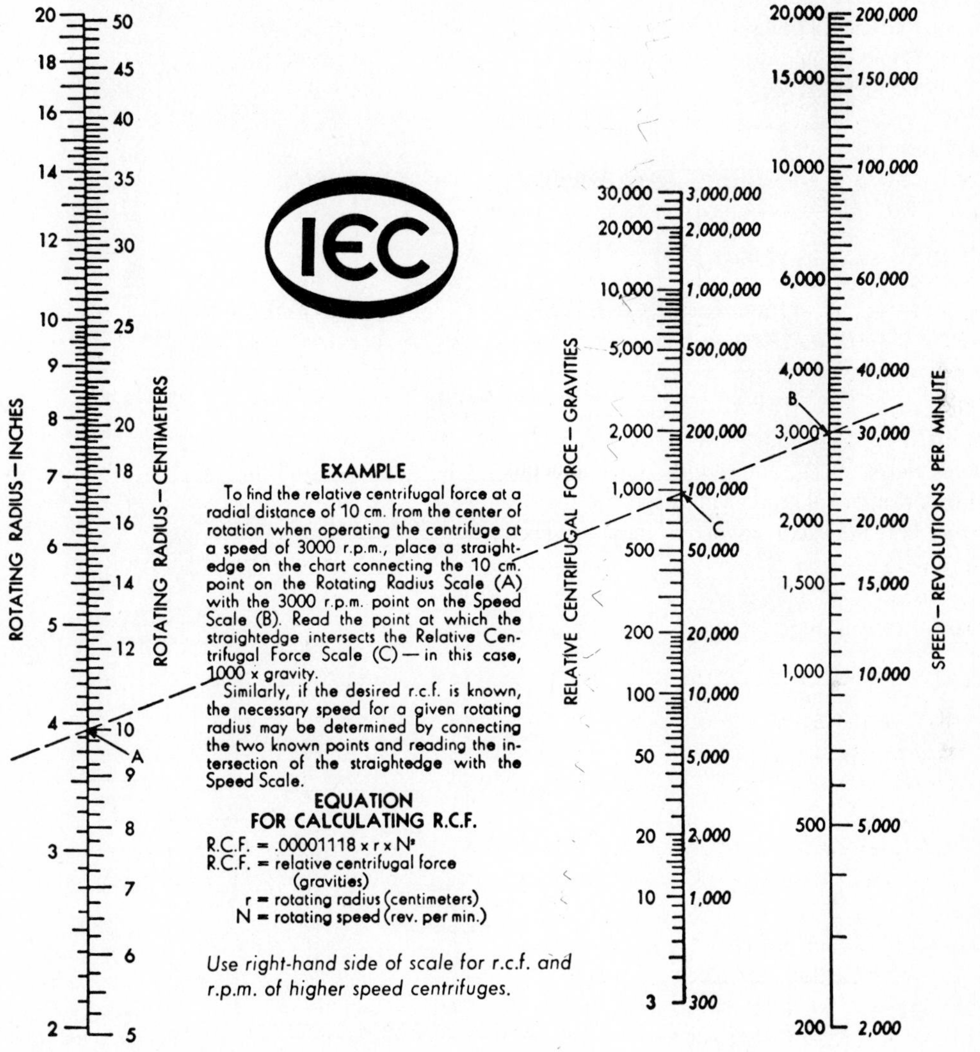

ROTATING RADIUS—INCHES
ROTATING RADIUS—CENTIMETERS
IEC
EXAMPLE
To find the relative centrifugal force at a radial distance of 10 cm. from the center of rotation when operating the centrifuge at a speed of 3000 r.p.m., place a straightedge on the chart connecting the 10 cm. point on the Rotating Radius Scale (A) with the 3000 r.p.m. point on the Speed Scale (B). Read the point at which the straightedge intersects the Relative Centrifugal Force Scale (C)—in this case, 1000 x gravity.
Similarly, if the desired r.c.f. is known, the necessary speed for a given rotating radius may be determined by connecting the two known points and reading the intersection of the straightedge with the Speed Scale.
EQUATION FOR CALCULATING R.C.F.
R.C.F. = .00001118 x r x $N^2$
R.C.F. = relative centrifugal force (gravities)
r = rotating radius (centimeters)
N = rotating speed (rev. per min.)
Use right-hand side of scale for r.c.f. and r.p.m. of higher speed centrifuges.
RELATIVE CENTRIFUGAL FORCE—GRAVITIES
SPEED—REVOLUTIONS PER MINUTE
A
B
C


*Fig. 16-2.* Nomograph for computing centrifugal force. (Courtesy International Equipment Co., Division of Damon.)

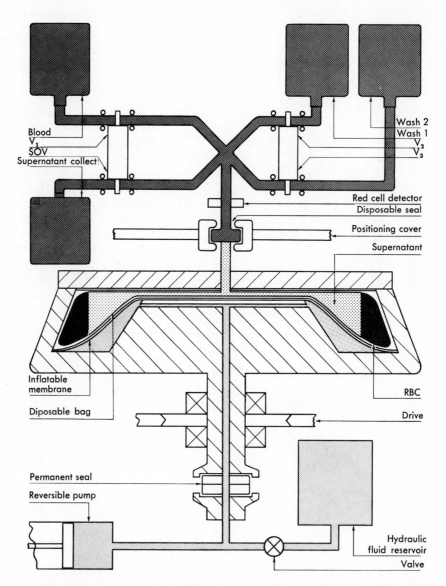

*Fig. 16-3.* Blood cell–washing scheme of IBM Model 2991 Blood Cell Processor. (Courtesy IBM.)

9. Any spills or spatters of patient samples should be promptly cleaned with a suitable disinfectant to avoid aerosols and dust that can spread disease organisms.

10. Speed of rotation should be checked periodically by using a tachometer, and, where appropriate, functional checks (such as packing checks for hematocrit centrifuges) should be performed periodically.

11. When timers are used, their accuracy should be verified from time to time.

*Special-purpose centrifuges.* Several special-purpose centrifuge systems are available. *Refrigerated centrifuges* are required for some enzymes analyses as well as other temperature-sensitive procedures. A compressor unit is provided in the base of the centrifuge, and the bowl of the centrifuge is maintained at a temperature low enough to more than compensate for the heat of air friction. Although they are necessarily moderately expensive, there is nothing complicated about them.

Various *cell washers* and continuous-flow *plasma* and *blood cell separators* are on the market. These are centrifuges equipped with pumps, valves, and sensors to allow them to cycle through the various steps of separating discarding and washing. The blood cell–washing scheme of the IBM 2991 Blood Cell Processor is presented in Fig. 16-3 as an example. The rationale of each of these instruments may seem complicated, but, once examined in detail, they are really fairly simple.

## Recorders

With the increasing use of microprocessors with electronic digital displays to show a final calculated, adjusted report, the use of mechanical recorders has decreased considerably. There are many types available, and only a general idea of their operation is presented here. We are primarily concerned with devices for making on a chart certain phenomena as a function of time. There are two mechanisms involved. The first is the chart-drive motor that feeds the paper under the writing pen at a constant speed. The second is the pen drive that translates the incoming electric signal (from the photometer or thermistor that is being monitored) into a displacement of the pen corresponding to the signal size (Fig. 16-4).

The chart drive is a simple electric motor geared to move the paper forward. Fig. 16-5 is an ex-

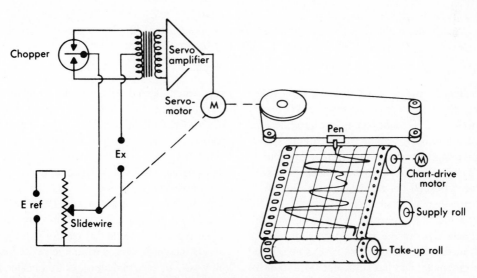

*Fig. 16-4.* Schematic diagram of recorder operation. (Courtesy Sargent-Welch Scientific Co.)

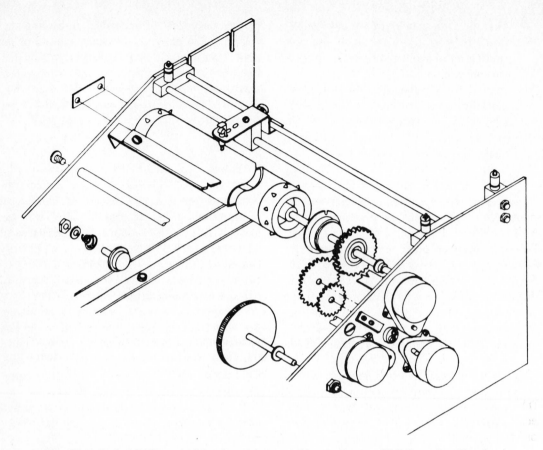

*Fig. 16-5.* Exploded diagram of the chart-drive assembly of a Sargent SRG Recorder. The clear, detailed sketch illustrates how carefully the manual is assembled to allow the untrained person to maintain and repair this type of equipment. (Courtesy Sargent-Welch Scientific Co.)

ploded diagram of the paper drive of a recorder. Different chart speeds may be supplied by one of two mechanisms. Some recorders provide one motor and a clutch assembly for changing speeds by engaging gear trains with different gear ratios. Other instruments use a separate small motor for each speed desired, as can be seen in Fig. 16-6.

The pen displacement may be done in any of several ways. Two general types will be considered here. One of the simplest types is used in the galvanometric recorder. The input signal is fed to a galvanometer that has sufficient force to move a pen or stylus. In effect, these recorders work very much like a d'Arsonval meter movement with a writing pen at the end of the meter needle. Most electrocardiographic machines use galvanometric recorders, and the record is burned into a plasticized paper by a hot wire or stylus. Some recorders that operate in this way describe an arc when the pen moves either up or downscale, since this is the way the tip of a pointer moves. Paper with curved time lines is used to correct the arc error. For some types of records this pattern is no particular disadvantage. Other galvanometric records employ various mechanical tricks to translate the arc-shaped movement into a straight line.

The most common type of pen displacement in laboratory recorders is that of the servo potentiometer. This is an automatic null-balancing device. The recorder has a reference source, such as a mercury cell or a Zener diode, that supplies a reference voltage against which the signal is measured. The error signal between the two currents is fed to the servo amplifier. The amplified current, in turn, drives the potentiometer to its null point and, at the same time, moves the pen a distance relative to the correction made.

By adding resistance to either side of the measuring circuit, the zero setting can be moved to the right or the left; by adjusting the bias to the servo amplifier, the span can be increased or decreased. The error signal is usually direct current and must be chopped for good amplification without drift. An electrical filter is placed in the input line to screen out extraneous signals of high frequency that would cause noise in the recording.

In evaluating a recorder, there are a number of terms used that apply only (or primarily) to recorders. A review of these terms may help to explain differences between instruments.

The *input signal* is the current that is to be measured. The *input span* is the voltage range that the recorder is capable of recording. Most general-purpose recorders have an *input-selector switch,* which allows the use of any number of different input spans. The input selector is a resistor substitution bank that permits selection of the resistor needed to accommodate the desired signal. The *chart speed* is the speed with which paper is moved forward under the pen and is usually measured in inches per minute. Most general-purpose recorders allow several choices. *Pen response* is the speed with which the pen moves and is usually measured in terms of the time it takes the pen to move from one edge of the paper to the other when an input signal greater than the input span is used. *Deadband* is the amount that the input signal can be varied without moving the pen. *Accuracy,* usually expressed in percent, is the limit that errors will not exceed when the instrument is used in accordance with the manufacturer's instructions. *Interference* is any unwanted current or voltage occurring in the instrument. *Common mode* is interference appearing between the measuring circuits and ground. *Null balance* is the situation in which the error signal between the input and the reference does not exceed the deadband. *Span* is the algebraic difference between the ends of the scale values. *Range* is the span expressed in terms of the values of the ends of the span.

*Reproducibility* is the measure of the instrument's ability to return to the same point on the scale when the same input signal is applied. *Normal mode* is the spurious voltage that occurs between the measuring terminals. *Step-response time* is the time required for the pen to come to rest after an abrupt signal change. *Input divider* is a resistor or resistors installed in such a way that only a specific portion of the signal is measured. For additional information on terminology of recorders, refer to the literature of various recorder manufacturers. Texas Instruments' Bulletin No. 007, from which many of the above definitions were taken, is particularly helpful.

Many recorders have the capability of recording either a linear signal or a log signal and are called *linear-log recorders.* Normally a signal (from a photometer, for example) will displace the pen a given distance for each millivolt of signal. In many cases it would be very handy if absorbance units (which are log values) could be used on the recorder paper as a straight-line function so that concentrations would be immediately obvious. (If this is not entirely clear, the discussion of Beer's law in Chapter 7 may give some help.) The recorder may be able to make this translation. Linear-to-log and log-to-linear converters, using integrated circuits electronically calculate the required information.

*Integrators.* Most recorders are equipped with integrators. These are extremely convenient in gas chromatography and electrophoresis scanning, as indicated in discussion of these techniques. In such situations the quantity of some component is determined by multiplying the amplitude of the signal from a detector by the length of time the signal

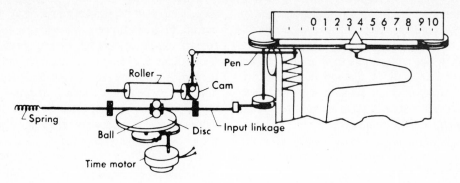

*Fig. 16-6.* Mechanical principle of the Disc Integrator. (Courtesy Disc Instruments, Inc.)

is produced. If both the flow rate of a gas in a tube and the time this rate of flow continues are known, it is easy to calculate the volume, for example. Both the rate of flow and the time interval might vary in a random manner. If this information were charted on a recorder, the increase in flow would produce a peak on the chart paper. The height of the peak would represent the rate of flow, and the width would represent its duration in minutes. Hence the area under the curve would represent the quantity of gas that had passed through the tube. An integrator is a mechanical or electrical device for translating the area under the curve to unit values.

*Mechanical integrators.* Most mechanical integrators work on the principle of the Disc Integrator, pictured in Fig. 16-6. This type of integrator can be understood if the disc, which is moving at a constant rate of speed, is thought of as the platform of a merry-go-round. If a miniature man were to pedal a tricycle at the outer edge of the platform fast enough to stay opposite the ticket booth, he would have to pedal very fast. If he were closer to the center, he could pedal much more slowly, and if he were in the exact center of the platform, he could stay in the same position with no effort. The speed with which the tricycle wheels turned would be a function of the tricycle's position on the merry-go-round platform. The ball in the illustration may be compared to the tricycle wheel. Its position is determined by the position of the pen on the chart paper. The spiral-in and spiral-

out cam is a device to push the integrator pen up and down on the edge of the paper each time the ball turns. This device is purely mechanical and has been relatively trouble free.

*Electronic integrators.* Modern recorders use electronic integrators. These consist of very accurate capacitors that store a representative portion of the output signal and then discharge into circuits, which record this current fraction as an event, such as a pen stroke. This capacitor discharge may be recorded as blips on the edge of a recorder paper, as digits on a dial, or as some other form of record. Electronic integrators possess the advantages of having very few moving parts and being trouble free.

Integrated circuits can be used to process electronic signals and integrate the area under curves. Microprocessors are then used to manipulate the collected information as the situation demands. If the actual graphic display is not needed, the recorder may be eliminated entirely and the data processed, integrated, and reported as a digital display. It is possible, using electronic devices now available, to sense the valley denoting the end of a peak, measure peak height, measure slope, and sense irregularities with a high degree of accuracy and reliability. Hence the need for the rectilinear recorder with its mechanical problems is fast declining.

*X-Y plotters.* X-Y plotters are recorders that record points on a graph as functions of two parameters. Time is usually not one of these parameters. Two pen-drive motors are required. One moves the pen along the abscissa while the other moves it along the ordinate of the graph. Such a system might plot the interrelationship of vibration frequency of a motor versus speed, or air temperature versus moisture content.

## Tissue-processing equipment

Tissue-processing equipment is in use in practically every hospital laboratory. Technicon Corp. has been the leader in this field since its inception over 40 years ago. Lipshaw Manufacturing Co., Fisher Scientific Co., and others also produce devices of this kind. The instruments are all purely mechanical arrangements to move tissue samples or fluids from place to place according to a predetermined time sequence. Small motors, gear assemblies, levers, and microswitches are the components that cause these to function. A few minutes of close observation will usually suffice for understanding the mechanics of any part of the system when it is open for observation. Problems usually involve the failure of microswitches or small motors. Occasionally lack of lubrication or long use may cause wear of a gear train or bearing, but in general these devices are well designed and capable of many years of hard service without excessive wear.

Technicon Corp.'s Autotechnicon Ultra adds heating or reagents, better agitation, and vacuum to the mechanics of the well-known models. There is no significant problem with this system other than minor ones mentioned earlier.

## Knife sharpeners

Knife sharpeners are in use in nearly every histology laboratory. Although they are extremely simple devices, they seem to give trouble occasionally. There are several common designs. They are of either the flat-surface type or the honing-wheel type. The first moves the knife in a very concise position back and forth over a glass honing plate to which honing compound has been applied. Some provision is made for turning the knife occasionally, either automatically or manually. This process obviously produces a straight bevel on the knife. The wheel type of sharpener presents the knife edge to a honing wheel, which may be glass or smooth metal, to which honing compound is applied. This type of sharpener gives the bevel a slightly concave characteristic, which some microtomists prefer. Obviously, when a knife has been sharpened on one type sharpener, a great deal of time is required to reestablish the new bevel on the other type of machine. It should be equally obvious that changing the bevel angle can be disastrous and should be done only if absolutely necessary. Any significant change in the bevel should be done by the manufacturer or another service facility completely knowledgeable concerning microtome knife reconditioning.

Abrasive compound is designed to cut away metal. Its accidental presence in bearings and gears is certain to cause unusual wear, and care should be taken to keep it away from moving parts. Lubrication should be done regularly. Electric parts should be kept dry. All these points would seem to be obvious, but problems such as these contribute greatly to the maintenance of equipment of this kind.

There is much variation between instruments in the use of abrasives, oils, and soaps in the sharpening process, and the only admonition appropriate is that the manufacturer's directions should be followed implicitly unless experience and careful observation have shown it safe to deviate from them. The same might be said about such details as turning cycles and bevel settings.

## Balances

Anyone working in a laboratory regularly has been exposed to many types of balances, and the principle of operation of some types is simple and obvious. In recent years a few new devices have been introduced in this area, and it seems worthwhile to make some mention of them. *Substitution balances* have come into common use. In these balances a weight in an air-damping chamber at one end of a beam is exactly balanced by a group of removable weights at the other end. When a sample is added to the latter end, weights are removed mechanically to maintain a constant balance. The weights removed represent the weight of the sample. Some of these balances have a small lens with a scale mounted in the beam in such a position that a slight imbalance moves the shadow of the scale into position along a pointer to indicate small errors in substitution. The air-damping chamber consists of a vane mounted around the weights in the nearly airtight chamber. As the weight moves, air slowly leaves the chamber, allowing the weight and vane on the beam to gradually assume the proper balance position. Magnetic damping is also used on some balances. Although the readout dial may be illuminated or an electric light may project the scale to show the imbalance and magnetic damping may be used, the substitution balance itself is still mechanical. In work on a balance of this kind, care in handling weights and protecting the ruby knife edges must be exercised, just as in a classic analytical balance.

Another concept is the *electrobalance,* which is capable of very accurate weighing of very small samples. The sample is weighed from a light metal beam attached to an electromagnetic coil that is suspended in a stronger electromagnetic field. Current through the field is automatically adjusted to counteract the torque caused by the object being weighed. The correcting electric current is calibrated against standard weights. The balance is quite versatile; different spans can be chosen to provide accurate weighings from tenth of a milligram to a few grams. Several sources of weighing error are eliminated in this instrument. The Cahn Division of Ventron Instruments Corp. has been a leader in developing electrobalances.

### Pipetters and dilutors (Fig. 16-7)

A large number of devices for pipetting accurately measured quantities of fluid are now available. These vary from the hand-gun type mentioned in the discussion of the Bio-Quest Fibrometer, through the syringe variations, to highly automated repetitive pipetters for moving tubes in a rack or drum and adding predetermined amounts of fluid to each. Two remarks might be appropriate here.

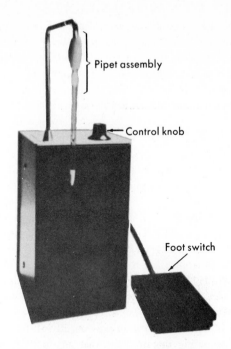

*Fig. 16-7.* Dade Dilutor. This is one of the most consistently accurate dilutors in its price class. (Courtesy Dade Reagents, Division of American Hospital Supply Corp.)

In general these devices are as good as their *seals.* Around the plunger, displacement element, or other device there must be some type of seal to contain the fluid that is generally being displaced under some positive pressure. Constant use eventually causes wear or damage to these seals, and they begin to leak. Even glass on glass and stainless steel on glass are eventually subject to this kind of wear. Small pieces of broken glass, sand, or other material can cause jamming and possibly considerable damage. Stainless steel or heavy Teflon seems to be the most durable.

The accuracy of any test is totally dependent on the accuracy of measurement of the sample and the reagents used. It should be apparent that measuring accuracy must be absolutely ensured at all times. Since all pipetters and dilutors are subject to wear, error, and failure, some regular program of checking sample and reagent delivery must be maintained. A classic means of checking accuracy is to weigh the amount of water delivered. Adjustment should be made for temperature. Since this method is tedious and time consuming, various alternatives have been developed. Any method that compares the volume delivered to the volume of an accurate glass volumetric pipette is adequate. This can be done by comparing dye dilutions, radioactive nuclides, flame photometry standards, or similar material. Some companies have produced kits to make the task easier. Some degree of accuracy should be established as the tolerable limit of error.

## Osmometry and osmometers

In most clinical laboratories and particularly in those involved with testing patients with renal disease, osmometry has become common. *Osmolality* is a measure of the total number of particles dissolved in a solution without regard for their homogeneity, molecular weights, particle size, or specific gravity. This solution concentration determines the osmotic pressure that would exist between the solution and a pure solvent (which in biological systems would be water). The standard of measurement is the *osmol,* which is one gram molecular weight of nonionizable material per kilogram of solvent. One milliosmol is, of course, one thousandth of an osmol. *Osmolarity* is occasionally used synonymously with osmolality, but there is a slight difference in definition, since osmolarity refers to solute per *liter* (volume) rather than per kilogram (weight).

These terms would seem to relate to the osmotic pressure of fluids, and it is indeed this physiologically important function that interests us. It proves to be impractical, however, to actually make this measurement using a membrane between two fluids, so other means are found to obtain the same information. There are four colligative (that is, logically related) *properties* that can be measured and mathematically related: osmotic pressure, vapor pressure, freezing point, and boiling point.

As solvent is added to water, the osmolality increases. At the same time, the solution will freeze at a lower temperature, boil at a lower temperature, and become a vapor at a lower temperature. Hence, any one of the properties could be mea-

sured and related mathematically to each of the others.

Specific gravity, total solids, or the refractive index do not give the same information as osmolality, since they are all concerned with the mass of the solute. Osmolality has specific value, since it is closely related to the colligative properties of body fluids, and it is these properties that determine thirst and stimulate diuresis and retention of water through their action on the osmoreceptors of the body.

The osmolality of serum depends, in large part, on sodium. The serum sodium in milliequivalents per liter times 2.1 should give the approximate milliosmols if the patient is normally healthy. Increases and decreases in serum sodium usually, but not always, cause changes in the osmolality. Abnormal osmolalities of serum should be immediately checked for sodium, sugar, and urea to determine the nature of the disturbance.

The ratio or serum to urine osmolality should be between 1:3 and 1:4 in the first morning urine. A urine value of less than 600, after overnight fluid deprivation, strongly suggests renal disease.

As can be seen from these random notes, the measurement of osmolality in serum is a screening procedure that quickly and easily points up certain abnormalities that might be missed without the testing of several parameters.

Most commercially available devices depend on the measurement of *depression of freezing point,* since the freezing point of a liquid is dependent on its solute concentration. Fiske Associates, Inc., has pioneered in the development of osmometers. A Fiske Osmometer is shown in Fig. 16-8. This model has become something of a standard for the industry, and the company has produced excellent newer models.

When a solution is cooled rapidly, it may not form ice even though the temperature is far below its freezing point. If a crystal or some impurity is added or if the solution is disturbed, ice formation quickly follows. An unfrozen solution that is colder than its normal freezing point is called a *supercooled liquid.*

When supercooled water produces ice, the tem-

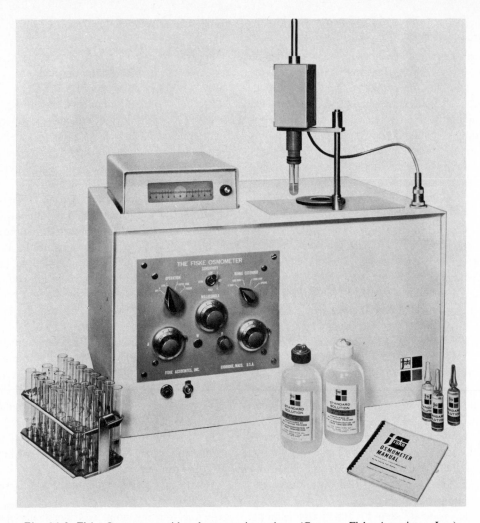

***Fig. 16-8.*** Fiske Osmometer with galvanometric readout. (Courtesy Fiske Associates, Inc.)

perature rises rather quickly to 0° C because crystal formation of water produces heat. This temperature change is not instantaneous, since crystal formation is not an instantaneous process. The freezing point (0° C for water) is an *equilibrium point,* and the temperature will stay constant there for a few minutes.

The Osmometer is a device that supercools urine or serum, causes it to crystalize, and measures its freezing point by locating the equilibrium-point

plateau. The freezing point, however, is read in milliosmols of solute rather than degrees of temperature.

The sample of serum or urine is placed in position, with the sensing probe tips immersed in the liquid. The sensing probe contains a tiny thermistor through which a small current is passed. As the temperature changes, the current is monitored by a galvanometer. The sample and probe are lowered into the coolant, where the refrigerator

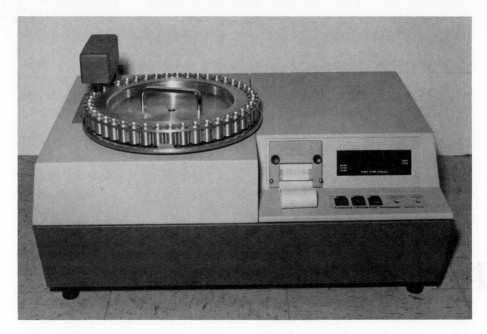

***Fig. 16-9.*** New Cryomatic Osmometer. (Courtesy Advanced Instruments, Inc.)

unit rapidly supercools the sample. A vibrator is activated, causing crystalization, and the temperature is watched on the galvanometer readout until the equilibrium-point plateau is reached. At this point resistance is applied to the Wheatstone balancing bridge to bring the galvanometer into balance. The resistance applied is relative to the temperature of the probe, which, of course, indicates the freezing point and osmolarity of the sample.

In general it could be said that the instrument contains a refrigeration unit with circulating pump, a temperature probe that activates a galvanometer, a vibrator, and a Wheatstone bridge. There is also a precooling tank for lowering the temperature of the sample before the test.

Although these comments are an oversimplification of this well-designed instrument, it should provide the student with some comprehension of the Osmometer's construction.

In operating the instrument, the student should follow the instruction of the manufacturer in de-

tail, since this is a very exact procedure.

The Fiske Osmometer is well built and relatively trouble free. There is little about the instrument that should give trouble in normal use.

Fig. 16-9 shows an automated osmometer, the Cryomatic (Advanced Instruments, Inc.), that will automatically test up to 44 samples without operator attention and print out the result on a paper tape. Time required is about 2 minutes per tape. This is a very new and relatively expensive instrument.

Another company, Precision Systems, also produces excellent freezing-point osmometers. The Osmette Model 2007 and the Osmette A are rugged and reliable instruments.

The Model 5100C Vapor Pressure Osmometer (Wescor, Inc.) (Fig. 16-10) produces an instrument that operates on an entirely different principle. A very small (5 $\mu$l) sample is absorbed onto a small disc of filter paper and placed in a tightly closed chamber. A hygrometer is used to measure the dew point within the chamber. The dew point

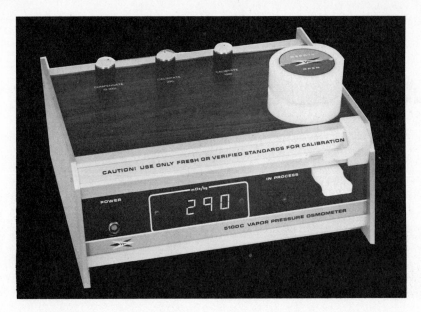

*Fig. 16-10*. Wescor Vapor Pressure Osmometer. (Courtesy Wescor, Inc.)

is an explicit function of vapor pressure. The exact measuring technique used in the Model 5100C is electronically sophisticated and is patented.

## Automation in microbiology

Bacteriology has been the last discipline of the medical laboratory to accept automation. Until recently very little had been done to eliminate or simplify the tedious process of subculturing organisms onto various inhibitory and enrichment media. The process has always been expensive in time and materials, and considerable knowledge of the subject is required.

A number of simple devices have found their way into use, but now major changes are taking place that will revolutionize the bacteriology laboratory, speed diagnosis, and ultimately reduce patient care costs.

Much of the progress has come about because of developments in media composition and packaging that have made the use of electronic detection devices possible. As with all other areas of instrumentation, the computer has also been involved. A number of exciting new instruments

have been announced. In the following pages a few of the instruments that have gained wide acceptance are presented.

The Pfizer Autobac I (Pfizer Diagnostics Division) is an efficient instrument for testing the sensitivity of an organism to various antibiotics (Fig. 16-11). Colonies of the organism to be tested are suspended in eugonic broth. When the broth tube is attached to a specially designed cuvette, the suspension can be made to flow evenly into thirteen test chambers. Twelve of these test chambers contain antibiotic discs. The remaining chamber is used to allow uninhibited growth of the organism. Up to 30 of these special cuvettes can be placed in an incubator shaker where, within 3 to 5 hours, growth will progress through about three generations. At the end of this time period, the cuvettes are read through a photometer, where the turbidity of each antibiotic-inhibited culture is compared with the uninhibited chamber. The photometric information is then translated to growth levels designated as *resistant*, *intermediate*, or *susceptible*.

A disc dispenser is available that can charge a

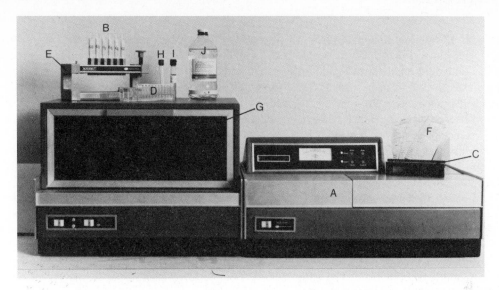

**Fig. 16-11.** Pfizer Autobac system. *A,* Photometer; *B,* cartridges of discs; *C,* printer; *D,* cuvette; *E,* disc dispenser; *F,* report forms; *G,* shaker-incubator; *H,* standards; *I,* inoculating tube; *J,* broth culture medium. (Courtesy Pfizer Diagnostics Division.)

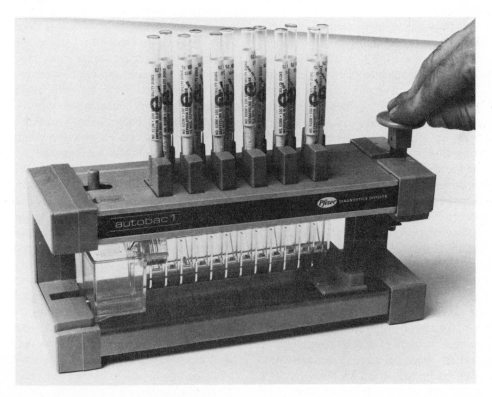

**Fig. 16-12.** Pfizer Autobac antibiotic disc dispenser showing cuvette in place to receive discs. (Courtesy Pfizer Diagnostic Division.)

cuvette with 12 different antibiotic discs when a plunger is depressed (Fig. 16-12). If a large number of sensitivity tests are to be done, additional incubator-shaker modules can be added. Since the readings and printed cycle are quite fast, a very large number of cultures could be tested in a day if sufficient incubator units were added.

Results obtained using the Pfizer Autobac are quite comparable to those found by the Kirby-Bauer method, and the sensitivity testing requires only 3 to 5 hours. This is an improvement of nearly one full day over the normal sensitivity testing methods. Human error is reduced, and considerable work time is saved. The instrument, in routine use, has proved to be easy to operate and free from maintenance problems. The entire system is shown in Fig. 16-12. A procedure that will allow the instrument to be used to determine minimal isorrheic concentrations (MIC) of antibiotics is also available.

Abbott Diagnostics Division produces an instrument for antibiotic sensitivity testing and MIC determinations, which works on a principle similar to that of the Autobac. The rationale and operation of the MS-2 Antimicrobial Susceptibility Testing System are somewhat different, however. In this instrument, growth is monitored, during the initial incubation/agitation period, by an LED and light detector. As soon as log phase growth begins, the culture broth is transferred to the test chambers containing the antibiotic discs. Here the turbidity of each chamber is monitored at 5-minute intervals, and the photometric information is translated into a susceptibility report. The company reports that a method of performing minimal inhibitory concentrations will be available.

Johnson Laboratories, Inc., has produced a system called *Bactec,* which works in a different way to detect bacterial growth. Glucose and certain other substances are tagged with the carbon isotope $C^{14}$. Almost all organisms metabolize glucose with the formation of at least some trace of carbon dioxide. When the tagged glucose is used, $C^{14}O_2$ is produced, and it can be drawn out of a sealed culture bottle and detected. If there is no growth, no gas will be produced.

Various configurations of the Bactec have been in use for several years. Growth is sometimes detected in 4 hours, allowing antibiotic sensitivty to be completed within the first day. In fulminating septicemias the saving of time can mean the saving of a life. The time spent in examining blood cultures for growth, streaking subcultures, and preparing and reading stained smears is largely saved by this instrument, and most laboratories feel that it has quickly repaid its cost.

Growth is accelerated by the use of a shaker/incubator. All culture bottles are sampled repeatedly at predetermined intervals. Most of the configurations of the instrument provide a mechanism for moving the bottles sequentially into sampling position. In large laboratories the saving of time has been quite considerable, and isolation of organisms has increased slightly.

A method that has excited a great deal of interest has involved the examination of the metabolic products of various bacteria by gas chromatography. Some of the first work was done on the gases released by anaerobes grown on certain media. More recently careful work has demonstrated that many, if not most, bacteria produce gases or volatile acids that are characteristic enough to identify them when studied by gas chromatography. Body fluids of animals infected by some bacteria can be shown to contain characteristic substances that are diagnostic. Virus infections in some cases can even be occasionally demonstrated in this way. Certain characteristic volatile acids and alcohols are the chief chemical components that can be identified by gas chromatography in this technique. This approach, although still experimental, would seem to offer considerable promise. The project seems huge now, but it indicates possibilities of growing, extracting, and chromatographing in an automated device and of identifying organisms, by computer, using gas chromatograms along with other detectable characteristics. Fig. 16-13 shows the AnaBac Gas Chromatograph designed specifically for bacteriology.

The most innovative and promising new approach to the automation of bacteriology is prob-

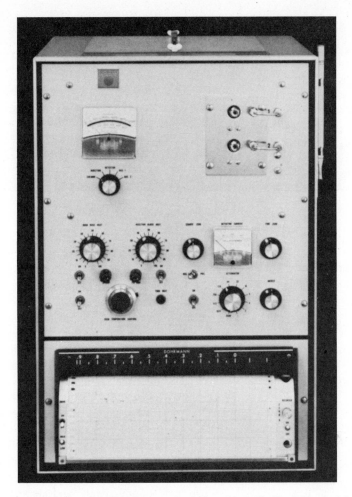

*Fig. 16-13.* AnaBac Gas Chromatograph, designed specifically for bacteriology.

ably the Vitek AutoMicrobic System AMS-120 (Fig. 16-14). The system is built around an ingenous test card system (Fig. 16-15). These disposable, plastic cards each have a number of wells connected by channels arranged in such a way that the wells can be filled through a common injection port. The wells contain specific nutrients, biochemicals, or antibiotics arranged in patterns by which the organism being cultured can be identified or its antibiotic sensitivity defined. After incubation, the test cards are monitored by a card reader that measures the transmittance of light through each well. Growth in each case produces turbidity, which reduces the transmitted light.

The entire system consists of six separate modules. The test card, in a plastic holder, with inoculum tubes is first placed in the *diluent dispenser module*. Here the proper dilution is made to ensure standard growth conditions. Next, the card in its holder is transferred to the *filling module* where it is first placed under a vacuum and then filled as air pressure is gradually returned to normal, pushing solution into the wells. Next, the card is placed in a *sealer* where the injection port is heat sealed.

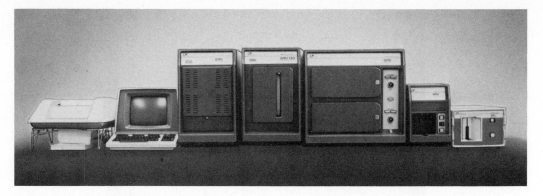

*Fig. 16-14.* The Vitek AutoMicrobic System, AMS-120. (Courtesy Vitek Systems, Inc.)

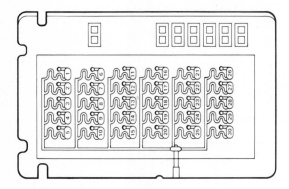

*Fig. 16-15.* Outline of a typical test card used by the Vitek AutoMicrobic System. Note that 26 media are inoculated by injecting the inoculum through one port. (Courtesy Vitek System, Inc.)

The cards are next transferred to the *reader-incubator,* which is the heart of the system. Here a pattern of photodiodes, located behind each well, read the light transmitted by LED light sources located in front of the wells. Each card is rotated through the reading devices for 15 minutes after which it is succeeded by the next card. Information from the reader is transmitted to the *computer-control module* where it is stored and analyzed. The minicomputer applies a rather sophisticated program to the collected growth information and identifies the organism and/or reports its sensi-

tivity pattern. In addition to analyzing the growth data, the computer also manages the system and provides messages of system malfunction. The *data terminal module* has a CRT, keyboard, and printer through which the operator communicates with the system. Information on any card, loading information, and system status can be requested at any time. A message function also reports problems on the CRT as they arise.

At the present time there are three configurations of test cards bearing 30, 20, and 16 test wells. These allow about 10 different diagnostic programs. The urine ID card will accept a diluted urine specimen and will report the approximate "colony count" and identification of any of nine common urinary tract pathogens. Other cards require isolated organisms and can identify the more common enteric and vibro organisms, yeasts, and some other organisms. Several antibiotic sensitivity panels are also available. Identification of organisms is often possible in under 12 hours, and in most, laser identification and sensitivity can both be reported in less than 24 hours.

The enteric organisms are the most readily handled by this system, although yeasts and some gram-positive organisms are also readily identified. The system is now in use in many places, and its utility is being extended rapidly. Obviously any system that can do the enteric organisms would greatly reduce the bacteriology workload, but the AMS-120 promises to do considerably more when its entire potential is realized.

The AutoMicrobic System is available in 60-, 120-, and 240-sample capacities. As additional research is done on new application for this approach to the automation of bacteriology, we can expect great changes in the time required for diagnosis of bacterial infections and in the way bacteriology is practiced.

Other studies have been involved with automated techniques for separating the bacteria in a mixed culture using size and electric charges. If this technique proves practical, the same characteristics that allowed separation may prove useful as criteria for identification.

Many other studies are progressing in such areas as the measurement of heat-produced bacterial growth, the plotting of growth curves, using absorbed and scattered light, and the release of radioactive materials form media variously tagged to demonstrate metabolic characteristics of diagnostic significances.

From all these projects and studies, it seems certain that the means to automate much of the tedium of microbiology will certainly be found and that feasible systems will be produced in the next few years.

Laboratories, being places for study and examination, will never be completely automated. There will always be new horizons for exploration and new information to examine and collate into the body of knowledge with which work is done. But it seems inevitable that a great deal of the study of human exudates, transudates, and tissues occupying us today will certainly be automated and computerized in the near future.

# CHAPTER 17

# Quality control and standards

Medical laboratories exist to provide analyses that can be used in patient diagnosis or treatment. The only product the laboratory provides is a report that is quantitative or descriptive or both. If the report is inaccurate or unreliable, the purpose for the laboratory's existence is defeated, and when the report is sufficiently misleading, it may do considerable harm. Errors are much more common that we generally realize or care to admit and are almost certain to occur routinely unless a well-organized program of error avoidance is put in place. This sort of program is generally referred to as quality control or quality assurance. In this chapter the various aspects of quality control are considered, and measures that apply more particularly to instrumentation are examined. Federal regulations and the standards imposed by the Joint Commission on Hospital Accreditation list some specific procedures and practices that should be followed. These are discussed and the logic of the regulation or standard explained.

## Validity of medical laboratory reports

If we were dealing with products such as dishes or nails, quality control would be somewhat more simple, since the final product must meet relatively simple standards and minor quality defects would cause little damage. Much of the quality control in such cases can be done at the end of production, and the product can be accepted or rejected. For medical laboratory reports, this is impossible, since only a few quality judgments can be made by looking at the report and the information is usually used before there is a chance to evaluate its qual-ity. An error in any step in the production of the report can cause a serious error in its validity that may not be apparent.

The ultimate reason for quality control of laboratory work is obviously to ensure the best care of the patient. If the decimal point is omitted in the blood sugar report of a diabetic patient who has a blood sugar of 50.0 mg/dl and the report is read as 500 mg/dl, insulin might be administered that could lead to the patient's death. Our responsibility is obviously to ensure that this sort of error does not happen and that each report reflects the patient's condition accurately, reliably, and promptly so that diagnosis and treatment can be carried out in the most effective and expedient manner.

It can be argued that the quality control normally performed actually exceeds this requirement and that we are looking for 2% errors when an error of 5% or 10% might not have an appreciable effect on the patient. Since this argument may, in some cases, have some validity, it is considered here.

One argument for such apparent over-control is that it is impossible to know in all cases what degree of accuracy may prove useful. The family physician may be unable to interpret variations of 10% in a test, but a specialist may immediately spot some significance in such a variation. The practice of medicine is such that each laboratory worker is unable to truly appreciate and understand all the physiologic, pathologic, and pharmacologic data implicit in each report that is rendered.

There is also a persuasive argument that we should all strive for excellence for its own sake.

Many things are now possible in medicine simply because someone proved that a higher degree of accuracy, precision, or specificity could be achieved. For example, 20 years ago cholinesterase measurement was a rather imprecise technique generally used only for detecting the effect of poisons such as parathion. Because of the increased accuracy and precision developed, it can now be used as a very sensitive indicator of small physiologic changes resulting from various other stimuli.

## Cost of quality control

It must be admitted, however, that the cost of "ultimate" quality control may be unrealistically high. If we are reassured by running two controls rather than one, is it not likely that a third control would further improve the chances of accuracy? How much control is enough? In the present climate of cynicism concerning regulation, various standards and regulations are being challenged. The cost of quality control supplies and labor is a substantial part of total cost. Most laboratories estimate that one third of their workload is made up of quality control specimens, and the cost of reference and standard materials is considerable. A reasonable balance is needed. Unfortunately, those who perform the most rigorous quality control probably need it least, and those who object most loudly to required controls may need them most. It is for this reason that standards of performance or regulation are important.

## Variables affecting quality control

Effective quality control needs to anticipate all possible variables that might affect the test report. The following list is representative of the potential sources of error that may affect the laboratory tests:

Patient identification
Specimen labeling
Specimen collection technique
Specimen preservation and storage
Mixing or sampling
Reagent quality (including water)

Instrument performance
Instrument calibration
Electric supply
Transposition of data
Standard and reference quality
Calculation
Choice of test method
Pipetting or weighing
Timing and timer accuracy
Temperature

The obvious point is that no simple program of quality control can anticipate all possible errors. The need is not so much for a rigid system as for an attitude and state of mind that compels each analyst to question everything about his own performance. Since this attitude is not universal and since even the best workers have lapses, some rules that help avoid the more common errors are needed. These rules must be invariably followed and must become such a part of work habits that they are automatically followed.

## Application of quality control procedures

Quality control rules must be clearly defined and publicized to all laboratory workers. Some mechanism must be adopted to ensure that they are always followed. To be effective, procedures should be written into the laboratory's policy and procedure manuals, and a system of reviewable records of compliance should be initiated. A regular review of such records not only guarantees that the quality control measures are being followed, but often provides supervisors with useful data for problem solving.

Quality control begins with the specimen itself. Proper identification procedures for the patient and sample should be written in detail. The manner in which the patient is prepared and the sample drawn should be described. If significant, preservatives, refrigeration of specimens, limits of stability, and other details of preservation, storage, and handling must be explained. Such instructions should be circulated to all who are involved such as nurses, physicians, ward secretaries, and couriers.

The procedure by which the specimen is to be analyzed should be clearly and completely described. In order to include all relevant details, a standard format should be followed. The National Committee for Clinical Laboratory Standards has proposed tentative guidelines for a standard format.* Any format that is adopted should include at least the following:

Principle of the test
Equipment required
Reagent source and preparation
Sample required
Technique of analysis
Calibration and quality control
Calculations
Normal and/or significant values
Notes about problems and interferences
Literature references for the method

When complete details are lacking, variations begin to appear, and precision and accuracy are lost. All new personnel who will perform the test should be required to read the method in detail before they begin to work.

Obviously, the method used must be a proven, published method, or enough data must be available to establish its accuracy, precision, and specificity. Any changes from a published method should be clearly explained and justified with appropriate data.

### Accuracy of measurement

The measurement of samples and reagents must be accurate. Measuring glassware of guaranteed accuracy is necessary, and it must not be damaged in any way that would impair its accuracy. Automatic pipettes, dilutors, syringes, and burettes should be rechecked on a regular basis to ensure their accuracy. The accuracy of measuring devices that comprise a part of an automated system should not be assumed. Several methods have

---

*Tentative guidelines for clinical laboratory procedure manuals, Publ. No. L2-T is available from The National Committee for Clinical Laboratory Standards, 771 East Lancaster Ave., Villanova, Pa., 19085.*

been proposed for checking the accuracy of measuring equipment. The amount of water delivered from a pipetter can be weighed and its volume calculated. Other methods involve diluting a dye sample from the pipetter with an accurately measured amount of diluent and comparing its optical density with that of a standard curve. Other dilution and comparison techniques have been devised using flame photometer standards and radioactive isotopes. Some procedure must be used that compares the delivery of the measuring device with some accurate standard.

The accuracy of pipetters may depend on the way they are used. Two people using the same device may get different results because of slight variations in technique. Sometimes the performance of different workers must be compared and their techniques observed to discover the source of pipetting errors. The same might be said of such procedures as mixing, cleaning, purging, and transferring.

### A few equipment rules

It is not unusual for an analytical instrument to be blamed for one of the errors discussed. When instrument performance is suspected, it is wise to consider all of the elements that might affect test results before instrument problems are considered.

Instruments and analytical systems used in the laboratory vary greatly in their principle of operation and complexity. There are many different pieces of equipment, and new ones are frequently introduced. Adaptation to these may be time consuming and troublesome. A number of general rules may be applied that can make the process simpler and more problem free. These general rules may also contribute considerably to quality control.

**Understanding the equipment.** No new piece of equipment should be operated before the operator understands what it does and how it functions. It is impossible to make reasonable judgments about such factors as temperature, timing, carry-over, and contamination without a clear understanding of the principle of operation of the equipment.

Operators' manuals generally provide most of the necessary information, and they should be studied carefully before tests are run. Obviously, more complex equipment requires more detailed study.

***Regular performance checks.*** Before an instrument is used each day, the necessary steps should be taken to ensure that it will perform properly. The nature of the equipment will determine what these steps might be. Certainly it should be clean and in good condition. If there are reagents or expendable supplies used, these should be checked. Very often the checking of some electrical function is required. This may require the actual checking of voltages as on the Coulter Model S Counters, or proper function may be simply observed. Temperature may be critical, If it is, the operating temperature should be observed and made a matter of record. Often the instrument must be zeroed or blanked or checked for background to ensure that no value is indicated in the absence of a sample. Many devices require operation through a cycle to ensure that all systems are functional and to prime pumps and fill lines and chambers. Others may require changing of membranes or charging with reagents. With computer-associated systems, certain programs or information may need to be furnished. All of such requirements should be combined into a start-up procedure, and the appropriate steps followed and checked off or recorded each day. Simple, small equipment naturally does not require an involved start-up procedure, but even centrifuges and baths should be conscientiously checked for proper function.

***Calibration.*** Calibration is important. This simply means ensuring that the measuring device is accurately reporting what it was meant to measure. Thermometers should be checked periodically against a certified thermometer or one of guaranteed accuracy. Timers should be compared with some accurate timepiece. Spectrophotometers should be checked against a standard calibrating filter, and gamma counters should be calibrated with a standard energy source. All calibrating procedures should be recorded.

***Preventive maintenance.*** Preventive maintenance refers to all those functions that may be regularly done to avoid downtime for repairs, adjustments, or restocking. This may include lubrication, retubing, changing membranes, and replacing small parts. For each instrument, there should be a description of these activities, and their frequency should be defined. A record should be kept that explains what was done on each date. Even very simple devices should be observed from time to time for proper condition and function. Frayed cords, defective switches, and worn parts should receive prompt attention.

Correct calibration or function of instruments should not be assumed just because test results seem to be right. Each element that can be checked should be tested independently of the test to be done.

***Reference samples.*** A clear statement of the laboratory's policy and procedures relating to quality control should include an explanation of the use of reference samples. Reference samples are assayed sera that chemically resemble patient samples. They may be commercially prepared and assayed sera, commercially prepared material that has been assayed by the laboratory or properly prepared and assayed pools of patients' samples. It is recommended that at least three levels be used to establish the linearity of the procedure through the expected range of patient values. Ideally, these should be run with each test run and must be run at least once on each day of testing. At least one level must be included in each run.

These reference sera are used to provide data of precision, which can indicate any unusual problem with the testing procedure. In order for them to serve a purpose, limits of acceptability must be established and observed. Whenever these limits are exceeded, the procedure must be considered to be out of control, and no results should be reported until the problem is resolved. It is useful to prepare a list of steps that might be taken to evaluate and correct the problem so that time is not lost in guessing and aimless activity. As soon as the problem seems to be corrected, the reference materials should be repeated. The test sequence should not be considered to be in control until reference test values fall within the established limits of acceptability. When limits are exceeded, some record should be made of the problem and of the steps that were necessary for its correction. A review of the records of problems and their correction at the end of a month may prove instructive and helpful.

### Limits of acceptability

Limits of acceptability are best established by using a rule of probability. It has been established mathematically that 95% of all test results will fall within two standard deviations (SD) of the average value of a test.

Each month all of the values obtained for each control are recorded and SD calculated as indicated in the example in Table 9.

If the value obtained from testing the reference serum falls outside ± 2 SD, there is a 95% probability that the test is out of control because of some component of the test system such as reagent or reference quality, sampling, temperature, or instrument function. These and other related matters should be carefully checked for possible error.

There is a 5% statistical chance that the method is in control, of course, if the result is between 2 and 3 SD away from the mean, but this should happen only 5 days in over 3 months, and if the deviation is repeated on successive days, it is highly probable that a problem exists. Most laboratories have a policy of rechecking each result that exceeds ±2 SD if at all possible, but a policy that recognizes the statistical possibility of values between 2 and 3 SD is certainly acceptable.

The quality control policy should also deal with

**Table 9.** Calculation of standard deviation*

| Observed value | Difference from mean | Square of difference |
|---|---|---|
| 98 | 1.4 | 1.96 |
| 101 | 1.6 | 2.56 |
| 103 | 3.6 | 12.96 |
| 97 | 2.4 | 5.76 |
| 99 | .4 | .16 |
| 100 | .6 | .36 |
| 102 | 2.6 | 6.76 |
| 96 | 3.4 | 11.56 |
| 101 | 1.6 | 2.56 |
| 97 | 2.4 | 5.76 |
| 103 | 3.6 | 12.96 |
| 99 | .4 | .16 |
| 98 | 1.4 | 1.96 |
| 101 | 1.6 | 2.56 |
| 100 | .6 | .36 |
| 96 | 3.4 | 11.56 |
| 97 | 2.4 | 5.76 |
| 99 | .4 | .16 |
| 100 | .6 | .36 |
| 102 | 2.6 | 6.76 |
| 1989 ÷ 20 = 99.4 (mean) | | 93 (Total of squares) ÷ 20 = 4.65 |
| | | $\sqrt{4.65}$ = 2.16 (SD) |
| | | 2.16 × 2 = 4.32 |
| | | 99.4 ± 4.32 (Range of 95% probability) |

accuracy and should relate to allowable deviation from the assay value assigned to the reference material. (The assay value and the laboratory's mean may not be the same.) Some judgment by the laboratory director or supervisor may be needed after the test methodology and the experience of other analysts with the method, equipment, and reference material are considered.

Plotting reference test results on a Levy-Jennings graph helps visualize results and makes the recognition of trends, bias, and other aberrations much easier (Fig. 17-1). Such plots should not be considered as window dressing but should be appreciated as tools that make quality control simpler.

It should be remembered that the 2-SD range is calculated from the statistics of the previous month. It establishes a probability range but does not tell anything about absolute precision. If the SD is divided by the mean, a coefficient of variation (CV) is obtained. This, expressed as a percent, is a true measure of precision. It is helpful to compare the coefficient of variation with that of other laboratories and other available methods. Some judgment needs to be made by the laboratory director as to whether this degree of precision is acceptable as it relates both to patient care and to analytical practice.

## Correlation of methods

The quality control policy of the laboratory should also recognize the need to correlate the results of different testing methods. It is not uncommon for laboratories to use two or more methods of testing a single substance. For example, glucose determinations may be done on a profiling

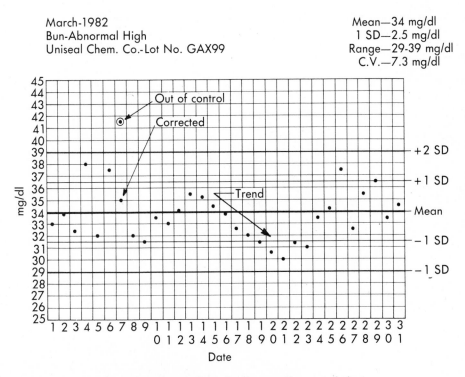

March-1982
Bun-Abnormal High
Uniseal Chem. Co.-Lot No. GAX99

Mean—34 mg/dl
1 SD—2.5 mg/dl
Range—29-39 mg/dl
C.V.—7.3 mg/dl

*Fig. 17-1.* Sample Levy-Jennings quality control chart.

instrument when the patient is admitted, and subsequent tests during the night may be done with a glucose analyzer. Both instruments may be giving appropriate quality control data, but because of different methods and reference material, the two may not agree with each other. In studying the correlation of various methods, it is important to check for agreement at extremely high and low levels, since these are the results that would be significant when sick patients are tested. If reasonable correlation cannot be achieved, it may be necessary to quote different normal ranges and to alert the medical staff to the differences found.

### Quality control for new methods

When new methods or equipment are introduced, it is necessary to establish accuracy and precision before the change is made. Enough testing should be done to calculate mean values and SD in order to judge future performance. The coefficient of variation should also be calculated so that the new methodology can be compared with the old and other available ways of testing.

The best quality control system is one that is easy to use and to interpret. When multiple reference controls are used and complex rules applied, the day-to-day functioning of the system may become difficult. The purpose of reference controls is simply to provide the basis for making the decision that the test is or is not in control. That decision should be easy, quick, and unequivocal.

The best quality control policy is of little value unless it is regularly and carefully observed and reviewed. This cannot be done unless careful records are kept. Ultimate responsibility for quality control rests with the supervisors and the director of the laboratory.

# CHAPTER 18

# Care, maintenance, and repair

The foregoing chapters should have given some insight into the principles and ideas behind the equipment in use. A thorough understanding of electricity and electronics could involve study for many months, and any single chapter of this book could be the subject for a book or a small library. It is hoped that students have now attained some appreciation of the instruments they use. The important problem of keeping valuable equipment working is yet to be considered.

Laboratory equipment has changed a great deal since the first edition of this book was printed in 1967. At that time, it was not only possible but advisable for laboratory workers to thoroughly understand their equipment and to perform many simple repairs. Electronics has been revolutionized by semiconductor devices. Specialized diodes—zeners, thermistors, LEDs, and a dozen others—have become common. Transistors have been adapted to perform a large range of functions, and solid-state crystals have been fashioned into fantastic integrated circuits the size of a grain of wheat that can be designed to perform complex calculations using algorithms. Sensitive and sophisticated transducers are able to detect nearly any type of physical change and convert it to an electrical force that can be quantitated. Ion-selective electrodes have been developed to the point where they can accurately measure many elements. Solid-state devices have been engineered into those marvelous devices called microprocessors and computers that can sort, count, calculate, and perform quantitative judgments to a truly remarkable extent with a speed that defies imagination. All these marvels have been miniaturized and engineered into instruments that are fast, accurate, convenient, and remarkably small. Thanks in large part to solid-state electronics, these devices are, for the most part, trouble free and easy to maintain.

It has become very difficult to diagnose problems that pertain to the technical detail of these instruments, and the temptation is to plug them in and accept the fact that they work until the time when they obviously do not. It seems that a great deal is lost when this philosophy is accepted. It is in our natures to want to know why and how; we begin to lose creativity, judgment, and initiative as we accept our inability to understand the things with which we work. This chapter is dedicated to the idea that common sense, logic, and initiative are still necessary and important. Specific diagnoses of problems are presented following a general review of troubleshooting including problem recognition, identification, and correction.

## Steps in problem solving

*Problem recognition.* An instrument malfunction cannot be identified or corrected until it is apparent to the instrument operator that there is a problem. As basic and self-evident as this may seem, many malfunctioning instruments continue to produce inaccurate results because the instrument operators are not aware that a problem exists. Instrument malfunctions manifest themselves in many ways. Symptoms of instrument probelms are sometimes very apparent and sometimes very subtle.

The accuracy of laboratory test results is jeopardized more by subtle than by the readily apparent instrumental problems. Readily apparent problems include malfunctions that make a required analytical determination impossible, for example, a burned out light source in an optical counter, atomic absorption spectrophotometer, or spectrophotometer; a burned out galvanometer light bulb in a galvanometric readout in a spectrophotometer or osmometer; a blown fuse; a ruined photodetector in any photometric instrument; depletion of fuels and/or reagents required for instrument function; or an unplugged power cord.

Problems expressed subtly require the alert, keen perception of an operator who is able to make fine distinctions between normal and abnormal instrument response characteristics. When these indistinctly expressed malfunctions are not detected, test result inaccuracies unfortunately may be accepted as valid. And therein lies the dangerous consequence of instruments being operated by poorly trained, unconscientious, unthinking robots. Examples of subtle malfunctions include slight misalignment of the optical system in spectrophotometric instruments, dirty or damaged optical surfaces in optical analytical instruments, contamination of required fuels and/or solutions for instrument operation, damaged or worn electrical potentiometers, and alteration of reference voltages in potentiometric analytical instruments.

*Problem identification.* Once the effect of a problem is perceived, the cause or causes of that problem must be identified. Problem identification is, therefore, the matching of cause and effect. Experienced instrument operators may readily relate a specific faulty response to its cause because of the frequency with which they have previously observed that malfunction. The continued exposure of the operator to characteristic instrument responses and their identification produces a mental index of cause-effect relationships. (This index should be written out so that the less experienced may benefit). Thus, the expression "experience is the best teacher" applies to troubleshooting.

However, not all practicing technical laboratory personnel have this "index of experience" on which to rely. Therefore, each malfunction may be a new problem to solve. The apprehension of facing a new problem can be replaced gradually with the self-assurance that comes from being able to apply knowledge to problem solving in a logical, stepwise fashion. The familiarity of the problem solving approach diminishes or eliminates the uneasiness produced by the unknown.

The logical steps to be followed in troubleshooting are state the perceived problem, list its possible causes (that is, formulate hypotheses), and then proceed to prove or disprove each hypothesis. Stating the problem caused by readily apparent malfunction is easy—for example, the light bulb went out in the spectrophotometer. More difficult are the subtle problems. These subtle problems present a constant challenge to the conscientious instrument operator. It is for identification of these malfunctions that persistent monitoring and vigilance are required. Calibration and quality control checks are the monitoring devices used for detection of subtle malfunctions or for forewarning of possible instrument problems. Preventive maintenance is a means of avoiding problems. Preventive maintenance procedures are well worth the time and effort invested, since the direct result is the avoidance of instrument problems that are detrimental to the speed and accuracy with which clinical laboratory analyses are performed. Calibration, quality control, and preventive maintenance are all too frequently approached with a "ho hum" attitude. However, these procedures are extremely important in indicating the presence of a subtle problem (for example, the warping of the photosensitive surface of a photovoltaic cell is best detected with a calibration check).

Possible causes of a problem should be listed in order of most to least probable. In the example of the spectrophotometer light bulb going out, the most probable cause would be a burned out bulb, followed by no current available to the bulb. The second possibility has a number of probable explanations: the power switch is off or the plug is not plugged into the power outlet (both of which are frequently responsible for inoperative instruments), a fuse is blown, the light bulb leads are not securely connected to the circuit connections, or no current is available from the power outlet. Additional causes of symptoms manifested by malfunctioning instruments are listed in most instrument operation manuals. If the most probable causes are proved not to be responsible for a problem, then these more comprehensive lists are very useful.

The procedure followed in proving or disproving hypothesized causes of a problem depends heavily on common sense. In the example of the light bulb in the spectrophotometer, a quick visual check of the bulb will determine whether it is burned out. If the bulb is not burned out, further investigation is required. By observing whether other electrically operated parts of the circuit are functioning, the operator can determine whether the problem is limited to the bulb or has affected the entire circuitry of the instrument. (For example, if the "on-off" indicator light is on, a cooling fan is working, and the galvanometer light is on, then the problem is not a "no-power-to-the-circuit" problem.) If all electronic functions of the instrument are inoperative, then the following checks should be made: "on-off" switch in "on" position, power line plugged into power outlet, fuse not blown, and current available at the power outlet (check with a simple indicator light or a voltmeter, or ask an electrician). Frequently, one of these obvious, easily checked, probable causes is found to be responsible for the malfunction.

If all the obvious causes are eliminated as the responsible problem, additional circuit analysis procedures may be required. Even the electronics novice can visually check a circuit for melted, scorched, or damaged components. The odor of overheated components is also a good indicator of a problem within a circuit. Voltage and signal waveform checks require the use of an oscilloscope; voltage checks require only a voltmeter. Competence in the use of these test instruments and experience in obtaining electrical readings from circuits provide the needed expertise to follow the simple test point measurements given in many instrument manuals.

***Problem correction.*** Problem correction also should be the responsibility of the instrument operator. Two options are available. First, the operator may decide that the minor repair and/or replacement needed for correction of a malfunction is within his or her capabilities. Second, the operator may conclude that additional troubleshooting or malfunction correction requires additional expertise. With this conclusion, expert assistance should be obtained.

Of utmost importance is the expedient, effective repair of malfunctioning clinical laboratory instruments. The malfunction must be recognized and identified promptly. A judgment must be made as to the level of expertise required for its repair. And, finally, an honest evaluation of one's own abilities must be made to determine whether an expert should be called on to correct the malfunction.

### Diagnoses of problems

In the second edition of this book, a chapter entitled "Shop Talk and Horse Sense" was included with some misgivings. Surprisingly, there were many favorable comments about this section, which considered simple, logical, little things that embarrass and confound intelligent people. Much of it seems relevant, and a section is reproduced here as it appeared originally.

Many of the devices in the laboratory are small, simple instruments such as pumps, heaters, dilutors, and simple spectrophotometers. These should be understood by qualified laboratory personnel, and their failure or malfunction should be diagnosable and in many cases repairable. Often solutions to problems with simple equipment involve calm good sense more than profound knowledge. When confronted with an instrument that does not work, consider the following:

1. Are you sure it is *plugged in?* Maybe the janitor pulled the plug.
2. Are you sure the *overload breaker* in the breaker panel is not thrown out? Try a desk

lamp or a test light in the receptacle to be sure there is electricity available.

3. If there is no electricity at the plug, find the *breaker box* that furnishes your area of the building. It is probably a small metal door in the hallway close by.

4. In older buildings there may be screw-in fuses in the box. They are rated as to the number of amps they will carry. You can tell if the *fuse is blown* by looking at the mica front window. If it is smoked up and the little metal band under it is melted, the fuse is blown and must be replaced.

5. Do not replace the fuse or reset the breaker until you have looked around for the *cause* of the fuse blowing. It may have been a direct short from a broken wire or some obvious defect. It could also be from too much load on the line (for example, too many heating devices). If no immediate cause is found, unplug as many items as possible, replace the fuse, and reconnect the devices one at a time until the new fuse blows. This will tell you which item is responsible for the overload. By taking everything else off the line and trying again, you can tell if the total load was too much for the fuse or if there was an electrical problem in the device last reconnected.

6. More than likely you will find rocker-type circuit breakers in the panel, instead of fuses of the older, screw-in type.

7. Rocker-type breakers have a small element that heats and expands when overloaded, throwing out the breaker and thus cutting off electricity to that circuit. When they are depressed to the right, they are usually "on" (depending on the mounting). At any rate they will be marked.

8. When breakers throw out, you cannot always easily tell by glancing at them. They may be pushed only slightly up from the "on" position. If you run a finger down the line of breakers, the one that is out will be slightly raised. Immediately after a circuit breaker throws out, it may feel warm or even hot. Other breakers that are heavily loaded may also feel warm, however,

9. To put the circuit back in use, push down on the off (or out) side and then depress the on (or in) side as far as it will go. If it throws out again and you cannot locate the problem, call an electrician.

10. If the instrument is still dead although plugged in and there is electricity in the line, check the instrument's fuse. Usually the fuse holder is a little black or brown knob close to the point where the power cable goes into the instrument. Some fuse holders have a cover with a milled edge that can be easily removed with the fingers. Others are threaded and must be screwed out, whereas still others have a bayonet lock that requires only a half-turn. Some fuse covers require a screwdriver to turn. The fuse holder is spring loaded so that the fuse will usually spring out, and one end may be clamped to the fuse cover.

11. Look at this small glass *minifuse* to see whether it is smoked up and whether the metal band or wire inside is melted. If it is a tiny wire, it may burn up completely. If you are not sure whether it is burned out, check it with a multimeter or replace it with another fuse of the same rating. The rating is engraved in the metal band at one end.

12. To check the fuse with a meter, set the meter to ohms and turn the selector knob to the lowest setting, which is usually marked $\times 1$ (or simply *1*). Touch the two meter leads together. The needle should move to the right side of the meter. (This shows that you are in the proper meter setting.) Now touch the two meter probes to either end of the fuse. If the needle responds, the fuse is all right.

13. If the fuse is good and the instrument still does not respond, check lamps. If an exciter lamp is out, a photometer will obviously not respond. Try a new exciter lamp. If the instrument has a galvanometer lamp and it is out, no light will appear on the scale even though the exciter lamp is on. It is probably best to un-

plug the instrument while checking and changing lamps, to avoid the possibility of shock. Never work with an instrument's wiring while standing on a wet floor or leaning against metal surfaces unless you are sure it is disconnected. Do not forget to plug it in again before trying it.

14. If the instrument still does not respond, remove the cover and start hunting for obvious problems such as the following: (A) A blackened spot may indicate a short circuit. (B) A loose wire that goes nowhere may indicate a broken lead. See if you can tell where it should have been connected. If this is not apparent, do not just guess. This could cause damage. (C) Melted resin, smoke deposit, or a strong smell around a transformer or motor may indicate that it is burned out. (D) Look for resistors that are split open. Sometimes excess heat or humidity may destroy a resistor, leaving a circuit open. (E) Check for any rarely used switches on the back or inside the instrument that might cancel the function you are attempting to use. (F) With the multimeter on the ohms position, attach a lead to one prong of the power cable and touch the other lead to the point inside the instrument where the power comes in. Repeat with the other side of the cable. A little searching will show where terminals connect inside the instrument. One side of the power cord will almost certainly go to the fuse holder. If continuity cannot be demonstrated (if the needle will not move), there may be a break in the cable. While checking, it is a good idea to bend or flex the cable to be sure that the wires inside the insulation are not broken and only occasionally making contact. Also check between the two wires for shorts. (G) If a three-strand power cable is used, the round peg of the plug-in is the ground, and it is probably attached to the frame of the instrument. Check this for continuity with the ohmmeter also. (H) Attach the meter leads (still on ohms) to the two sides of the main power switch and throw the switch. The meter should deflect in the "on" position and return to the peg in the "off" position. (I) If the instrument has vacuum tubes, replace them, being careful to replace with the proper type of tube. (J) Switch the meter to ac volts and set it on 110 V or higher to see whether, with the instrument plugged in and turned on, you can measure 110 V (more or less) at the point where the power cord enters the instrument. If you can, follow the two lines along to see how far you can trace the current. You may be able to find the defective element in this way after you have had a little experience and know the instrument. Be careful not to shock yourself or produce a short by touching two hot points with the same probe. Handle the probes on the insulated portion only. If the problem has not been solved by this time, you should turn the instrument over to a qualified repairman.

15. When a meter responds erratically and the controls do not produce a smooth response, the problem may be in a faulty potentiometer. Try turning the control, as evenly as possible, from one end of its travel to the other. If the meter needle does not respond smoothly, the pot may be defective. Try tapping the control knob with the ball of your finger and notice whether the meter needle remains relatively steady. If not, this is an additional indication of a defective pot. Try this latter test in several positions of the control knob. The defect of the pot may be at only one point. A pot is not difficult to change after a little practice with a soldering iron. Be sure to replace with the proper type of pot. The size indicates the wattage, whereas the ohms and the percent accuracy are usually stamped on the back. Be sure to note which lead goes to which contact of the pot. If you have wired it backward, the meter will move in the wrong direction when the knob is turned. Also, be sure that all contacts are tightly soldered and that no loose drops of solder have fallen where they can cause shorts.

16. Soldering is not difficult, and you can become reasonably proficient, with a little practice. For instrument work a small *pencil-type iron* is to be preferred over a *solder gun*. The latter heats more quickly but produces more heat than is needed and is harder to get into small places without causing damage to delicate parts. Remove as much of the old solder as conveniently possible. Hook the wires to be soldered into the solder holes or otherwise secure them. Place the tip of the iron on the point to be soldered so that both the wire and the contact are heated. Touch the solder to the iron at the point of contact and let the solder fuse completely before withdrawing the iron. If the contact is not hot enough, the solder will not bond to it and a "cold-solder joint" may be made; this could result in a poor electrical connection. Avoid using an excess of solder and dripping hot drops of the metal onto other parts. A resin-cord solder of about no. 20 G or 22 G is right for this sort of work. The soldering iron should not be left plugged in for extended periods of time. *Retinning* the tip of the iron occasionally helps to keep it in good shape. This is done by melting a drop of solder on the point and quickly wiping it over the hot surface with a piece of waste.

17. When electric motors will not function, the following checks may be made: (A) Is electricity getting to the motor? Check whether the motor is plugged in, check the line circuit breaker, the instrument fuse, etc., as noted earlier. (B) Check whether the motor can be turned freely by hand. (C) If it can, unplug the device and check the *brushes*. They are accessible through small plastic caps on either side of the motor. Be sure that plenty of carbon is left on the brushes, that the brushes are actually touching the *armature* (is the lower edge worn shiny?), and that the spring or wire making electric contact in the brush holder is not broken. The brush should fit snugly in the brush holder. If it is so loose that the brush is worn off at an angle, it is probably the wrong size brush. If the brush does not slide easily into the holder, it may fail to feed down against the *commutator* as the carbon is worn away. This may be due to the brush being too large or to a deposit of carbon building up in the brush holder. Carbon may be cleaned out with a cotton-tipped applicator soaked in carbon tetrachloride or some similar solvent. Dry out any excess solvent. Special solvents for cleaning motors are available. (D) If the motor turns but not easily, there is a good chance that a *bearing* has become so dry that it is impeding the motor and could result in burning the motor out. Work light oil into the bearings as well as possible and turn the motor back and forth on its bearings until the bearings are completely free and the motor will turn easily by hand. Try it under power to see whether the problem has been solved. Next time, oil the bearings before they get dry. (E) If the motor cannot be turned by hand, a bearing is probably "seized" or "frozen" from lack of lubrication and possibly too much heat. An attempt can be made to work the bearing loose with lubricants and a little carefully exercised force. If this does not work, the motor must be torn down and the bearings replaced. If the bearing has been frozen and under power for very long, it is possible that the motor is badly burned and will require extensive repair or replacement. (F) If the motor turns freely and the brushes are in good shape, it is quite possible that there is a break in either the *field coil* or *armature winding,* and the motor will need to be sent to a shop for rewinding. (G) If the motor hums but does not move or moves only slightly, there may be a short, which condition will also require rewinding. (H) If the motor runs very noisily and occasionally hangs up, the bearings may be badly worn. To check end play, with the motor in a vertical position (as in a centrifuge), lift the shaft as much as possible and let it drop a few times. A little play with just a faint click can be heard as the shaft falls back

into place. A barely perceptible end play is necessary for the motor to run smoothly. If considerable play exists or if a definite metallic clank can be heard, the bearing is probably getting rather badly worn. Some motors have a single ball bearing at the lower end of the shaft with a take-up screw beneath it for adjusting out any end play. If this does not exist, the motor will have to be removed and the bearings replaced. To check the top bearing, grasp the top of the shaft (or the centrifuge head) and attempt to work it from side to side. If any play is felt, the bearing is worn. If a definite metallic clank can be heard, the bearing is in bad condition and should be replaced before the motor binds and causes damage to the windings. Keep in mind that some motors are mounted on rubber grommets and the whole motor may move when you attempt to move the shaft in its bearings. (1) It is always possible that a switch, a rectifier, Variac, or some other component has failed. By using the multimeter and a little reasoning, you may possibly locate such a failure, but in any case a repairman may very possibly be needed to make the repair.

18. Heating equipment rarely fails except when cords are broken or switches defective, but heat control is often a problem. Heating elements seem to last about as long as the device in which they are installed. The thermostat may be a different matter. There are several types of thermostats. The type that actually makes and breaks the current to the heater through the thermostatic elements is very often subject to failure. The points may become so corroded and burned that contact can no longer be made. Burnishing the contacts with emery cloth may restore them temporarily. New points or a new thermostat may have to be installed. If the points arc and get hot enough to weld together, current will continue to flow until a fuse blows or the device actually burns. This type of thermostat is fortunately seldom used now. A more common type relies on a microswitch actuated by the thermostatic element, to make and break the circuit. These switches fail occasionally. In most cases the switch makes an audible click when switching occurs. If you cannot cause the switch to click by depressing and releasing its plunger, it is probably bad. It can be checked with an ohmmeter as described if there is any doubt about it. These switches are usually easy to replace if the correct replacement can be found. In water baths the sensing element (often a fluid-filled capsule and capillary) lies in the bottom of the bath. Corrosive reagents used around the bath may corrode the capillary until it leaks. The sensing element must then be replaced.

19. Laboratory power lines are often overloaded, since planners often do not realize the considerable amount of electricity used by the dozens of laboratory devices. Although there is usually at least one electrician or plant engineer who worries about such things, it is wise to keep an eye on overload problems. One danger signal is excessive heat at the circuit breaker panel. If a circuit is heavily loaded, that particular breaker will be hot, and, if the circuit if very much overloaded, the breaker will throw out occasionally. Sometimes it is possible to physically move some high-consumption devices to other circuits, or the electrician may move some circuits from one breaker to put them on a less-used position in the breaker box. When the entire lab load begins to be too heavy for the system supplied, voltage may drop. This may cause many serious problems with laboratory equipment. Voltage can be checked at the wall plug with a voltmeter. One of the wires at the receptacle is the hot wire, and the other is essentially zero. For current to be quite adequate, the voltage difference between the two should be 117 V or close to it, and fluctuation should not occur. Recording voltmeters are available to monitor voltage over a period of time if

this seems desirable. Most laboratory instruments will compensate fairly well for drops to about 100 V, but some will not. A lower drop may cause motors to stall and burn. Surges of very high voltage, occasionally associated with overloading, can be very damaging to some components, including vacuum tubes. Voltage measured from the hot line to the ground line (the round hole of the receptable on a three-wire system) should read essentially the same as the voltage from the high wire to the low wire. If there is no reading at all, the ground line is not grounded and the electrician should check it. When power requirement exceeds the potential of the system, unused 220 V lines may be split out to provide two 110 V circuits, or lines may be run in from adjacent areas.

20. The person responsible for the care and maintenance of laboratory equipment is seldom able to keep up with all the potential problems. If he develops an awareness of equipment and constantly looks and listens for items needing attention, he may be able to avoid many breakdown situations. The tools should be closely available, and loose screws should be tightened, dry bearings lubricated, dirty contacts cleaned, etc. as a normal part of housekeeping.

21. A listing and a diagrammatic representation of the symbols used in wiring diagrams are presented on pp. 351 to 353. As experience is gained, you can pick up some comprehension of diagrams that will enable you to follow through some wiring plans and better understand their function and their potential problems. Some diagrams are presented throughout the book both for their practical value and for practice work. Study these in comparison with the instrument involved to gain more understanding of wiring diagrams.

22. There are no instant electronics or instrument experts. Only experience, observation, and interest can develop the abilities necessary to cope with instrument failure. It is hoped

that the information contained herein will help students acquire some understanding and interest.

23. The following tools and supplies are suggested for any reasonably active laboratory.

*Tools*
Pliers—needle-nosed and ordinary
Wire cutter and stripper
Vise-grip wrenches
Files—crosscut, rattails, and triangular
Set of small end wrenches
Set of screwdrivers–small to large, and off-set screwdriver
Philips screwdrivers
Set of Allen wrenches
Small vise
Small soldering iron
Flashlight
Multimeter
Test lamp
Small knife
Hemostats
Small hammer

*Supplies*
Solder
Spool of 18- or 20-gauge hook-up wire
Electrician's tape
Emery paper
Epoxy cement
Spade terminals or other types
Fuses for all instruments
Brushes for all motors
Didymium filter that will fit into appropriate spectrophotometer
Spare vacuum tubes for instruments in use
Replacement lamps for all instruments on hand
3-in-one oil and centrifuge lubricant
Instruction manuals for all instruments
Any repair or replacement parts recommended by manufacturer
Collection of miscellaneous hardware—nuts, bolts, etc.

## *Care and use of meters*

A multimeter such as the VOM or VTVM is strongly recommended as a working tool in the clinical laboratory. These instruments are rugged and well built, but certain sensible precautions must be taken when using them.

It should be obvious from the description of the d'Arsonval movement that meters incorporating this movement are sensitive to mechanical shock. They should never be handled roughly. Taut-Band meter movements, which incorporate some features of the galvanometer, are used in many multimeters. These are considerably more rugged than those using a rotating shaft on a jewel.

The switches on the front of the instrument tell which parameter and what range you will read. If 115 V is applied to the meter with the range switch set on 3 V, the tiny coil in the meter movement may be completely burned up and the instrument ruined. A fuse if provided to keep this from happening. (To discover the fuse one may have to remove the instrument from its case). Usually the fuse is soldered to its leads to reduce the internal resistance of the meter). Always set the range switch higher than the expected value and decrease the settings as necessary to read accurately.

Voltage is measured in parallel; that is, the leads can be contacted to the circuit at two points and the difference in potential between the two points will be indicated on the dial.

To measure amperage with the ordinary VOM, the current must be passed through the instrument. In other words, the instrument must be in series in the circuit that is to be measured; so the circuit must actually be broken at some point to allow the meter to be connected.

When measuring ohms, one is passing the current from a battery in the multimeter through the resistance one wishes to measure. If the battery deteriorates so much that one can no longer zero the meter when the leads are connected, one obviously cannot get an accurate reading. Care must be taken that an old corroding battery does not leak and damage the circuits of the meter. An alkaline or mercury battery is less likely to produce this problem.

When measuring a resistance in a circuit, be sure that one end of the circuit is open so that you are not measuring resistance of more than one pathway at a time. Never try to measure resistance when current is passing through the circuit.

Be sure to read the instructions that come with your VOM or VTVM and become familiar with the instrument before starting to use it.

Do not store the instruments with the switch set to read ohms. If the lead wires make contact, the battery may be discharged as it sits on the shelf.

## *Maintenance and repair service*

As equipment becomes more sophisticated and automated, it becomes less possible for medical laboratory personnel to perform adequate repairs. Indeed, the maintenance problem is one that is shared with society in general. Cars, radios, TVs, and refrigerators become less amenable to simple repair, and each year shows a larger proportion of the national work force involved in service and less in production. Also, the problem of getting competent repair is often next to impossible. Several solutions may be suggested. One of the simplest, intended to avoid serious repair problems, with down time, is to insist that all personnel who use equipment carefully read operating and maintenance instructions. All steps in care and maintenance should be posted (if complicated or detailed) and should be followed in all cases. Deviations from normal instrument performance should be noted and investigated. A record should be kept of repairs, calibrations, and maintenance procedures.

It is now mandated, by accrediting agencies and third-party payers, that detailed records must be kept of instrument performance, including dates of calibration and repair. Each year the records required become more specific and detailed. At least two types of records should be kept on *all* equipment. First, the record of performance must be kept by the person responsible for its use. This

```
                         HISTORY  OF  MAINTENANCE                                    PAGE  56
                         ON  LABORATORY  EQUIPMENT
                       JANUARY, 1973  THRU  APRIL, 1973

ITEM EQUIPMENT                                                        YR OF   YR OF   COST OF
NO.  NAME                   MANUFACTURE      MODEL-NO.   SERIAL-NO.   PURCH.  DEPR.   EQUIPMENT

089  FLAME PHOTOMETER       RADIOMETER       FLM 251     228          1971            $      .

DATE        MAINTENANCE PERFORMED ON EQUIPMENT                    WORK HOURS      PRICE OF PARTS

 2/07/0     25  CLEAN COMBUSTION CHAMBER AND RELATED ITEMS.         02.5          $   6.10
            26  OPERATIONAL CHECK.
            30  CALIBRATION.
            32  CLEAN OR REPLACE DUST & AIR FILTERS- VISUAL EXAM.
            47  MECHANICAL REPAIRS.
            54  CLEANING.
            55  OPERATIONAL ADJUSTMENTS.

03/29/73    30  CALIBRATION.                                        05.0          $    .00
            54  CLEANING.
            55  OPERATIONAL ADJUSTMENTS.
04/06/73    25  CLEAN COMBUSTION CHAMBER AND RELATED ITEMS.         00.2          $    .00
            26  OPERATIONAL CHECK.
            30  CALIBRATION.
            32  CLEAN OR REPLACE DUST & AIR FILTERS- VISUAL EXAM.
```

***Fig. 18-1.*** Computer printout of instrument maintenance record.

record would provide temperature checks of heating and cooling devices, calibration corrections and dates of such devices as colorimeters, calibration checks of measuring equipment such as pipetters, and verification of function of mechanical devices such as rotators and shakers. Second, a property record should record the date and price of purchase, name of manufacturer, and the dates and details of repair or maintenance procedures. Most devices should be placed on some type of schedule for periodic cleaning, repair, and calibration. Laboratories with any considerable quantity of equipment may elect to use a computer schedule and record of repair such as that shown in Fig. 18-1.

## *Clinical laboratory standards*

The National Committee for Clinical Laboratory Standards (NCCLS) has been actively involved in establishing a degree of uniformity among manufacturers in specifying instructions for the installation, operation, care, maintenance, and repair of instruments. Standards and guidelines are established jointly by experts representing government, professional disciplines, and industry. A number of published NCCLS Approved Standards for Instrumentation are presently available from NCCLS. *Preparation of manuals for installation, operation, and repair of laboratory instruments (NCCLS Approved Standard ASI-1)* identifies for manufacturers and users the specific information that must be available to permit sound decisions on instrument selection. Requirements are itemized within the general areas of installation and environmental requirements, operating and maintenance manuals, warranties, and field repair manuals. *Power requirements for clinical laboratory instruments and for laboratory power sources (NCCLS Approved Standard ASI-5)* offers recommendations for detection and monitoring of power fluctuations as one effective way of minimizing instrument performance problems. A detailed list of operator training, installation, preventive maintenance, and repair for proper service of an instrument that should be provided by the manufacturer is presented in *Guidelines for service of clinical laboratory instruments (NCCLS Tentative Standard TSI-6)*. Presently an effort is underway to develop guidelines for uniformity in manufacturers' information on instrument performance, appropriate quality control, and required maintenance. These NCCLS publications constitute a collection of valuable information regarding instrumentation that should prove helpful to manufacturers in preparing their communications, to users in selecting and operating their instruments, and to inspectors in reviewing instrument records.

It is entirely necessary to have access to some maintenance and repair capability. Most hospitals now have electronic repair sections with some level of competence with certain types of laboratory devices. The more sophisticated equipment will probably require the services of factory-trained service personnel from the manufacturer or vendor. Such services are usually available under warranty or service contract.

It is always necessary to have available a person with electronics background, trained to do some repairs and knowing what steps to take when the matter is beyond his competence. Finding the right persons and establishing their limitations in a realistic manner may be a problem. Vocational schools and junior colleges are beginning to train people with a fair competence in instrumentation. The supply is improving, as is the quality of training. The person being introduced into this role should

have immediate access to all manuals and operating instructions. Once he has familiarized himself with the equipment, he should set up an *adequate* and *realistic* inventory of repair parts (with help from a knowledgeable technologist). A regular schedule for checks and maintenance should be set up and followed.

Sometimes a local repair shop that is adequate to the situation can be found. In larger cities this is generally possible. In smaller towns it may be a problem. Radio and TV repairmen are generally not too helpful unless they are willing to take the time to learn laboratory equipment and be available when needed.

Recently several large companies have undertaken to train and equip persons to meet the laboratory-wide or even hospital-wide repair problems. Honeywell Corp. and other companies have set out to provide repair centers in many areas of the United States. These centers are able to repair any hospital equipment and have a complete library of maintenance and repair information on common equipment and a reasonable stock of repair parts.

Most equipment is warranted in some way for a year. Larger equipment can then be put under a maintenance contract with the manufacturer in most instances. To make an adequate judgment about the reasonableness of a maintenance proposal, one must have some idea about such factors as past repair costs and the existence of viable alternatives. The more expensive a system is, the more critical it is that it can be kept in service. Some large companies have had real problems with equipment that was reasonably good because their backup was inadequate.

## Environment

As equipment becomes larger and more complex, the environment becomes increasingly important.
1. Most solid-state circuits are sensitive to extreme changes in temperature. Adequate temperature control is imperative.
2. Dust and dirt around mechanical and electrical

# WHEN ALL ELSE FAILS

## READ THE DIRECTIONS

*Fig. 18-2.* (Courtesy Cahn Division, Ventron Instruments Corp.)

equipment is both dangerous and apt to cause malfunctions.

3. Corrosion and shorts are caused by moisture and spillage of acids, alkalies, and other corrosive chemicals.

4. All equipment should be plugged into a wall receptacle. Do not use extension cords, multiple (octopus) plugs, or other temporary wiring.

5. All circuits must be grounded. Wall receptacles should provide for a three-pronged receptacle. The ground terminal should be checked to be quite certain that it is indeed connected to an adequate ground and that is has *no* electric potential.

6. Circuits should be checked at the instrument site to determine whether adequate voltage is maintained when a full working load is imposed on the line. If there is any indication for it, the sine wave pattern of the ac supply should be checked to be sure there is no distortion.

7. There should be no exposed wiring in work areas, and covers should be kept on equipment to protect it and the operator, unless repair or maintenance is actually being performed.

8. Work areas around equipment should be kept clear and free of trash, debris, and stored supplies. Floors should be clean and dry. Traffic should be kept to a minimum.

All these precautions are necessary to the optimal performance of the equipment and the safety of the operator.

## Summary

The medical laboratory represents a considerable investment in equipment and a large ongoing payroll and overhead expense. A thorough appreciation of equipment, its application, maintenance, repair, and replacement is crucial. It is hoped that the time spent with this book has been profitable.

# *APPENDIXES*

# Glossary of terms

*absorbance (A)* Optical density of a substance expressed as negative log (base 10) of percent transmittance.

*alphanumeric* Including both alphabetical and numerical information.

*ampere (A)* Unit of electric current; amount that will flow through resistance of 1 $\Omega$ when potential of 1 V is applied.

*amplifier* Electrical circuit for amplifying or increasing strength of a signal; this is normally done by vacuum tubes or transistors; amplifier circuit is usually single system within entire circuitry of instrument; there may be more than one amplifier circuit (for example, a preamp circuit, signal amplifier, and high-voltage amplifier) is one instrument.

*analog* Physical variable, such as a photosignal, that is analogous to value being measured by system generating the signal.

*analog-to-digital (A-to-D) converter* Circuit or device for converting an analog signal to digits so that it can be expressed as a decimal number.

*angstrom unit (Å)* Unit of length approximately 0.1 nm; identified as equal to wavelength of red line of cadmium.

*anion* Ion bearing negative charge; hence, ion that is attracted to anode.

*anode* Electrode having positive charge, to which stream of electrons will flow; also called *plate* in vacuum tubes.

*armature* Moving part of motor, generator, relay, or other magnetic circuit; commonly called *rotor*.

*background* Extraneous signal not related to parameter being measured.

*band pass* Section of spectrum allowed to pass through monochromator; Coleman 6C has band pass of 35 nm; Spectronic 20 has 20 nm band pass; Beckman DU can work effectively in some areas well under 5 nm.

*barrier-layer cell* Common type of photogenative or photovoltaic cell.

*BCD output* Binary coded digital information is in a form that will allow most printers to print digital values without further signal conversion.

*Beer's law* Physical law that describes behavior of light; Beer's law states that intensity of light transmitted through chemical solution is inversely proportional to molar concentration of solution and that relationship is logarithmic. Not all solutions obey Beer's law, and most vary at extreme concentrations.

*bias* Voltage applied to grid of vacuum tube to control flow of electrons between cathode and anode; grid voltage controls amplification factor of vacuum tube.

*binary* Having to do with number two; binary system used in computers allows only two choices in each situation—positive or negative, first or second, up or down, etc.

*bit* Single digit of computer information, which can be stored on one magnetic position.

*blaze angle* Angle of the grooves in the face of a diffraction grating; blaze angle determines which area of the spectrum is least distorted.

*bolometer* Instrument for measuring very small changes in radiated heat.

*bridge* Arrangement in which electrical measuring device is connected or bridged between two sides of circuit; bridge often arranged so as to measure resistance changes (see *Wheatstone bridge*); in physiological measurement resistance transducers and bridge arrangements of this sort are common.

*byte* Grouping of bits, of computer information, of a given size; may be thought of as a computer "word."

*capacitance* Measure of capacity for storage of electric charge; read in farads.

*capacitor* Electrical component with capacity of storing electrical energy for release at later time; stored energy is measured in farads; two conducting surfaces with known capacitance are separated by resistor of known resistance.

*carousel* A circular conveyor that presents samples or tests in a sequential pattern depending on their relative positions near the circumference of the conveyor.

*cathode* Negative electrode; emits electrons; often referred to as *emitter*.

*cation* Positive-charged ion that would be attracted to cathode or negative pole.

*chopper* Component for converting direct current into alternating current with minimum of distortion; this may be done mechanically, electronically, or, in case of photocurrents, by interrupting light path.

*coefficient of extinction* Term sometimes used to denote optical density of a solution at a given wavelength under various conditions. Since it is ambiguous, its use is discouraged.

*collimate* To arrange into organized column or beam.

*collimator* Lens or other device for collimating energy into organized beam or path; in radioisotope work, lead shield allowing radiation to pass in only one pathway or in several more or less parallel pathways.

*colorimeter* Device for measuring color intensities; usually refers to filter colorimeter, which defines transmitted light in terms of color characteristics of filter used.

*common mode* Potential difference between the measuring circuit and ground; hopefully it is constant.

*Compton effect* Effect produced when a gamma ray collides with an electron, causing dissipation and scattering of the transmitted energies.

*computer language* Machine-readable codes by which the computer can be instructed as to what manipulations to perform; *low-level languages* are *assembly* or *machine languages* that devices can immediately follow; *higher-level languages* such as Fortran, Cobol, and ASCII are closer to standard English and require more complex equipment to use.

*conductance* Reciprocal of resistance, measured in terms of mho.

*continuous-flow analyzer* Analyzer in which the sample is moved along through consecutive analytical steps in a flowing stream; primarily, the Technicon Auto-Analyzer systems.

*coulomb* Unit of electric charge, equal to $6.28 \times 10^{18}$ electrons.

*CPU* Central processing unit of a computer.

*curie* Measurement of radioactivity, equal to $3.7 \times 10^{10}$ disintegrations per second; this is a rather large unit, and the millicurie (one thousandth) and microcurie (one millionth) are more commonly used.

*current* Flow of electrons; when current measurement is referred to, it is in terms of amperes (that is, total number of electrons).

*dark current* Current flowing through light-measuring cell or tube when no light is striking its sensitive surface; most light-measuring instruments (except those with photogenerative cells) have control for cancelling out effect of dark current on readout of instrument; photogenerative cells have no appreciable dark current.

*d'Arsonval movement* Moving-coil movement that is heart of most ammeters; current to be measured is passed through coil that is delicately mounted between poles of magnet; electric field thus produced opposes magnetic field, producing torque, which moves coil and attached pointer clockwise; small spring attached to coil reorients it when no current is flowing.

*deadband* Range of voltage or amperage through which the input signal can vary without moving the recorder pen.

*diffraction grating* Surface bearing delicately etched or superimposed gridwork of very fine lines capable of scattering or diffracting light waves in such a way as to form spectrum.

*digital readout* Device for converting increments in electric current into digits in multiples of ten and decimal values.

*diode* Vacuum tube or transistor having only two electrodes or elements; since plate is always positive in relation to cathode, this arrangement allows only part of alternating current flowing in one direction to pass, since all electrons go from cathode to anode (that is, toward positive pole); other half of cycle is rejected and may be passed through another diode and inverted; two outputs then become direct current of regularly varying voltage (see Chapter 4).

*direct current (dc)* Electric current in which electrons flow only in one direction; negative-charged electrons flow toward positive pole.

*discrete analyzer* Analyzer in which the sample maintains its identity in a separate, discrete reaction vessel or vessels throughout the analysis.

*electrochemistry* Study of interrelations of electricity and chemical change.

*electromagnetic spectrum* Spectrum of frequencies possessing radiant energy, including gamma rays, x-rays, ultraviolet light, visible light, infrared heat waves, microwaves, and radio waves.

*electromotive force (EMF)* Potential difference between terminals or materials; measured in volts.

*electron* Smallest effective unit of electrical energy; theories differ over whether it possesses mass or is simply energy; quantum theory seems to indicate it does possess mass ($9.1 \times 10^{-28}$ gram).

*electron volt (eV)* Very fine measurement of power, equal to energy of 1 electron accelerated through potential difference of 1 V, or $1.6 \times 10^{-16}$ erg.

*encoder* Device for transferring coded information from one medium to another.

*end point reactions* Reactions in which the final change is measured after a given time, following a specific experimental protocol; the total change is significant rather than the rate of change.

*error signal* Difference between two opposing electrical impulses.

*exciter lamp* Source of light energy used in measurement of color intensity and fluorescence in colorimeters, photometers, fluorimeters, etc.

*extrinsic conduction* Conduction in a semiconductor due to the impurities added to the crystal to enhance conduction.

*farad* Unit of capacitance, equal to 1 C under pressure of 1 V.

*feedback* Use of fraction of output signal to make a correction electronically.

*FET* Field-effect transistor; a transistor designed to permit direct current to be amplified without being chopped.

*filter* In electronics, filter is component, such as induction coil, that eliminates or controls ripple or eliminates undesirable frequencies.

*flip-flop circuit* Circuit that may reverse direction of current flow each time it is brought into use to prevent polarization; in computers, term refers to components able to assume two different stable states in order to store information of binary nature.

*flow cell* The cuvette, in continuous-flow analysis, where the stream carrying individual tests passes for colorimetric determination.

*fluorometer* Instrument for measuring fluorescent light or light excited by stimulation of substance with light of lower wavelength.

*frequency* Number of times event occurs per time interval; for example, *cycles of alternating current per second is frequency of alternating current;* often expressed in hertz (Hz).

*gain* Expression of amplification factor of amplifier circuit or element; primarily dependent on grid bias.

*galvanometer lamp* Lamp used to provide light image reflected by galvanometer mirror.

*galvanometer* or *string galvanometer* Ammeter in which moving coil (see *d'Arsonval movement*) is suspended on thin string or wire that offers very little resistance to movement; more sensitive than ordinary ammeter; usually coil has small mirror attached that reflects beam of light (rather than pointer) to scale to indicate current value.

*gamma energy* Radiant energy having a wavelength of less than 1 Å, usually produced by nuclear transitions, as in radioactive isotopes.

*ground* Contact to earth, with zero potential.

*ground state* Normal state of an atom, in which no electron is in an elevated energy state.

*half-life* Time required for a radioactive substance to lose one half of its radioactivity.

*half-life, biological* Time required for half of a radioactive substance to disappear from a physiological system to organism by excretion, without regard to physical half-life.

*half-life, physical* Time required for an isotope to lose half of its radiant energy; radioactivity is lost exponentially; therefore not all energy is lost in two half-lives.

*hardware* In computer terminology, the actual instrument and devices forming the computer system.

*heat filter* Filter that allows light waves to pass but deflects or absorbs heat waves.

*heat sink* Metal radiator provided to dissipate heat around such components as power transistors.

*henry* Unit of inductance.

*hertz (Hz)* Unit of frequency per second.

*hollow cathode lamp* Vapor lamp having a cathode charged with a specific element or elements; emission of the hollow cathode lamp will be the same as the emission of the element when heated in a flame; used in atomic absorption spectrophotometry.

*ideal black-body radiator* Surface that would not reflect any light energy of any kind; statistically significant but nonexistent.

*impedance* Total opposition to flow of alternating current, which is offered by circuit or component; in complicated circuit its calculation can become quite complex because it often varies with frequency and is sum of number of variables; impedance is measured in ohms and is represented by letter $z$ in formulas.

*incident light* Light falling on sample.

*inductance* Resistance to change in current, caused by counter potential of field of induction; measured in henries.

*induction* Production of magnetic field around current-carrying conductor or production of current in a parallel wire.

*infrared (IR)* Region of spectrum having longer wavelengths than red light; these wavelengths are invisible; usually considered to be from about 700 to 5,000,000 nm or 0.5 cm; they may produce heat.

*input* Information that is received by an instrument or component, such as light striking phototube or photoelectric current fed to meter.

*integrated circuit* Component containing several semiconductor crystals in a configuration allowing that single component to perform multiple electronic functions.

*intrinsic conduction* Conduction in a semiconductor crystal that is due to naturally occurring carriers in the pure crystal.

*ion* Atom or molecule with electrostatic charge.

*ionization* Dissociation of any substance into its constituent ions.

*isolating transformer* Transformer used primarily to assure that the secondary current is protected from changes in the primary.

*isosbestic point* Wavelength at which two solutions of equal concentration have equal optical density.

*isotope* Two or more forms of the same element.

*kinetic reaction* Reaction in which the rate of reaction or change is the significant variable; primarily enzyme reactions.

*Lambert's law* Physical law that states that transmitted light decreases exponentially as absorbing medium increases arithmetically in thickness.

*LED* Light-emitting diode; semiconductor diode capable of converting electrical energy into light; now widely used in digital readout devices.

*limits of reliability (colorimetry)* With most types of colorimeters and spectrophotometers, concentrations of solutions showing more than 85% T, or less than 20%, give unreliable readings; limits will vary considerably with instrument, cuvettes, and handling of sample in question.

*linear-to-log converter* Device or circuit for converting linear numbers into log numbers. Since Beer's law indicates that concentration has a linear relationship to the log of the %T, this converter, in effect, makes it possible to read out photoelectric information in terms of concentration.

*mechanical zero* Device on most galvanometers and ammeters for mechanically adjusting meter to read zero with no current flow.

*mho* Unit of conductance: reciprocal of ohm.

*millimicron (m$\mu$)* 10 Å or 1/10,000,000 ($10^{-7}$) cm; wavelength of light is often expressed in millimicrons; also called *nanometer*.

*mnemonics* Shortened forms of words that are used in communicating with the computer.

*molar absorptivity ($\epsilon$)* Absorbance of 1-molar solution when viewed in 1 cm light path.

*monochromatic light* Light of one color; composed of narrow band of wavelengths.

*monochromator* Filter, prism, or diffraction grating, along with slit and/or other parts necessary, that separates out narrow band of light, essentially of one color.

*MOS detectors* Detectors of radiation, using the sensitivity of metal oxide semiconductors for radiant energy.

*nanometer (nm)* Millimicron; newer and preferred terminology.

*nephelometer* Instrument for measuring light reflected or scattered by particles in solution.

*neutral-density filter* Filter capable of reducing total light transmitted without absorbing light of any given wavelength more than another.

*noise* In electronics, any unwanted electrical disturbance that interferes with signal one is attempting to read.

*nuclide* Any nucleus plus its orbital electrons.

*ohm ($\Omega$)* Unit of resistance used in electrical measurements; amount of resistance in which 1 V maintains current of 1 A; a 1-meter column of mercury 1 mm in diameter provides resistance of about 1 $\Omega$.

*optical density* Characteristic of solution, defined in terms of ability to absorb light energy; it is log of reciprocal of transmittance; term is nearly synonymous with *absorbance;* since absorbance is somewhat more explicit, it is preferred.

*ordinate* Of graph, chart, or recording, its vertical axis.

*parallax error* Error caused by looking at meter needle at angle that makes pointer seem to be higher or lower on scale; parallax-correcting meters have mirrored panel on scale; if needle image is obscured by needle, there is no parallax error.

*parameter* Variable to be measured or considered in given situation.

*percent transmittance (%T)* Ratio of transmitted light to incident light, expressed as a percentage.

*periodic* Recurring in a definite sequence, as atoms recur in the same arrangement to form a crystal.

*phase* When two or more currents have same frequency and polarity, they are said to be "in phase."

*photoconductive cell* Component that does not conduct appreciable quantity of current in dark but transmits well when illuminated; resistance is inversely proportional to light.

*photocurrent* Current produced by photodetector when it is exposed to light energy.

*photodetector* Device that uses photoelectric effect to detect light energy.

*photoelectric effect* Effect produced when a gamma ray transmits all of its energy to an electron, which in turn produces a photocurrent analogous to the energy of the gamma ray.

*photogenerative cell* or *photovoltaic cell* Component made up of metal base (often iron) covered with layer of oxide or selenide capable of producing small direct current when exposed to light; electrons flow from coating to metal base through external circuit; actual construction somewhat more complex, but function remains quite simple; electricity produced is proportional to incident light; this is not linear but approaches linearity through working range.

*photomultiplier tube* Phototube with cathode, usually nine dynodes (each providing step-higher voltage), and anode; arrangement provides successive steps of amplification to original signal from cathode; mica shield prevents electrons from jumping to wrong dynode; photomultiplier tubes provide as high as 2,000,000 amplication factor.

*photon* Unit of measurement of light energy.

*photosignal* Electric signal generated or modified by light-detecting device.

*phototube* Vacuum or gas-filled tube with cathode capable of emitting stream of electrons when exposed to light and provided with appropriate plate voltage; with all other conditions constant, current is directly proportional to illumination; much larger current can be obtained with phototube than with photocell.

*polarography* Electronic measurement of the gain or loss of electrons in a chemical reaction.

*potential* Difference in EMF, or voltage difference between two bodies or portions of circuit.

*potentiometer* or *pot* Variable resistance.

*power* Change in energy per second; in electricity, usually expressed in watts (see *watt*).

*power supply* Electric circuit or component designed to provide proper voltages, amperages, and frequencies to operate systems of instruments; may include transformers, batteries, diodes, capacitors, filters, etc.

*precision* Measure of repeatability, irrespective of accuracy.

*premix burner* In flame photometry, a burner in which only the thoroughly nebulized portion of the sample is burned, as it is drawn from an atomizer chamber in which heavier droplets fall out.

*prism* Piece of glass cut in such manner as to diffract light to form spectrum of good quality.

*program* In computer science, the set of instructions telling the computer what steps to take to accomplish a desired function.

*programmer* Person who converts problems from human-readable form to a program the computer can understand.

*quantum efficiency* In fluorescence measurement, relationship between the incident light and the emitted light.

*radiant energy* Energy of electromagnetic waves.

*radionuclide* Radioactive nuclide.

*raster pattern* Pattern produced by a scanner detector as it crosses a field, moves over a short distance, and returns on a line parallel and close to its previous excursion.

*ratio recording* Characteristic of a spectrophotometric instrument rendering it capable of recording ratio of light transmitted through reference tube to light transmitted through sample at each wavelength, without manual correction.

*recorder* Instrument for converting electric or physical signals to a graphic record; many types; most relate time as one coordinate to electrical impulse (such as absorbance from a spectrophotometer) as other coordinate.

*relative centrifugal force (RCF)* Measure of centrifugal force, expressed in relation to gravity; calculated by multiplying the square of the revolutions per minute $\times$ radius in cm $\times$ 0.00001118.

*relay* Electrically operated switch by means of which weak current may be made to open or close much heavier circuit.

*resolution (colorimetry)* Ability of a colorimetric instrument to faithfully record small bands of spectral absorption or transmission.

*root mean square (rms)* or *effective voltage* In sine wave, square root of sum of squares of infinite number of moment voltage is effective voltage.

*scintillation detector* Instrument for detecting radiation; radiation from radioactive isotope is absorbed by phosphor crystal that emits very small flashes of short duration that are detected by photomultiplier tube and amplified.

*servomechanism* Self-correcting feedback device; usually input signal is matched to reference signal, and error signal drives motor or other device to perform some function such as change of position, temperature, or other environmental factor or equalization of reference and input by slide-wire mechanism, with readout as analog of parameter providing input.

*Severinghaus electrode* The electrode used to measure $P_{CO_2}$ by measuring the change in pH of a buffer as it is affected by absorbed carbon dioxide passing from blood to buffer across a semipermeable membrane.

*shunt* Secondary channel or bypass for current; in meter, for example, shunt carries larger fraction of current around measuring movement.

*signal* Information (usually electric in nature) arising from systems or situation under measurement and analagous to change that is to be measured.

*signal-to-noise ratio* Ratio of extraneous current variations to variations of current being measured.

*slit width* Width of slit or opening through which section of spectrum falls on sample; determines band pass when other conditions remain fixed.

*software* Total of the coded instructions to the computer, necessary to make it functional.

*solenoid* Electromagnetically operated valve to control flow of liquids or gas.

*"spec" sheets* Specification sheets that give factual technical information in concise form. Most instrument specifications are given in uniformly acceptable terms and units of reference.

*spectral emission* Specific spectrum emitted by given light source; sun, for example, emits light generally accepted to be pure white light; other sources vary in spectral content; each element has characteristic spectral emission when heated to appropriate temperature.

*spectral scanning* Continuous sequential examination of solution with varying colors in light, to determine its absorbance at each wavelength; most conveniently done with the radio-recording spectrophotometer, which automatically corrects for varying phototube characteristics at different wavelengths.

*spectrophotometer* Colorimeter in which monochromatic light is provided by creation of spectrum and isolation of one small band of color.

*spectroscope* Instrument designed to produce spectrum from light source or from light reflected from object; such spectrum defines emitted or reflected light, thereby identifying substance under examination.

*spectrum* Continuously varying band of color observed when stream of white light is passed through prism, which separates various components of light into their respective wavelengths; recognizable colors, from shortest to longest wavelength, or violet, blue, green, yellow, orange, and red.

*stray light* Light, of scattered wavelengths, that passes (unwanted) through the cuvette of a photometer. The spectra of higher orders and small amounts of reflected light make up most of the stray light.

*supercooled liquid* Substance in its liquid state at temperature lower than its freezing point.

*taut-band suspension* Meter suspension in which moving coil is suspended on taut wire or other material in such a way that no friction is involved in its rotation.

*TC detectors* Thermal conductivity or "hot wire" detectors used in gas chromatography.

*thermal runaway* Unfortunate situation in which heat increases conductivity of a semiconductor, and increased current flow increases heat until the component is destroyed by excessive heat.

*thermistor* Device working on principle of impedance varying with temperature in circuit; output unit of thermistor circuit may be a thermometer scale indicating temperature or an electronic device of any kind that might be operated on error signal.

*thermocouple* Bimetallic device capable of generating current whose potential varies with temperature; may be constructed to measure very small temperature changes in physiological situations.

*thermoregulator* Component that responds to change in temperature by opening and closing relay to put in motion heating or cooling device to correct change.

*total-consumption burner* In flame photometry, a burner in which all of the aspirated sample passes into the flame.

*transducer* Component designed to convert some physical signal—pressure, temperature, movement, etc.—into transmissible signal, usually electric in nature.

*transformer* Component designed to change voltage supply to voltage desired; step-up transformer increases voltage; step-down transformer diminishes voltage; change of voltage is effected by setting up induction current in coil parallel to coil carrying supply voltage; new voltage depends on relative number of turns of wire in coils.

*transistor* Solid-state component capable of most functions of vacuum tubes.

*transmittance (T)* Ability of solution to pass or transmit light of selected wavelength; usually expressed in percentage of light transmitted; this value has reciprocal relationship to absorbance.

*turbidimetry* Measurement of cloudiness or turbidity of solution by amount of light it is able to transmit or disperse.

*turnkey operation* Computer system in which the responsibilities for programming and operational details are the responsibility of the vendor.

*ultraviolet (UV)* Region of spectrum having shorter wavelengths than violet light; outside the visible range and generally considered between 5 and 400 nm (between x-rays and violet light).

*Venturi* T-shaped tube for producing suction in side arm by rapid passage of stream of liquid or gas through straight portion.

*volt (V)* Unit of electromotive force (pressure) that will send 1 ampere through 1 $\Omega$ of resistance.

*voltage stabilizer* Device for preventing large fluctuations in current supplied to instrument; these vary from simple stabilizing transformers to complex electronic power supplies.

*voltaic* Producing difference in potential by chemical action or contact.

*watt (W)* Unit of electric power equivalent to work performed when 1 V moves 1 A; this is 1 joule per second.

*wavelength (λ)* Distance between crests of consecutive waves of any type; might apply to light, sound, radio waves, x-rays, etc.

*Wheatstone bridge* Arrangement of four opposing resistances by which resistance can be measured; first pair of resistances acts to bring two currents to comparable levels; one of remaining resistors is unknown, and fourth is variable; if all resistor values are known, this device may be used to calculate voltage or amperage by applying Ohm's law.

*zener diode* Semiconductor diode designed to carry a very specific current when reverse-biased at a given voltage. Generally used to control current very accurately.

*zener voltage* Voltage required to cause a zener diode to conduct when reverse-biased; also called "breakdown voltage"; indicated as $V_z$.

# *Periodic table of elements*

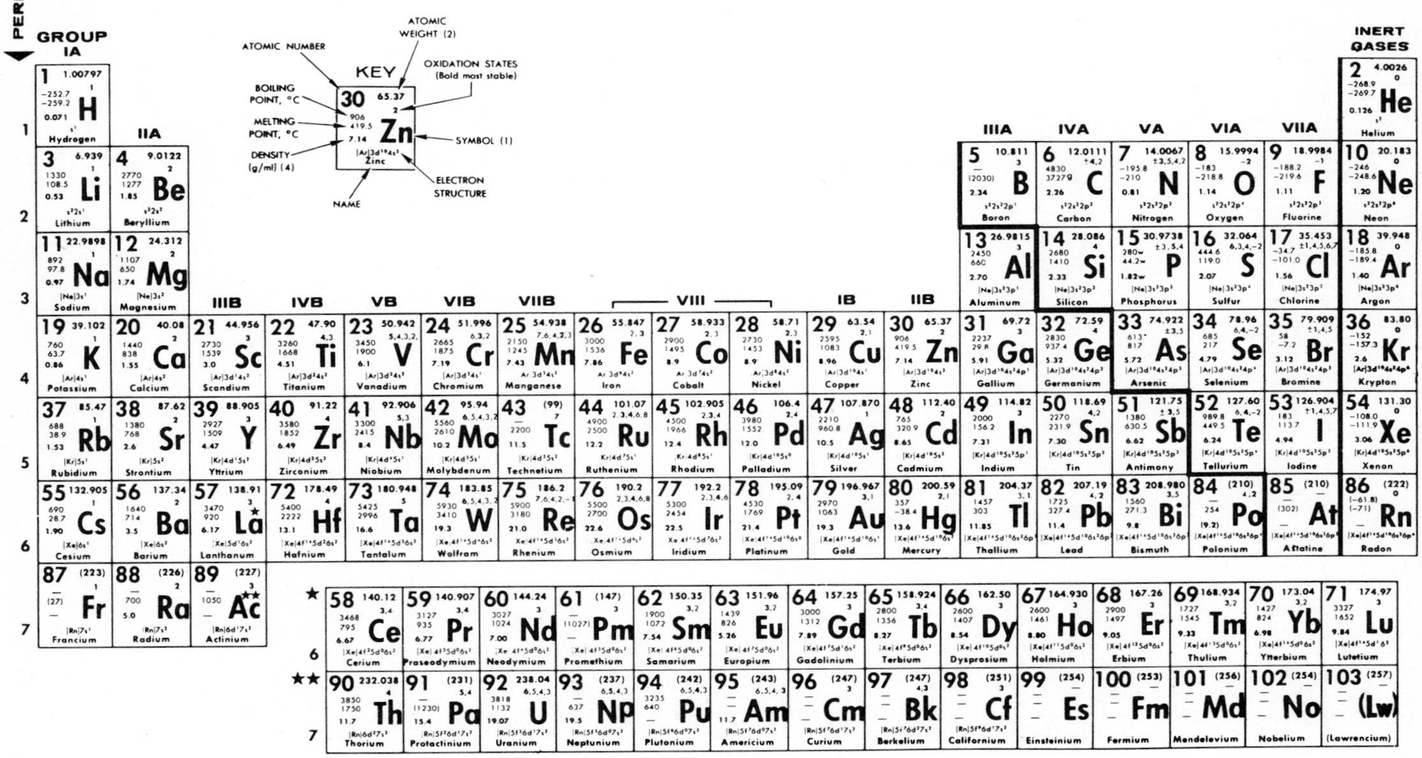

GROUP IA

PERIOD

**KEY**

ATOMIC NUMBER
ATOMIC WEIGHT (2)
OXIDATION STATES (Bold most stable)
SYMBOL (1)

30  65.37
±2
906
419.5
7.14
Zn
[Ar]3d¹⁰4s²
Zinc

BOILING POINT, °C
MELTING POINT, °C
DENSITY (g/ml (4))
ELECTRON STRUCTURE
NAME

| GROUP | IA | IIA | IIIB | IVB | VB | VIB | VIIB | | VIII | | IB | IIB | IIIA | IVA | VA | VIA | VIIA | INERT GASES |
|---|---|---|---|---|---|---|---|---|---|---|---|---|---|---|---|---|---|---|
| | | | | | | | | | | | | | | | | | | 2 He |

Period 1: 1 H (1.00797), 2 He (4.0026)

Period 2: 3 Li, 4 Be, 5 B, 6 C, 7 N, 8 O, 9 F, 10 Ne

Period 3: 11 Na, 12 Mg, 13 Al, 14 Si, 15 P, 16 S, 17 Cl, 18 Ar

Period 4: 19 K, 20 Ca, 21 Sc, 22 Ti, 23 V, 24 Cr, 25 Mn, 26 Fe, 27 Co, 28 Ni, 29 Cu, 30 Zn, 31 Ga, 32 Ge, 33 As, 34 Se, 35 Br, 36 Kr

Period 5: 37 Rb, 38 Sr, 39 Y, 40 Zr, 41 Nb, 42 Mo, 43 Tc, 44 Ru, 45 Rh, 46 Pd, 47 Ag, 48 Cd, 49 In, 50 Sn, 51 Sb, 52 Te, 53 I, 54 Xe

Period 6: 55 Cs, 56 Ba, 57 La★, 72 Hf, 73 Ta, 74 W, 75 Re, 76 Os, 77 Ir, 78 Pt, 79 Au, 80 Hg, 81 Tl, 82 Pb, 83 Bi, 84 Po, 85 At, 86 Rn

Period 7: 87 Fr, 88 Ra, 89 Ac★★

★ 58 Ce, 59 Pr, 60 Nd, 61 Pm, 62 Sm, 63 Eu, 64 Gd, 65 Tb, 66 Dy, 67 Ho, 68 Er, 69 Tm, 70 Yb, 71 Lu

★★ 90 Th, 91 Pa, 92 U, 93 Np, 94 Pu, 95 Am, 96 Cm, 97 Bk, 98 Cf, 99 Es, 100 Fm, 101 Md, 102 No, 103 (Lw)

# *Units of electricity*

*ampere (A)* Practical unit of electric current: amount of current that will flow through resistance of 1 Ω when potential of 1 V is applied across resistance; amperage in formulas is I.

*coulomb (C)* Charge containing $6.28 \times 10^{18}$ electrons; 1 C passing a point in 1 second is 1 A.

*farad* Unit of capacitance; circuit, or capacitor, is said to have capacitance of 1 farad when charge of 1 V per second across it produces current of 1 A.

*henry* Unit of inductance; circuit, or inductor, is said to have self-inductance of 1 henry when counter electromotive force of 1 V is generated by rate of change of current of 1 A per second.

*hertz (Hz)* Unit of frequency per second.

*mho* Unit of conductance; reciprocal of resistance; that is, relation between conductance $G$ and resistance $R$ is given by:

$$G = \frac{1}{R} \text{ mho}$$

*ohm (Ω)* Practical unit of resistance; amount of resistance that will permit 1 A to flow at potential difference of 1 V. Usually designated on diagrams by Ω; in formulas **R,** for resistance, is used.

*volt* Practical unit of electromotive force (EMF) or electrical potential; potential that will cause current of 1 A to flow through resistance of 1 Ω; abbreviation is **V;** voltage or EMF in formulas is **E.**

*watt* Unit of electrical power defined as work performed when 1 V moves 1 A; abbreviation is **W.**

***Table 10.*** Accepted nomenclature for photometry

| Preferred nomenclature and symbols | Definition | Other terms used |
|---|---|---|
| Absorbance (A) | $\text{Log}_{10}(1/T) = -\log_{10}T = 2 -\log_{10} \%T$ | Optical density (OD) Density Extinction Absorbancy |
| Absorptivity (a) | Absorbance per unit concentration and thickness; i.e., specific absorbance | Extinction coefficient Specific absorption Absorbance index |
| Molar absorptivity | Absorptivity in moles per liter per light path; concentration in moles per liter and thickness in centimeters (usually 1 mole per liter in 1 cm light path) | Molar extinction coefficient Molar absorbancy index |
| Angstrom unit | Approximately $10^{-10}$ meter | Å or A |
| Frequency | Cycles of energy per unit of time | |
| Far UV | Radiant energy between 10 and 200 nm | |
| Near UV | Radiant energy between 200 and 380 nm | |
| Visible light | Radiant energy between 380 and 780 nm | |
| Near IR | Radiant energy between 780 nm and 2.5 $\mu$m | |
| Middle IR | Radiant energy between 2.5 and 25 $\mu$m | |
| Far IR | Radiant energy between 25 and 400 $\mu$m | |
| Transmittance (T) | Ratio of radiant energy transmitted by sample to radiant energy incident on sample under identical conditions | Transmission Transmittancy |
| Percent transmittance | Transmittance expressed as percent | %T |

***Table 11.*** Greek alphabet as symbols*

| | | | | | | |
|---|---|---|---|---|---|---|
| A | Alpha | | | N | Nu | |
| $\alpha$ | Alpha | | | $\nu$ | Nu | Frequency |
| B | Beta | | | $\Xi$ | Xi | |
| $\beta$ | Beta | Van Slyke buffer value, beta particle | | $\xi$ | Xi | |
| $\Gamma$ | Gamma | | | O | Omicron | |
| $\gamma$ | Gamma | Gamma radiation | | $o$ | Omicron | |
| $\Delta$ | Delta | Symbol of finite change | | $\Pi$ | Pi | 3.14 |
| $\delta$ | Delta | | | $\pi$ | Pi | 3.14 |
| E | Epsilon | | | P | Rho | |
| $\epsilon$ | Epsilon | Molar absorptivity or coefficient of extinction | | $\rho$ | Rho | Density |
| | | | | $\Sigma$ | Sigma | Sum of |
| Z | Zeta | | | $\sigma$ | Sigma | Standard deviation, also used for wave number |
| $\zeta$ | Zeta | | | | | |
| H | Eta | | | T | Tau | |
| $\eta$ | Eta | | | $\tau$ | Tau | |
| $\Theta$ | Theta | | | $Y$ | Upsilon | |
| $\theta$ | Theta | Angle of diffraction | | $\upsilon$ | Upsilon | Velocity or speed |
| I | Iota | | | $\Phi$ | Phi | |
| $\iota$ | Iota | | | $\phi$ | Phi | |
| K | Kappa | | | X | Chi | |
| $\kappa$ | Kappa | | | $\chi$ | Chi | |
| $\Lambda$ | Lambda | | | $\Psi$ | Psi | |
| $\lambda$ | Lambda | Wavelength | | $\psi$ | Psi | |
| M | Mu | | | $\Omega$ | Omega | Ohm |
| $\mu$ | Mu | Micrometer or micro | | $\omega$ | Omega | Energy per reciprocal centimeter |

*Greek letters are used widely in the sciences as symbols. The same letter may have different meanings in different disciplines. A few of the very common usages are indicated above.

***Table 12.*** Prefixes

| Multiple or submultiple | | | Prefix | Symbol |
|---|---|---|---|---|
| 1 000 000 000 000 | $10^{12}$ | | tera | t |
| 1 000 000 000 | $10^9$ | | giga | g |
| 1 000 000 | $10^6$ | | mega | m |
| 1 000 | $10^3$ | | kilo | k (or K) |
| 100 | $10^2$ | | hecto | h |
| 10 | $10^1$ | | deka | dk |
| 0.1 | $10^{-1}$ | | deci | d |
| 0.01 | $10^{-2}$ | | centi | c |
| 0.001 | $10^{-3}$ | | milli | m |
| 0.000 001 | $10^{-6}$ | | micro | $\mu$ |
| 0.000 000 001 | $10^{-9}$ | | nano | n |
| 0.000 000 000 001 | $10^{-12}$ | | pico | p |

# Electrical symbols

Several of the more commonly used electrical symbols appear on this and the following page. There are, of course, many others. Some draftsmen use symbols that are slightly different from those shown here. Using these, however, you will find simple diagrams easy to follow. As you become more experienced you will recognize additional symbols, and practice will greatly increase your comprehension. If some diagrams are confusing or individual circuits seem hopeless, do not become discouraged. Follow the general outline and fill in the details as you puzzle them out.

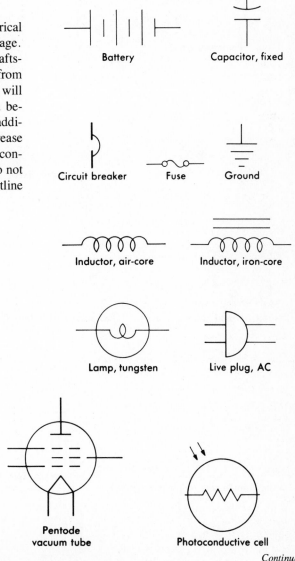

Battery        Capacitor, fixed

Circuit breaker    Fuse    Ground

Inductor, air-core     Inductor, iron-core

Lamp, tungsten     Live plug, AC

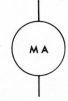

Meter (lettering in center tells type)

Pentode
vacuum tube

Photoconductive cell

*Continued.*

351

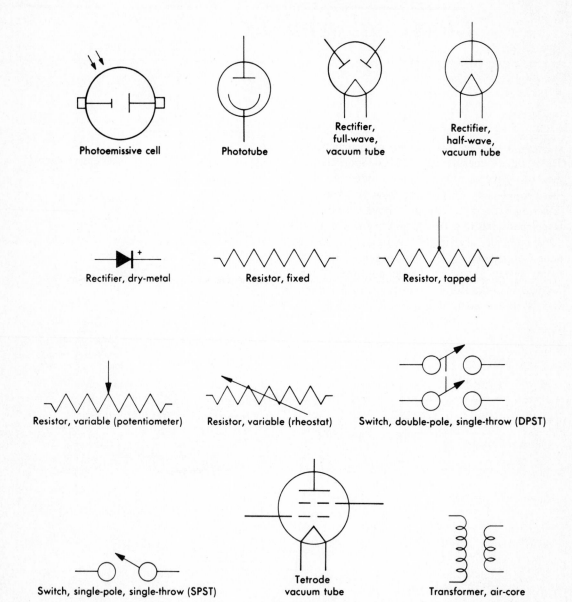

Photoemissive cell

Phototube

Rectifier,
full-wave,
vacuum tube

Rectifier,
half-wave,
vacuum tube

Rectifier, dry-metal

Resistor, fixed

Resistor, tapped

Resistor, variable (potentiometer)

Resistor, variable (rheostat)

Switch, double-pole, single-throw (DPST)

Switch, single-pole, single-throw (SPST)

Tetrode
vacuum tube

Transformer, air-core

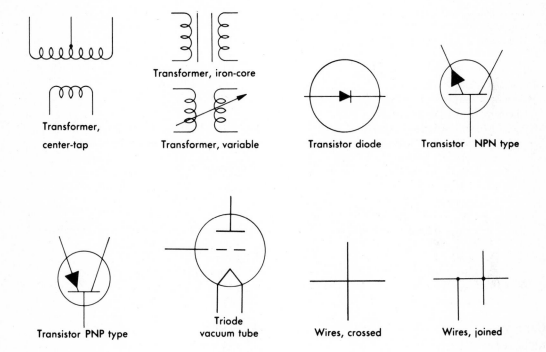

Transformer, center-tap

Transformer, iron-core

Transformer, variable

Transistor diode

Transistor NPN type

Transistor PNP type

Triode vacuum tube

Wires, crossed

Wires, joined

# *Metric system*

### Length

Millimeter (mm) = Meter ÷ 1000
Centimeter (cm) = Meter ÷ 100
Decimeter (dm) = Meter ÷ 10

*Basic unit = Meter (m)*

Decameter (dkm) = Meter × 10
Hektometer (hm) = Meter × 100
Kilometer (km) = Meter × 1000
Myriameter (mym) = Meter × 10,000
1 mm = 0.0394 in
1 cm = 0.3937 in
1 dm = 3.937 in
1 m = 39.37 in
1 dkm = 32.81 ft
1 hm = 328 ft 1 in or 109 yd 13 in
1 km = 32.8 ft 1 in or 0.62 mi
1 mym = 6.2 mi
2.54 cm = 1 in
30.48 cm = 1 ft
0.914 m = 1 yd
1.609 km = 1 mi

### Capacity

Milliliter (ml) = Liter ÷ 1000
Centiliter (cl) = Liter ÷ 100
Deciliter (dl) = Liter ÷ 10

*Basic unit = Liter\* (l)*

Decaliter (dkl) = Liter × 10
Hektoliter (hl) = Liter × 100
Kiloliter (kl) = Liter × 1000

### Cubic capacity

1 ml = 0.06 cu in
1 cl = 0.6 cu in
1 dl = 6.1 cu in
1 l = 61.02 cu in
1 dkl = 0.35 cu ft
1 hl = 3.53 cu ft
1 kl = 1.31 cu yd
1.67 cl = 1 cu in
2.85 dkl = 1 cu ft
0.76 kl = 1 cu yd

### Liquid capacity

1 ml = 0.27 fluidram or 0.0338 fl oz
1 cl = 0.338 fl oz
1 dl = 3.3815 fl oz or 0.21 pi
1 l = 2.1134 pt or 1.0567 qt or 0.2642 gal
1 dkl = 9.091 qt or 0.264 gal
0.02957 l = 1 oz
0.473 l = 1 pt
0.946 l = 1 qt
3.785 l = 1 gal

### Dry capacity

1 dl = 0.18 pt
1 l = 1.816 pt or 0.9081 qt or 0.1135 pk or 0.028 bu
1 dkl = 18.162 pt or 9.081 qt or 0.14 pk or 0.28378 bu
1 hl = 2.84 bu
0.55 l = 1 pt
1.101 l = 1 qt
8.809 l = 1 pk
35.238 l = 1 bu

---

\*Liter = 1000 cu cm (approximately 1 qt). Liter implies cubic capacity, so it is *not* prefixed by *cubic*. In the metric system, dry and liquid measures are identical.

## Area

Sq centimeter (sq cm) = 0.0001 centare (ca) or
$$1 \text{ ca} \div 10,000$$

*Basic unit = Centare (ca) = 1 sq m*

Are (a) = 1 ca × 100
Hectare (ha) = 1 ca × 10,000
Sq kilometer (sq km) = 1 ca × 1,000,000
1 sq mm = 0.00155 sq in
1 sq cm = 155 sq in
1 sq m or ca = 10.764 sq ft or 1.196 sq yd
1 a = 119.6 sq yd
1 ha = 2.47 acres
1 sq km = 0.3861 sq mi
6.451 sq cm = 1 sq in
0.093 sq m = 1 sq ft
0.836 sq m = 1 sq yd
4047 sq m = 1 acre
2.59 sq km = 1 sq mi or 640 acres

## Volume

Cu centimeter (cu cm) = 0.000001 cu m or
$$1 \text{ cu m} \div 1,000,000$$
Decistere (ds) = 0.1 cu m or cu m ÷ 10

*Basic unit = Stere (s) = 1 cu m*

Decastere (dks) = 10 s or 1 cu m × 10
1 cu mm = 0.000061 cu in
1 cu cm = 0.061 cu in
1 cu dm = 61.02 cu in or 0.035 cu ft
1 ds = 3.53 cu ft
1 cu m or 1 s = 35.31 cu ft or 1.31 cu yd
1 dks or 10 cu m = 353.1 cu ft or 13.1 cu yd
16.387 cu cm = 1 cu in
0.028 cu m = 1 cu ft
0.765 cu m = 1 cu yd

## Weight and mass

Milligram (mg) = Gram ÷ 1000
Centigram (cg) = Gram ÷ 100
Decigram (dm) = Gram ÷ 10

*Basic unit = Gram (g)*

Decagram (dkg) = Gram × 10
Hectogram (hg) = Gram × 100
Kilogram (kg) = Gram × 1000
Quintal (q) = Gram × 100,000
Metric Ton (MT) = Quintal × 10
1 mg = 0.015 grain
1 cg = 0.154 grain
1 dg = 1.543 grains
1 g = 0.035 oz
1 dkg = 0.353 oz
1 hg = 3.527 oz
1 kg or 1000 g = 35.275 oz or 2.2046 lb
1 q or 100,000 g = 220.46 lb
Ton
0.907 MT = 1 short ton
2000 lb
1.016 MT = 1 long ton
2240 lb
Hundredweight (cwt)
45.359 kg = 1 short cwt
100 lb
50.802 kg = 1 long cwt
112 lb
28.349 g = 1 oz
453 g = 1 lb
0.453 kg = 1 lb
0.907 MT = 1 short ton
1.016 MT = 1 long ton

# *Manufacturers' addresses*

For convenience the following company names and addresses are provided. All these companies are manufacturers of instruments discussed or mentioned earlier. More information on many technical matters relating to these instruments is available through the manufacturers' technical manuals, operating manuals, seminars, and training courses. Many of the companies have provided illustrations, consultations, data, and advice, for which we wish here to express our deep appreciation.

Abbott Laboratories
Diagnostics Division
North Chicago, Ill. 60064

Abbott Scientific Products Division
820 Mission St.
South Pasadena, Calif. 91030

Advanced Instruments, Inc.
1000 Highland Ave.
Needham Heights, Mass. 02194

American Instrument Co., Inc.
8030 Georgia Ave.
Silver Springs, Md. 20910

American Monitor Corp.
P.O. Box 68505
Indianapolis, Ind. 46268

American Optical Corp.
Analytical Instrument Division
200 S. Garrard Blvd.
Richmond, Calif. 94804
Scientific Instrument Division
Buffalo, N.Y. 14215

Ames Co.
Division Miles Laboratories, Inc.
Elkhart, Ind. 46514

Antek Instruments, Inc.
6005 N. Freeway
Houston, Tex. 77022

Artek Systems Corp.
275 Adams Blvd.
Farmindgale, N.Y. 11735

B-D Spear Medical Systems
123 Second Ave.
Waltham, Mass. 02154

Baird Atomic, Inc.
125 Middlesex Turnpike
Bedford, Mass. 01730

Baker Instruments
270 Marble Avenue
Pleasantville, N.Y. 10570

J.T. Baker Instruments
540 New Haven Ave.
Milford, Conn. 06460

Bausch & Lomb
820 Linden Ave.
Rochester, N.Y. 14625

Beckman Instruments, Inc.
2500 Harbor Blvd.
Fullerton, Calif. 92634

Becton, Dickinson & Co.
Bio-Quest Division
Cockeysville, Md. 21030

Bio/Data Corp.
3941 Commerce Ave.
Willow Grove, Pa. 19090

Bio-Dynamics, Inc.
9115 Hague Rd.
Indianapolis, Inc. 46250

Brinkmann Instruments, Inc.
Cantiague Rd.
Westburg, N.Y. 11590

CAPCO
Clinical Analysis Products Co.
599 N. Mathilda Ave.
Sunnyvale, Calif. 94086

Chemetrics Corp.
P.O. Box 8521
San Mateo, Calif. 94402

Clay Adams
Division of Becton, Dickinson & Co.
299 Webro Rd.
Parsippany, N.J. 07054

Clinical Analysis Products Co.
599 N. Mathilda Ave.
Sunnyvale, Calif. 94086

Coleman Instruments
Division of Perkin-Elmer Corp.
2000 York Road
Oak Brook, Ill. 60521

Corning Scientific Instruments
Medfield, Mass. 02052
Coulter Electronics, Inc.
590 W. 20th St.
Hialeah, Fla. 33010

Dade Reagents
Division of American Hospital Supply Corp.
1851 Delaware Parkway
Miami, Fla. 33152

Damon/IEC Division
300 Second Ave.
Needham Heights, Mass. 02194

Digital Equipment Corp.
146 Main St.
Maynard, Mass. 01754

Disc Instruments, Inc.
2701 Halladay St.
Santa Ana, Calif. 92705

Diversified Numeric Applications
Division of AVNET, Inc.
9801 Logan Ave., South
Minneapolis, Minn. 55431

Dow Diagnostics
P.O. Box 68511
Indianapolis, Ind. 46268

Eastman Kodak Co.
343 State Street
Rochester, N.Y. 14650

E.I. duPont de Nemours & Co.
Wilmington, Del. 19898

Electro-Nucleonics, Inc.
368 Passaic Ave., P.O. Box 803
Fairfield, N.J. 07006

Elementary Principles, Inc.
P.O. Box 1606
Orlando, Fla. 32802

Ericsen Instruments
Ossining, N.Y. 10562

Farrand Optical Co., Inc.
Commercial Products Division
535 S. Fifth Ave.
Mount Vernon, N.Y. 10550

Fisher Scientific Co.
711 Forbes Ave.
Pittsburgh, Pa. 15219

Fiske Associates, Inc.
Quaker Highway
Uxbridge, Mass., 01569

Gam Rad, Inc.
16825 Wyoming Ave.
Detroit, Mich. 48221

Gelman Instrument Co.
600 South Wagner Rd.
Ann Arbor, Mich. 48106

General Diagnostics Division of Warner-Lambert Co.
Morris Plains, N.J. 07950

Geometric Data
999 West Valley Rd. Wayne, Pa. 19087

Gilford Instrument Laboratories, Inc.
132 Artina St.
Oberlin, Ohio 44074

Harleco
60th & Woodland Ave.
Philadelphia, Pa. 19143

Helena Laboratories
P.O. Box 752
Beaumont, Tex. 77704

Hewlett-Packard Co.
175 Wyman St.
Waltham, Mass. 02154

Honeywell, Inc.
Industrial Division
1100 Virginia Dr.
Fort Washington, Pa. 19034

Honeywell, Medical Systems Center
600 Second St. NE
Hopkins, Minn. 55343

Hycel, Inc.
P.O. Box 36329
Houston, Tex. 77036

Hyland, Division of Travenol Laboratories, Inc.
3300 Hyland Ave.
Costa Mesa, Calif. 92626

IBM Corp.
Blood Cell Processor
P.O. Box 10
Princeton, N.J. 08540

Infotronics, Inc.
8500 Cameron Rd.
Austin, Tex. 78753

Instrumentation Laboratory, Inc.
113 Hartwell Ave.
Lexington, Mass. 02173

International Equipment Co.
Division of Damon
300 Second Ave.
Needham Heights, Mass. 02194

International Technidyne Corp.
P.O. Box 2200
Menlo Park Station
Edison, N.J. 08817

Johnson Laboratories, Inc.
3 Industry Lane
Cockeysville, Md. 21030

Kimble Instruments Division of Owens Illinois, Inc.
P.O. Box 1035
405 Madison Ave.
Toledo, Ohio 43666

LKB Instruments, Inc.
12221 Parklawn Dr.
Rockville, Md. 20852

E. Leitz, Inc.
468 Park Ave. South
New York, N.Y. 10016

Lipshaw Manufacturing Co.
7446 Central Ave.
Detroid, Mich. 48210

Medical Laboratory Automation, Inc.
520 Nuber Ave.
Mt. Vernon, N.Y. 10550

Micromedic Systems
102 Witmer Rd.
Harsham, Pa. 19044

Millipore Corp.
Ashby Rd.
Bedford, Mass. 01730

Nuclear Data, Inc.
100 W. Gold Rd.
P.O. Box 451
Palatine, Ill. 60067

Ohio Nuclear, Inc.
6000 Cochran Rd.
Solon, Ohio 44139

Orion Research, Inc.
380 Putnam Ave.
Cambridge, Mass. 02139

Ortho Diagnostics Instruments
410 University Ave.
Westwood, Mass. 02090

Packard Instrument Sales Corp.
2200 Warrenville Rd.
Dowers Grove, Ill. 60515

Perkin-Elmer Corp.
723G Main Ave.
Norwalk, Conn. 06856

Pfizer Diagnostics Division
235 E. 42nd St.
New York, N.Y. 10017

Philips Electronic Instruments
750 S. Fulton Ave.
Mount Vernon, N.Y. 10550

Photovolt Corp.
1115 Broadway
New York, N.Y. 10010

Picker Corp.
12 Clintonville Rd.
Northford, Conn. 06472

Precision Systems
6 Cornell Rd.
Framingham, Mass. 01704

Radiometer
811 Sharon Dr.
Cleveland, Ohio 44145

Roche Analytical Instruments, Inc.
Nutley, N.J. 07110

Roche Medical Electronics, Inc.
Cranbury, N.J. 08512

Royco Instruments, Inc.
141 Jefferson Dr.
Menlo Park, Calif. 94025

Sargent-Welch Scientific Co.
10558 Metropolitan Ave.
Kensington, Md. 20795

Schoeffel Instrument Corp.
15 Douglas St.
Westwood, N.J. 07675

Searle Analytic, Inc.
Subsidiary of G.D. Searle & Co.
2000 Nuclear Dr.
Des Plaines, Ill. 60018

Sherwood Medical Industries, Inc.
1831 Olive St.
St. Louis, Mo. 63103

Smith Kline Instruments, Inc.
880 West Maude Ave.
Sunnyvale, Calif. 94086

Sony Corp. of America
47-47 Van Dam St.
Long Island, N.Y. 11101

Technicon Instruments Corp.
Tarrytown, N.Y. 10591

Tech/Ops Instruments
Distributors for Joyce Loebel
Northwest Industrial Park
Burlington, Mass. 01803

Texas Instruments, Inc.
P.O. Box 66029
Houston, Tex. 77006

Transidyne General Corp.
462 Wagner Rd.
Ann Arbor, Mich. 48106

Travenol Laboratories, Inc.
9299 Washington Boulevard
Savage, Md. 20863

G.K. Turner Associates
2524 Pulgas Ave.
Palo Alto, Calif. 94303

Union Carbide
Clinical Diagnostics
401 Theodore Fremd Ave.
Rye, N.Y. 10580

Varian Techtron
2700 Mitchell Dr.
Walnut Creek, Calif. 94598

Ventron Instruments Corp.
Cahn Division
7500 Jefferson St.
Paramount, Calif. 90723

Volu-Sol
P.O. Box 14097
Las Vegas, Nev. 89101

Wescor, Inc.
459 S. Main. St.
Logan, Utah 84321

Yallen Instruments, Inc.
160 Pleasant St.
Brocton, Mass. 02401

Yellow Springs Instrument Co., Inc.
Yellow Springs, Ohio 45387

# *BIBLIOGRAPHY*

Accreditation manual for hospitals, Chicago, 1982, Joint Commission on Accreditation of Hospitals.

Ackerman, P.G.: Electronic instrumentation in the clinical laboratory, 1972, Waltham, Mass., Little, Brown & Co.

Astrup, P., Jorgensen, K., Siggard-Anderson, O., and Engel, K.: The acid-base metabolism: a new approach, Lancet **1;** 1035, 1960.

Basic electronics for medical technologists, No. 1313, Houston, 1972, The American Society for Medical Technology and the ASMT Education & Research Fund, Inc. Publications.

Bauman, R.P.: Absorption spectroscopy, New York, 1962, John Wiley & Sons, Inc.

Bibbero, R.J.: Microprocessors in instruments and control, New York, 1977, John Wiley & Sons, Inc.

Boyce, Jefferson, C.: Microprocessor and microcomputer basics, New Jersey, 1979, Prentice-Hall, Inc.

Burns, P.: Identification of microorganisms using computer programs, unpublished master's thesis submitted for publication, 1972, Mississippi State University.

The journal of clinical laboratory automation, vol. 2, No. 2, E. Norwalk, Conn., March-April 1982, Appleton-Century-Crofts.

Clinical laboratory electronics, No. 1314, Houston, 1972, American Society for Medical Technology and the ASMT Education & Research Fund, Inc. Publications.

Cromwell, L., Weibell, F.J., Pfeiffer, E.A., and Usselman, L.B.: Biomedical Instrumentation and Measurements, Englewood Cliffs, N.J., 1973, Prentice-Hall, Inc.

Early, P.J., Razzak, A.M., and Sodee, D.B.: Textbook of nuclear medicine technology, St. Louis, ed. 3, 1979, The C.V. Mosby Co.

Ferris, C.D.: Guide to medical laboratory instruments, Waltham, Mass., 1980, Little, Brown & Co.

Hicks, R., et al.: Laboratory Instrumentation, New York, 1980, Harper and Row, Publishers.

Hodges, D.A.: Microelectronic memories, Sci. Am. Sept. 1977, pp. 130-145.

Holton, W.C.: The large-scale integration of microelectronic circuits, Sci. Am. Sept. 1977, pp. 82-94.

Jacobson, B., and Webster, J.G.: Medicine and clinical engineering, Englewood, N.J., 1977, Prentice-Hall, Inc.

Johnson, D.E., Hilburn, J.L., and Julich, P.M.: Digital circuits and microcomputers, New Jersey, 1979, Prentice-Hall.

Malmstadt, H.Y., and Enke, C.G.: Electronics for scientists, New York, 1962, W.A. Benjamin, Inc.

Meloan, C.E.: Instrumental analysis using physical properties, Philadelphia, 1968, Lea & Febiger.

Meloan, C.E.: Instrumental analysis using spectroscopy, Philadelphia, 1968, Lea & Febiger.

The National Committee for Clinical Laboratory Standards: Guidelines for service of clinical laboratory instruments; Power requirements for clinical laboratory instruments and for laboratory power sources; Preparation of manuals for installation, operation, and repair of laboratory instruments; Tentative guidelines for clinical laboratory procedure manuals, NCCLS, 771 East Lancaster Ave., Villanova, Pa., 19085.

Rayer, F.G.: Electronics and computers, New York, 1968, A.S. Barnes & Co., Inc.

Severinghaus, J.W., and Bradley, A.F.: Electrodes for blood $Po_2$ determination, J. Appl. Physiol. **13:**515, 1958.

Suprynowiez, V.A.: Introduction to electronics, Reading, Mass., 1966, Addison-Wesley Publishing Co., Inc.

Tammes, A.R.: Electronics for medical and biology laboratory personnel, Baltimore, 1971, The Williams & Wilkins Co.

Vesely, J., Weiss, D., and Stulik, K.: Analysis with ion-selective electrodes, New York, 1978, John Wiley & Sons, Inc.

White, W.L., Erickson, M.M., and Stavens, S.C.: Practical automation for the clinical laboratory, ed. 2, St. Louis, 1972, The C.V. Mosby Co.

Willard, H.H., Merritt, L.L., Jr., and Dean, J.S.: Instrumental methods of analysis, ed. 4, Princeton, N.J., 1965, D. Van Nostrand Co.

Yanof, H.M.: Biomedical electronics, Philadelphia, 1965, F.A. Davis Co.

# Index